ISGE Series

Series Editor
Andrea R. Genazzani

More information about this series at http://www.springer.com/series/11871

Roberta Diaz Brinton • Andrea R. Genazzani
Tommaso Simoncini • John C. Stevenson
Editors

Sex Steroids' Effects on Brain, Heart and Vessels

Volume 6: Frontiers in Gynecological Endocrinology

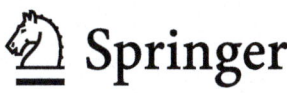 Springer

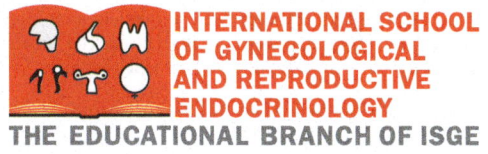
INTERNATIONAL SCHOOL
OF GYNECOLOGICAL
AND REPRODUCTIVE
ENDOCRINOLOGY
THE EDUCATIONAL BRANCH OF ISGE

Editors
Roberta Diaz Brinton
Center for Innovation in Brain
Sciencies-Department of Pharmacology
and Neurology
College of Medicine, University of Arizona
Tucson, AZ
USA

Andrea R. Genazzani
International School for Gynecological and
Reproductive Endocrinology
International Society of Gynecological
Endocrinology
Locarno
Switzerland

Tommaso Simoncini
Department of Clinical and Experimental
Medicine
Division of Obstetrics and Gynecology
University of Pisa
Pisa
Italy

John C. Stevenson
National Heart and Lung Institute
Imperial College London
London
UK

Copyright owner: ISGE (International Society of Gynecological Endocrinology)

ISSN 2197-8735   ISSN 2197-8743   (electronic)
ISGE Series
ISBN 978-3-030-11354-4   ISBN 978-3-030-11355-1   (eBook)
https://doi.org/10.1007/978-3-030-11355-1

This Springer imprint is published by the registered company Springer Nature Switzerland AG
The registered company address is: Gewerbestrasse 11, 6330 Cham, Switzerland

Contents

Neuroendocrine Changes of the Menopausal Transition

Andrea Giannini, Marta Caretto, and Tommaso Simoncini

The hypothalamic–pituitary reproductive axis undergoes considerable changes during the menopausal transition. These modifications are in part secondary to declining ovarian function, but several lines of evidence suggest that the brain undergoes independent functional modifications that are important for reproductive ageing [1]. According to this hypothesis, menopause may mirror puberty, a time at which a set of hypothalamic processes also influences the reproductive axis. Increases in pituitary-derived FSH can be identified in middle-aged women well before oestrogen declines or cycle irregularities are noticed. Similarly, changes in luteinizing hormone (LH) secretion patterns are found at this stage, with broader and less frequent pulses. Experimental work in rodents suggests that an age-related desynchronization of the neurochemical signals involved in activating GnRH neurons takes place before changes in oestrous cyclicity. Several hypothalamic neuropeptides and neurochemical agents (e.g. glutamate, noradrenaline and vasoactive intestinal peptide) that drive the oestrogen-mediated surge of GnRH and LH seem to dampen with age or lack the precise temporal coordination that is required for a specific pattern of GnRH secretion [2]. Disruption of this hypothalamic biological clock would lead to progressive impairment in the timing of the preovulatory LH surge, which would add to the poor ovarian responsiveness that is encountered at this reproductive stage. Endocrine changes during the transition. As discussed above, the endocrine changes of the late reproductive years depend on the combined dysfunction of the ovaries and the hypothalamus [3]. A shortened follicular phase and the associated increase in FSH levels are characteristic of early menopausal transition. This accounts for the shorter cycle intervals that are experienced by many women in this period of life. Cohort studies have demonstrated that shortened follicular phases are associated with accelerated ovulation, which occurs at a

A. Giannini · M. Caretto · T. Simoncini (✉)
Division of Obstetrics and Gynecology, Department of Experimental and Clinical Medicine, University of Pisa, Pisa, Italy
e-mail: andrea.giannini@unipi.it; tommaso.simoncini@med.unipi.it

© International Society of Gynecological Endocrinology 2019
R. D. Brinton et al. (eds.), *Sex Steroids' Effects on Brain, Heart and Vessels*, ISGE Series, https://doi.org/10.1007/978-3-030-11355-1_1

smaller follicle size. The prevailing explanation for this phenomenon is the loss of inhibin B production, which leads to increased FSH release and, therefore, to an 'overshoot' of oestrogen production. This would facilitate (and accelerate) the achievement of the LH surge [4]. With time, the age-related hypothalamic modifications determine a decrease in oestrogen sensitivity and the LH surge becomes more erratic. Follicles also become less sensitive to gonadotropins, which leads to luteal phase defects and anovulatory cycles, and, accordingly, to the first menstrual irregularities. Hypothalamic insensitivity to oestrogens also explains why menopausal symptoms—such as hot flushes and night sweats—commonly occur at this stage, when women have rather high levels of oestrogens, as well as why exogenous oestrogens are effective in reducing the symptoms. In summary, natural menopause is the consequence of lost ovarian function. This is the final step in a long and irregular cascade of events taking place both in the brain and in the ovaries.

This changing hormonal environment produces a cascade of CNS-related and peripheral symptoms of variable severity for an unpredictable amount of time.

Therefore, menopause is ultimately defined by ovarian follicular exhaustion; several lines of scientific evidence in humans and animals now suggest that dysregulation of estradiol feedback mechanisms and hypothalamic–pituitary dysfunction contributes to the onset and progression of reproductive senescence, independent of ovarian failure [5].

In this view, decline of HPO axis has a key role in determining several symptoms afflicting different aspects of women life and in reducing quality of life [6].

Hypothalamic–pituitary–adrenal axis (HPA) hyperactivity has been demonstrated in chronic diseases affecting nervous system disorders like depression [7]. The end products of HPA axis, glucocorticoids (GCs), regulate many physiological functions and play an important role in affective regulation and dysregulation. During menopausal transition, also androgen's tone may be impaired resulting in lack of energy, sexual arousal and satisfaction and long-term development of cognitive, metabolic and mood disorders. Despite DHEA's levels which markedly decrease throughout adulthood, an increase in circulating cortisol with advanced age has been observed in human and nonhuman primates [8]. In addition, unlike DHEA's concentrations that decline under conditions of chronic stress and medical illness, cortisol concentrations generally either rise or do not change, resulting in a decrease in DHEA-to-cortisol ratio. Therefore, it may be important to consider the ratio of both steroids in addition to their absolute concentrations. The resulting decrease in the DHEA/cortisol ratio may have drastic implications for many physiological processes, including learning and memory, a view that is supported by the finding that lower DHEA/cortisol ratios area associated with greater cognitive impairment [9]. However, the relationship between steroidal concentrations and cognitive impairment is still debated.

Alterations in thermoregulation are the leading hypothesized mechanisms underlying vasomotor symptoms [10]. Menopause is associated with a reduction in the thermoneutral zone of the body, meaning that minor increases in core body temperature can trigger an excessive thermoregulatory reaction and promote heat dissipation by peripheral vasodilation and sweating. The thermoregulatory circuit is composed of functional elements that are under catecholaminergic and/or serotonergic control, and the hypothalamus is ascribed a key role in the integration of thermal information and in the control of thermoregulatory reactions [11]. During perimenopause, hormonal cycles desynchronize, leading to erratic levels of sex hormones, which often peak and plummet. Thermoregulatory dysfunction might be a result of a maladaptation of the brain to this acyclicity, with alterations in the function of noradrenergic and serotoninergic pathways [12] that normally have a decisive role in stabilizing the thermoneutral zone. Indeed, vasomotor phenomena are more common in periods of amenorrhoea, which are characterized by fluctuations in oestrogen levels. The slow progression, reduction and final disappearance of vasomotor symptoms during menopausal transition suggest a readjustment of the brain to the different concentrations of require a variable amount of time, depending on the individual.

Although initial studies reported that LH pulses occur during hot flashes in postmenopausal women, a causative link was never found [13]. The emerging hypothesis linking these two events temporally involves the discovery that kisspeptin, neurokinin B and dynorphin (KNDy) neurons, which project to the preoptic thermoregulatory area, also regulate the hypothalamic gonadotropin-releasing hormone (GnRH) pulse generator, most likely by mediating oestrogen-dependent negative feedback of LH secretion. At postmenopause, KNDy neurons undergo hypertrophy, and the expression of the genes encoding neurokinin B and kisspeptin increases as a result of oestrogen withdrawal, leading to increased signalling to heat dissipation effectors in the CNS and to GnRH neurons [14].

There is also evidence in the literature that severe vasomotor symptoms are associated with activation of the hypothalamus–pituitary–adrenal axis, as increased urinary cortisol secretion has been reported during the late menopausal transition stage in women with severe vasomotor symptoms compared with women who have mild complaints, and higher salivary cortisol levels have also been associated with more frequent, severe and bothersome daily self-reported hot flashes. Higher circulating concentrations of cortisol and noradrenaline were also reported in women at the menopausal transition or the early postmenopausal stages who experienced vasomotor symptoms [15]. Increased cortisol might activate a stress response with a consequent increase in catecholamines, adrenaline and noradrenaline, which, in turn, induce vasodilation [16].

The biological mechanisms underlying the sleep difficulties that develop during menopausal transition are still unclear. Lower levels of inhibin B, a marker of the early menopausal transition, have been found to strongly predict poor sleep quality in women at late menopausal transition and at postmenopause, whereas higher mean urinary FSH levels, the hallmark of ovarian failure, have been associated with poor sleep quality in premenopausal and perimenopausal women [17]. In addition, a faster rate of increase in FSH levels has been associated with longer sleep duration, indicative of less restful sleep and more non-REM sleep.

Postmenopausal women also show an advanced onset of melatonin release compared with premenopausal women; therefore, advanced circadian phase might contribute to early morning awakening, a common complaint in menopausal women [18]. Furthermore, obstructive sleep apnoea might exacerbate these sleep difficulties in menopausal women. Reduced levels of progesterone, a respiratory stimulant, in perimenopausal woman might be the underlying cause of this nocturnal breathing disorder.

Oestradiol is believed to have a major role in cognitive performance as anatomical studies have demonstrated that the hippocampus and prefrontal cortex, which mediate episodic and working memory, express high levels of oestrogen receptors (ERs). In these areas of the CNS, oestradiol-dependent activation of ERs can modulate the synthesis, release and metabolism of neurotransmitters (such as serotonin, dopamine and acetylcholine) and neuropeptides [such as β-endorphin and neurosteroids, namely, allopregnanolone and dehydroepiandrosterone (DHEA)] and can also influence the electrical excitability, function and morphological features of the synapses. Thus, unstable levels of oestrogen during perimenopause might cause the transient cognitive deficits that are observed clinically at this time [19]. However, the link between circulating levels of oestradiol and cognitive impairment is not well established, and clinical trials evaluating hormone therapy in women at midlife have not shown improvements in cognition. It has been shown that the concomitant rise in LH levels that occur with ovarian failure might drive both cognitive dysfunction and loss of spine density in an independent manner. Indeed, animal studies have shown that lowering the peripheral levels of LH using leuprolide acetate, a GnRH agonist, improved cognition and spatial memory and increased spine density [20]. Persistently high levels of FSH and LH have been linked to Alzheimer disease in postmenopausal women, and it is hypothesized that these hormones might be responsible for increased production of amyloid-β, a main constituent of senile plaques. Indeed, pharmacological suppression of LH and FSH using leuprolide acetate reduced plaque formation in animal models of Alzheimer disease.

According to the oestradiol withdrawal hypothesis, migraine in women is triggered by the sudden decline in oestrogen levels that occur immediately before menses, during the menopausal transition or in the early postmenopausal period. There is accumulating evidence that changes in oestradiol levels in the brain might precipitate a kind of neurogenic inflammation that is characterized by vasodilation, release of pro-inflammatory mediators and plasma extravasation [21], leading to the typically reported throbbing and pulsing pain.

The most accredited likely biological hypothesis underlying changes in mood is that fluctuations in levels of steroid hormones, more than their decline, might trigger perimenopausal depression. It seems that the longer the duration of the menopausal transition, and therefore the longer the exposure to fluctuating hormones, the greater the risk of perimenopausal depression. In the Penn Ovarian Ageing Study, it was found that a more rapid rise in FSH levels before the FMP was predictive of a lower risk of depressive symptoms after the FMP, suggesting that a shorter menopausal transition protects against perimenopausal depression. A subset of perimenopausal women might have an increased sensitivity to changes in gonadal steroids, specifically oestrogens and progesterone, which in turn modulate neuroregulatory systems associated with mood and behaviour. In particular, fluctuating oestrogen levels might lead to dysregulation of serotonin and noradrenaline pathways in the CNS as oestrogen facilitates a number of actions of serotonin and noradrenaline, specifically by modulating receptor binding and the availability of these neurohormones at the synaptic level [22]. In an interesting theoretical model, fluctuations in progesterone-derived neurosteroids, particularly allopregnanolone, caused by changes in oestradiol and progesterone levels might underlie menopause-associated depressive symptoms. In particular, failure of the GABA-A receptor—the main target of neurosteroids—to adapt to changes in levels of allopregnanolone over the course of the menopausal transition might lead to depressive symptoms in vulnerable women, such as those with a history of premenstrual dysphoric disorder and/or postpartum depression [23]. The inability to maintain GABAergic homeostatic control might exacerbate the response of the hypothalamus–pituitary–adrenal axis to stress. Indeed, there is increasing evidence that dysregulation of the hypothalamus–pituitary–adrenal axis, which is correlated with oestradiol fluctuation, might be implicated in the pathophysiology of perimenopausal depression [24]. Moreover, very stressful life events seem to contribute greatly to the onset of depressive symptoms during the menopausal transition in the presence of oestradiol variability [25] (Fig. 1.1).

Natural transitional menopause is the consequence of gradual loss of ovarian function. This is the final step in a long and irregular cascade of events taking place both in the brain as well as in the ovaries. Genetic factors influence the timing of this process, but the key molecular pathways involved are yet unknown. Identifications of such factors would be invaluable to set new strategies to treat reproductive dysfunction and menopause-associated diseases.

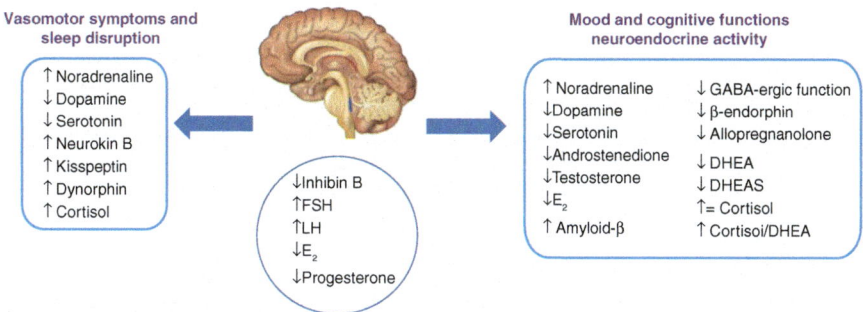

Fig. 1.1 Neuroendocrine changes across menopausal transition and biological basis of vasomotor and cognitive symptoms

References

1. Wise PM. Neuroendocrine modulation of the "menopause": insights into the aging brain. Am J Phys. 1999;277(6 Pt 1):E965–70.
2. Downs JL, Wise PM. The role of the brain in female reproductive aging. Mol Cell Endocrinol. 2009;299(1):32–8.
3. Butler L, Santoro N. The reproductive endocrinology of the menopausal transition. Steroids. 2011;76(7):627–35.
4. Santoro N, Isaac B, Neal-Perry G, et al. Impaired folliculogenesis and ovulation in older reproductive aged women. J Clin Endocrinol Metab. 2003;88(11):5502–9.
5. Woods NF, Mitchell ES. Symptoms during the perimenopause: prevalence, severity, trajectory, and significance in women's lives. Am J Med. 2005;118(Suppl 12B):14–24.
6. Woods NF, Smith-DiJulio K, Percival DB, Tao EY, Mariella A, Mitchell S. Depressed mood during the menopausal transition and early postmenopause: observations from the Seattle Midlife Women's Health Study. Menopause. 2008;15(2):223–32.
7. Weber MT, Maki PM, McDermott MP. Cognition and mood in perimenopause: a systematic review and meta-analysis. J Steroid Biochem Mol Biol. 2014;142:90–8.
8. Bromberger JT, Schott LL, Kravitz HM, et al. Longitudinal change in reproductive hormones and depressive symptoms across the menopausal transition: results from the Study of Women's Health Across the Nation (SWAN). Arch Gen Psychiatry. 2010;67(6):598–607.
9. Bromberger JT, Schott L, Kravitz HM, Joffe H. Risk factors for major depression during midlife among a community sample of women with and without prior major depression: are they the same or different? Psychol Med. 2015;45(8):1653–64.
10. Fogle RH, Stanczyk FZ, Zhang X, Paulson RJ. Ovarian androgen production in postmenopausal women. J Clin Endocrinol Metab. 2007;92(8):3040–3.
11. Freedman RR. Hot flashes: behavioral treatments, mechanisms, and relation to sleep. Am J Med. 2005;118(Suppl 12B):124–30.
12. McConnell DS, Stanczyk FZ, Sowers MR, Randolph JFJ, Lasley BL. Menopausal transition stage-specific changes in circulating adrenal androgens. Menopause. 2012;19(6):658–63.
13. Rossmanith WG, Ruebberdt W. What causes hot flushes? The neuroendocrine origin of vasomotor symptoms in the menopause. Gynecol Endocrinol. 2009;25(5):303–14.
14. Boulant JA. Role of the preoptic-anterior hypothalamus in thermoregulation and fever. Clin Infect Dis. 2000;31(Suppl 5):S157–61.
15. Woods NF, Carr MC, Tao EY, Taylor HJ, Mitchell ES. Increased urinary cortisol levels during the menopausal transition. Menopause. 2006;13(2):212–21.
16. Hale GE, Hitchcock CL, Williams LA, Vigna YM, Prior JC. Cyclicity of breast tenderness and night-time vasomotor symptoms in mid-life women: information collected using the Daily Perimenopause Diary. Climacteric. 2003;6(2):128–39.
17. Gordon JL, Rubinow DR, Thurston RC, Paulson J, Schmidt PJ, Girdler SS. Cardiovascular, hemodynamic, neuroendocrine, and inflammatory markers in women with and without vasomotor symptoms. Menopause. 2016;23(11):1189–98.
18. Freeman EW, Sammel MD, Lin H, et al. Symptoms associated with menopausal transition and reproductive hormones in midlife women. Obstet Gynecol. 2007;110(2 Pt 1):230–40.
19. Pines A. Circadian rhythm and menopause. Climacteric. 2016;19(6):551–2.
20. Andersen ML, Bittencourt LR, Antunes IB, Tufik S. Effects of progesterone on sleep: a possible pharmacological treatment for sleep-breathing disorders? Curr Med Chem. 2006;13(29):3575–82.
21. Short RA, Bowen RL, O'Brien PC, Graff-Radford NR. Elevated gonadotropin levels in patients with Alzheimer disease. Mayo Clin Proc. 2001;76(9):906–9.
22. Wober C, Brannath W, Schmidt K, et al. Prospective analysis of factors related to migraine attacks: the PAMINA study. Cephalalgia. 2007;27(4):304–14.

23. Avis NE, Brambilla D, McKinlay SM, Vass K. A longitudinal analysis of the association between menopause and depression. Results from the Massachusetts Women's Health Study. Ann Epidemiol. 1994;4(3):214–20.
24. Freeman EW, Sammel MD, Boorman DW, Zhang R. Longitudinal pattern of depressive symptoms around natural menopause. JAMA Psychiat. 2014;71(1):36–43.
25. Gordon JL, Girdler SS, Meltzer-Brody SE, et al. Ovarian hormone fluctuation, neurosteroids, and HPA axis dysregulation in perimenopausal depression: a novel heuristic model. Am J Psychiatry. 2015;172(3):227–36.

The Neurological and Immunological Transitions of the Perimenopause: Implications for Postmenopausal Neurodegenerative Disease

2

Gerson D. Hernandez and Roberta Diaz Brinton

2.1 Introduction

Menopause is characterized by reproductive senescence and is the final stage of a midlife neuroendocrine transition state in the female known as perimenopause. About 900 million women are between the age of 40 and 60 years in the entire world [1]. The majority of women will transition through perimenopause and reach menopause at a median age range between 50 and 52 years in industrialized countries [2, 3]. Clinically, functional changes in the reproductive symptoms are characterized by women typically noticing a lengthening of intermenstrual interval increasing from a normal interval of 25–35 days up to 40–50 days [4]. Although viewed as a reproductive transition, the symptoms of the perimenopause are largely a result of neurological and immunological transitions and are observed irrespective of cultures, races, and ethnicities [5–24].

Neurological symptoms that emerge during the perimenopause are indicative of disruption in multiple estrogen-regulated systems including thermoregulation, sleep and circadian rhythms, sensory processing, affect, and multiple domains of cognitive function. Many of these symptoms are also associated with risk of Alzheimer's disease (AD) [5]. The main symptoms that characterize the perimenopausal transition tend to cluster in occurrence and severity [25] and in many instances persist after menopause [13, 14]. The breadth of neurological symptoms during the perimenopausal transition include but are not limited to vasomotor symptoms (hot flushes and night sweats), depression, sleep disturbances, vaginal dryness, sexual

G. D. Hernandez · R. D. Brinton (✉)
Center for Innovation in Brain Science, College of Medicine, University of Arizona, Tucson, AZ, USA
e-mail: gersonhe@email.arizona.edu; rbrinton@email.arizona.edu

© International Society of Gynecological Endocrinology 2019
R. D. Brinton et al. (eds.), *Sex Steroids' Effects on Brain, Heart and Vessels*, ISGE Series, https://doi.org/10.1007/978-3-030-11355-1_2

Table 2.1 Brain regions and their corresponding estrogen-regulated functions affected during the perimenopausal transition

Brain regions	Functions	Estrogen receptors affected
Prefrontal cortex	Executive function and working memory	ER-β, ER-α
Basal forebrain	Learning and memory	ER-β, ER-α, GPER
Hypothalamus	Thermoregulation, balance, sleep, energy, appetite	ER-β, ER-α, GPER
Thalamus	Sensory integration	ER-β, GPER
Amygdala	Emotion and motivation	ER-β, ER-α
Hippocampus	Information processing, and short-term memory	ER-β, ER-α, GPER
Raphe nucleus	Serotonergic system: affect and mood	ER-β, ER-α
Locus coeruleus	Adrenergic system: attention, anxiety, and arousal	ER-β, ER-α
Posterior cingulate	Default mode network, working memory, task preparation	ER-β

dysfunction, joint pain, and cognitive changes, all of which are indicative of a disruption in multiple systems regulated by estrogen [4]. Their concurrent emergence during this transition indicates they likely share common controlling factors (Table 2.1), which is also evidence that multiple requirements must be fulfilled beforehand.

2.2 The Perimenopausal Transition

The variability in physiological and neurological symptoms increases during the perimenopausal transition. The female reproductive system, controlled by the hypothalamic–pituitary–ovarian–uterine axis, undergoes targeted accelerated changes relative to other systems that are otherwise healthy [26].

The Stages of Reproductive Aging Workshop (STRAW) criteria [4], an international collaborative effort, along with the Study of Women Across the Nation (SWAN), based on an ethnically diverse US population [27], have contributed to both the classification of the perimenopausal transition while simultaneously identifying the complexity of symptoms and the ethnic diversity of perimenopausal phenotypes. These well-defined endocrine features of the perimenopause have enabled a classification system that describes the stages of reproductive aging across the perimenopause to postmenopause transition [4].

Endocrinologically, during perimenopause, changes in the hypothalamic–pituitary–ovarian–uterine axis [28] result in fluctuations in the level of circulating hormones and irregular menstrual cycles which causes ovulation to occur irregularly. Follicle-stimulating hormone (FSH), luteinizing hormone (LH), and 17β-estradiol levels are highly variable across the stages of the perimenopausal transition. Levels of FSH and LH may rise during some cycles but return to premenopausal levels in subsequent cycles [29]. Moreover, the determination of FSH is complicated by the pulsatile pattern of secretion, and only when perimenopause is complete do FSH levels stabilize [4]. The concentrations of 17β-estradiol are also highly variable throughout perimenopause as levels can be both persistently low but can also be abnormally high [20]. 17β-estradiol stabilizes at a low level in late-stage perimenopause when cycling has ceased and the menopausal transition has been completed. This high variability in estrogen is exemplified by the four distinct trajectories that have been described in regard to its levels during the perimenopausal transition: a slow gradual decline, a flat low level, a rise with slow decline, and a rise with steep decline [30]. Trajectories of hormonal change were highly correlated to race and BMI [30]. Remarkably, cyclicity of progesterone appears to remain generally intact, whereas the level of progesterone can vary between normal values and high spikes of progesterone to undetectable levels [29]. Variability in hormone levels creates difficulties in relying upon a single hormone level at a single time point to rule in or rule out perimenopause [31]. Despite the well-characterized trajectory of perimenopausal stages, variability in stage duration, complexity of symptom profile, and symptomatic severity can differ dramatically across and within ethnic groups [32].

From the neuroendocrine perspective, insensitivity to estrogen is associated with reactive gliosis in the hypothalamus and ultimately cell death [33]. In vitro findings from rat primary hippocampal neurons showed that the concentration or the pattern of exposure to estrogen was the determining factor of neuronal viability: a low concentration of estrogen promoted neuronal survival and intracellular calcium homeostasis, whereas a high concentration was ineffective and increased vulnerability to neurodegenerative insults [34]. Other studies examining ovarian versus neuroendocrine contributions to reproductive senescence revealed that both ovary and brain are determinants of reproductive life. Interestingly, it was neuroendocrine brain responses that limited reproductive system function, as the ovarian transplants remained viable [33, 35]. These data indicate that reproductive senescence is driven by both the ovaries and the brain and that persistent high levels of estrogen from the ovaries as occurs during the perimenopause are a likely candidate mediating the neural switch to reproductive senescence.

2.3   The Estrogen Receptor Network

Neural structures controlling neurological functions affected during the perimenopausal transition are populated with multiple types of estrogen receptors [36–43]. To date there are three distinct estrogen receptors: estrogen receptors alpha and beta (ERα, ESR1, and ERβ, ESR2) and the G-protein-coupled estrogen receptor (GPER; aka GPR30). For estrogen to be a regulator of the neurological systems generating perimenopause-associated symptoms, the estrogen receptors should be found in the relevant brain regions. The abundance of estrogen receptors in the hypothalamic preoptic nucleus, which is the primary thermoregulatory center, is among the densest in the brain [36, 44]. Likewise, the suprachiasmatic nucleus of the hypothalamus which plays a central role in regulation of sleep and circadian rhythms is rich in estrogen receptors [44]. In brain regions critical to learning and memory, estrogen receptors are present in the prefrontal cortex, each of the subfields of the hippocampus, the amygdala, and the cingulate/retrosplenial cortex [36, 44]. The serotoninergic neurons of the raphe nucleus are positive for estrogen receptors [41, 45] as are the adrenergic neurons of the locus coeruleus [36].

Oophorectomy prior to menopause induces the neurological symptoms of the perimenopausal transition, whereas replacement with estrogen prevents or reverses neurological symptoms [26, 38, 46–48]. Progesterone, also produced by the ovaries, does not appear to have the same impact and in many instances antagonizes the neural action of estrogen [49–51]. The ovarian and neural hormone estrogen regulates multiple neurological systems and functions in brain through the estrogen receptor network. Its regulatory function across multiple functional domains ensures that the brain can effectively respond within a timeframe of seconds/minutes up to hours/days. Additionally, estrogen ensures that cells and networks can generate sufficient energy to fuel neurological demand. Changes in either the availability of estrogen or its receptor network can impact both intracellular signaling and neural circuit function. While the intricacies of estrogen receptors and signaling cascades are well characterized, the coordination across the network of estrogen receptors necessary for neural circuit function awaits detailed investigation.

At the cellular level, the distribution of estrogen receptors creates a network poised to integrate actions at the membrane, endoplasmic reticular, mitochondrial, and nuclear compartments. These receptive elements allow for rapid, intermediate, and long-term responses at the cellular and neural system levels to generate an estrogenic cellular and neural system phenotype. Because of a hormonal and paracrine delivery system, estrogen is able to simultaneously activate its network of receptors in different neural systems to thereby coordinate responses throughout the brain. The pattern of estrogen receptor location permits the sequential activation of estrogen receptors to initiate rapid response cascades followed by engagement of genomic networks for longer-term responses. Regardless of intracellular locale, all estrogen receptors are activated by the endogenous estrogen, 17β-estradiol.

At the mitochondria, ERβ can regulate mitochondrial function [52] and potentially induce mitochondrial gene expression [53]. ERβ is also detected in the zone where the mitochondria interface and communicate with the endoplasmic reticulum, a region termed mitochondria-associated membranes [54]. ERβ within mitochondria is uniquely positioned to regulate mitochondrial gene expression [55]. Placing ERβ within mitochondria, estrogen can regulate energy homeostasis throughout the cell. This is particularly relevant for neurons where ATP is critical for synaptic transmission. Seventy-five percent of all ATP generated in neurons is utilized to meet the energetic demand of the Na^+/K^+ pump which pumps both Na^+ and K^+ against their concentration gradient to reestablish the neuronal membrane potential necessary to respond to the next volley of action potentials. This function is particularly critical for high-frequency synaptic transmission associated with learning and memory function [38, 47].

In the nucleus, transcription of nuclear-encoded genes requires translocation of ERα and ERβ. Estrogen receptors will bind to its specific estrogen response element (ERE) sequence on the DNA or tether onto other transcription factors such as the activator protein 1 or specificity protein 1 to regulate gene expression [39]. A one-dimensional view of estrogen receptor regulation of gene expression is that these transcription factors only promote gene expression. However, this is an over simplification, as exemplified in the case of estrogen regulation of the bioenergetic system of the brain. In this system, both ERα and ERβ promote expression of nuclear-encoded genes required for glucose transport, metabolism, and mitochondrial function while simultaneously suppressing genes required for ketone body metabolism, inflammation, and β-amyloid generation [50, 55].

The range of estrogen receptor complexity is extended through splice variants of both ERα (ESR1) and ERβ (ESR2) which typically generate differences in function [56]. In the brain, three splice variants of ERα have been detected [57] and one variant for ERβ [58]. Relevant to this discussion are splice variants generated during the perimenopausal transition. Splice variants of ERα were detected in both hypothalamus and hippocampus of the human female brain. A particular variant, MB1, appeared in perimenopausal aged women and increased throughout the transition with greatest expression in the postmenopausal brain [59]. MB1 variant is expressed in neurons, astrocytes, and endothelia where it is associated with nitric oxide production required for vasodilation. ERβ splice variants are also expressed in select brain regions including hypothalamus, hippocampus, and cerebral cortex [60]. A well-characterized variant, ESR2, has 18 amino acids inserted into the ligand-binding domain which significantly reduces the binding affinity of 17β-oestradiol [56]. In animal studies, ERβ2 was induced following ovariectomy and was associated with reduced neurogenesis and behavioral indicators of depression. Expression of ERβ2 was reversible if estrogen was administered soon after removal of the ovaries whereupon which restored neurogenesis and reversed behavioral indicators of depression [61]. Delaying administration of estrogen was ineffective in reversing the expression of ERβ2 and the concomitant ovariectomy-induced decline in neurogenesis and increase in depressive behavior [61]. Expression of splice variants of ERα and ERβ with, in some cases, decline in binding affinity could partially account for the perimenopausal loss in sensitivity to estrogen [62]. In addition to splice variants, there are several ERα polymorphisms that increase the risk of AD specifically in women, particularly when associated with the APOE4 allele [63].

The estrogen receptor network forms the basis of the dynamic signaling that occurs in the brain during the perimenopausal transition and as such is a determining factor of future cognitive health. For many women, the brain can compensate for the change in estrogen and its receptors. For others, however, adaptive compensation is diminished or lacking or expressed in some but not all estrogen-regulated neural networks giving rise to the complex phenotype of neurological symptoms.

2.4   Estrogen Regulation of the Bioenergetic System

Estrogen, its receptor network, and the regulation of the brain bioenergetic system are probable candidates to network the network [26, 38, 47, 63]. Estrogen utilizes a complex selection of receptors and signaling pathways to activate and regulate molecular and genomic responses required for neurological function [63].

Regulating the bioenergetic capacity within and across neural circuits would simultaneously support the function of multiple circuits while concurrently creating an energetic connectome between and across neural circuits.

In the brain, estrogen promotes the entire bioenergetic system from glucose transport to glucose metabolism to mitochondrial respiration and ATP production [38, 47, 55, 64–66]. Within the bioenergetic system of the brain, there appears to be an estrogen-dedicated component as either loss of estrogen or reproductive aging result in a 15–25% decline across components of the system suggesting that the estrogen-regulated aspects are connected [65, 67]. Estrogenic control of the bioenergetic system in the brain was established by the classic endocrine strategy of removing the ovaries and replacing estrogen or vehicle. Removal of the ovaries in premenopausal rodents resulted in bioenergetic deficits comparable to those that occurred during reproductive aging with one exception [67, 68]. Further, biochemical, genomic, and bioinformatic data indicate a synergistic interaction between the estrogen and insulin signaling pathways in the brain [69].

During the perimenopausal transition in the rodent, the bioenergetic system in brain undergoes profound changes resulting in a persistent decline in glucose metabolism in brain. Brain hypometabolism was first evident by a decline in glucose uptake as detected by FDG-microPET, in the neuron specific glucose transport (GLUT 3), and in hexokinase activity. These were accompanied by an inactivation of pyruvate dehydrogenase, and complex IV activity [64], thus resulting in impairment of the mitochondrial energy conservation systems. Lactate transport and utilization decreased in parallel to the decline in glucose transport indicating that lactate, which is generated from glucose in astrocytes, did not serve as an alternative fuel source.

During the normal perimenopause to postmenopausal transition, oxidative stress and free radical damage to mitochondrial lipid membranes do not appear until the animals have transitioned through perimenopause to reproductive senescence. In contrast, endocrine and aging programs were combined in the ovariectomized females with simultaneous induction of hypometabolism, mitochondrial dysfunction, and oxidative stress [67, 68]. Peripherally, dysregulation of the metabolic system was evidenced by impaired glucose tolerance indicative of insulin resistance [68]. The adverse impact of ovarian hormone loss on the bioenergetic system was prevented by administration of 17β-estradiol at time of ovariectomy [55, 67, 68, 70].

In response to glucose deprivation, the perimenopausal brain shifts to an adaptive bioenergetic response indicative of long-term fasting: utilization of ketone bodies as an alternative energy fuel [64, 65, 71–73] as evidenced by a rise in peripheral ketone bodies and their neuronal and astrocytic monocarboxylate transporters and an increase in mitochondrial succinyl-CoA:3-ketoacid CoA transferase (SCOT) necessary to metabolize ketone bodies [64, 65, 73]. In addition to the use of peripheral ketone bodies as an alternative fuel was the disconcerting rise in proteins necessary to metabolize fatty acids in the brain. These proteins, CPT1 (carnitine palmitoyltransferase 1A) and HADHA (hydroxyacyl-CoA dehydrogenase/3-ketoacyl-CoA thiolase/enoyl-CoA hydratase), are respectively required for fatty acid transport into and metabolism by the mitochondria. The trifunctional enzyme HADHA converts long-chain fatty acids to acetyl-CoA, the primer for ketone body synthesis. Because neither cholesterol nor fatty acids cross the blood–brain barrier, an increased fatty acid metabolism in the brain is predictive of catabolism of brain-derived lipids, which, in the long term, has dire consequences for cell membranes and lipid-rich reservoirs such as myelin in brain [72].

In women, a shift in metabolism during the perimenopause is also apparent and has been associated with dysregulation of glucose metabolism and insulin resistance [27, 63]. Overall, the data from analyses in the brain indicate that the perimenopausal transition is an orderly and sequential process during which the brain undergoes an uncoupling of the estrogen receptor network from the bioenergetic system. The uncoupling of the estrogen receptor from the bioenergetic system in the brain is also associated with a release of suppression of enzymes required to metabolize ketone bodies in the brain. The loss of suppression allows for the emergence of an adaptive compensatory response in the brain necessary to utilize ketone bodies as an alternative fuel.

2.5 Perimenopause-Associated Neurological Conditions

Multiple studies of brain metabolism in women suggest an association between hypometabolism in the brain and neurological symptoms [51]. The data is predominantly derived from studies of postmenopausal women with few studies specifically targeting the perimenopausal transition. In the aggregate, these studies indicate that users of estrogen therapy have a different pattern of brain metabolism relative to nonusers. In women on estrogen therapy, glucose metabolism is preserved in brain regions promoting estrogen-dependent neurological functions. In nonusers, glucose metabolism declined in estrogen-dependent regions and increased in brain regions that are estrogen-independent. These findings illustrate again the adaptive capacity of the menopausal female brain and highlight the need for more detailed analyses of brain metabolism during the perimenopause in studies focused on genotypic and phenotypic characteristics.

Vasomotor symptoms—The most frequent and often defining feature of the perimenopausal transition is hot flushes which occur in 75–80% perimenopausal women and which can continue unabated for decades in ~5% of women [4, 74, 75]. Hot flushes can be the only symptom of the perimenopause experienced by women. However, in many women hot flushes are clustered with other neurological symptoms including memory impairment [13, 76], sleep disturbances, pain, and depression [25]. The clinical manifestations of a hot flush have been well documented and are characterized by the sudden onset of a disturbing and intrusive rise in body temperature intensively primarily experienced in upper body encompassing chest, neck, and head with visible flushing [75]. The hot flush is a transient event characterized by a rapid onset and dissipation within seconds to minutes but can also be prolonged in duration lasting 60 min. Hot flushes range from mild to severe, can occur with a frequency of 2–50 per day, and occur throughout the day and night with particular severity and frequency during the sleep cycle which can disrupt sleep and daily activities causing severe stress and anxiety [77].

The hypothalamus controls thermoregulation and thus is thought to initiate the hot flush in response to a rise in core temperature [78]. The prevailing conceptualization of the hot flush is a compression of the hypothalamic thermoneutral zone that leads to the episodic release of heat in response to a slight elevation in core body temperature [75]. While the hypothalamus is undoubtedly involved in the thermoregulatory response, functional MRI analyses indicate that the insula and anterior cingulate cortex were activated during hot flushes and were coupled to superior frontal gyrus activation with sweating [78]. Insular cortex activation is associated with the sensation of "rush of heat." These findings advance our understanding of the perimenopausal hot flush beyond the temperature regulatory zones of the hypothalamus to include an expanded neural network that includes subcortical and cortical structures.

Research in the field points toward an association of hot flushes with altered glucose metabolism [64, 79, 80]. Preclinical studies of bioenergetics in animal models of the perimenopausal and menopausal female brain indicate that a rise in skin temperature is coincident with onset of reproductive variability and senescence, decline in brain glucose metabolism, compromised glucose tolerance in the periphery indicative of insulin resistance, and utilization of ketone bodies and fatty acid metabolism in the brain [64, 65, 73]. Consistent with preclinical findings, FDG-PET imaging analyses in the human female brain indicate a decline in brain glucose metabolism during late perimenopause that continues into postmenopause [81]. In the SWAN study, hot flushes or night sweats were significantly associated with dysregulation in glucose metabolism indicated by significantly higher fasting blood glucose and HOMA score [80]. The relationship between estrogen and insulin receptors is well established in the brain and provides yet another link whereby decline in estrogen may contribute to dysregulated glucose metabolism in the brain [69]. Further evidence for metabolic dysregulation and the hot flush is the association between impaired adipokine profile and occurrence of hot flushes early in the perimenopausal transition [63, 82]. Lower adiponectin and higher leptin were associated with higher odds of hot flushes early, but not later, in the menopause transition. This adipokine profile paralleled BMI in this population of women who exhibited a stage-dependent relationship with hot flushes such that higher BMI was associated with higher odds of hot flushes early, but not later in the transition. Higher serum level of the inflammatory monocyte chemoattractant protein 1 (MCP-1) was associated with higher odds of night sweats regardless of menopause stage [82]. Collectively, the data indicate a strong association of hot flushes with impaired glucose homeostasis that is evident in both brain and the periphery [63].

Sleep disturbances—Insomnia is a prevalent symptom of the perimenopausal transition and is frequently associated with hot flushes, night sweats, depression, and cognitive deficits [25, 83, 84]. Interestingly, in the suprachiasmatic nucleus, a key node for diurnal rhythm, ERβ exhibits a diurnal rhythm which is evident in young and middle age rodents but not in the old [85]. In the SWAN study, prevalence of sleep disturbance varied with ethnicity with the highest prevalence (40%) in Caucasian women; intermediate prevalence (31–38%) in Chinese, Hispanic, and African American women; and lowest in Japanese women (28%) [84]. The SWAN data indicate that sleep difficulties are greatest during late perimenopause and persist into postmenopause, irrespective of vasomotor symptoms [84]. Brain imaging in perimenopausal women with sleep disturbances has not been conducted; however, an emerging body of data indicate long-term adverse consequences of sleep deprivation for brain structure and function [86]. Multiple studies have indicated an association between insomnia and reduced brain volume in regions that include the hippocampus and orbitofrontal and parietal grey matter [86]. Further, most prospective studies show poor sleep quality is associated with an increased likelihood of cognitive impairment and in some studies an increased risk of dementia [86]. Further, sleep deprivation is now recognized to induce β-amyloid accumulation in the brain [87].

Cognition—Subjective and objective memory deficits are well documented during the perimenopausal transition [14]. FDG-PET indicators of hypometabolism in brain regions required for learning and memory function have been reported for regional cerebral blood flow [88] and glucose metabolism [51, 81]. Hypometabolism was apparent in menopausal women over a 2-year period of observation in hippocampus, parahippocampal gyrus, temporal lobe [88], medial prefrontal cortex, and posterior cingulate cortex [51, 81]. Estrogen or hormone therapy prevented hypometabolism in each of these brain regions [51, 88] and preserved memory function [88]. In the study of regional cerebral blood flow, women on estrogen replacement therapy increased resting state cerebral blood flow over time in brain regions now recognized as part of the default mode network whereas nonusers did not [88]. Nonusers, however, increased cerebral blood flow to brain regions required for motor and spatial function [88, 89]. In perimenopausal hormone therapy users, enhanced activation in the hippocampus combined with decreased parahippocampal activation suggests that perimenopausal hormone therapy increased both state-dependent and recollective processes to promote verbal recognition performance [90]. Recent analyses of the default mode network in neurologically normal postmenopausal women at risk for AD indicated that women with higher blood insulin levels had diminished network connectivity relative to women with low insulin levels [91]. Protective metabolic effects of hormone therapy were most evident in women with lower insulin resistance, whereas it was ineffective in women with greater insulin resistance [92]. Performance in working memory paralleled the metabolic response to hormone therapy [92]. It is now well established that brain metabolism is critical to neurological function and that hypometabolism in the brain is evident decades prior to diagnosis of neurodegenerative diseases such as AD [93–95].

Depression—Perimenopausal women have a higher risk of depression compared to premenopausal women [12, 14, 15]. Short-term estradiol treatment in perimenopausal women that exhibited major or minor depression decreased their depression assessment scores [12]. Risk for major depression has been linked to variants of ERα: women homozygous for the ESR1 rs9340799 variant G had a 1.6-fold increased lifetime risk of major depressive disorder [96]. Timing of estrogen therapy appears to be critical in the effectiveness of treatment since depression scores were not improved in women who received estrogen treatment 5–10 years post perimenopause [10]. Brain metabolism in brain regions regulating depression and anxiety is complex with differing metabolic phenotypes in the pons (where the serotonergic raphe nucleus and locus coeruleus adrenergic systems originate) and frontal cortices [10, 97]. Relative to non-depressed women, depressed women exhibited hypometabolism in the pons and hypermetabolism in the middle and inferior frontal gyrus [97]. In non-depressed postmenopausal women in their late 60s, regional cerebral blood flow was increased in the left pons [88]. Although the long-term impact of perimenopausal depression remains to be determined, extensive epidemiological analyses indicate that depression is a risk factor for AD [98, 99].

2.6   Sex Difference and Risk of AD

The greatest risk factors for AD are age [100], the ApoE4 allele [101], and female sex [100]. Postmenopausal women constitute >60% of the affected AD population and are those who will bear the greatest burden of the disease [47, 102–104]. Farrer and colleagues two decades ago indicated that women with a single copy of the ApoE4 allele was sufficient to increase disease risk associated with two copies of the ApoE4 gene in men, suggesting a sex difference in the lifetime risk of AD in women [105]. This finding was confirmed later by Payami and colleagues who found that ApoE4 heterozygote men had lower risk than ApoE4 homozygotes [106]; there was not significant difference between epsilon4 heterozygote males and those without epsilon4. In contrast, epsilon4 heterozygote women had the same significant twofold increased risk as homozygote men [106]. Barnes et al. found an even greater sex difference in the impact of pathology and risk of AD [107]. Each additional unit of AD pathology was associated with a nearly three-fold increase in the odds of clinical AD in men compared with a more than 22-fold increase in the odds of clinical AD in women [107].

The earliest etiological factors that ultimately lead to late-onset AD, when prevention is still possible, remain unresolved for the primary casualties of the disease, postmenopausal women [5, 38]. While AD is not unique to the female, women constitute the majority of persons with the disease [108]. Discovery of high-risk AD phenotypes in women and their underlying mechanisms could potentially lead to the early identification of those at greatest risk of developing AD and interventions to prevent the disease.

2.7   Metabolic-Inflammatory Axis

Oxidation-reduction regulation connects the brain metabolism and neuroinflammation. Aging and neurodegenerative brains are found to be associated with chronic neuroinflammation primarily due to a dysregulation of the innate immunity, mainly driven by senescent microglia. Deficits in metabolic and mitochondrial function lead to the impairment of redox homeostasis, which is one of the major stimulators of the neuroinflammatory responses in aging and AD. The peripheral metabolism also plays an important role in the progression of neurodegeneration and is evidenced by the reciprocity between brain functioning and the systemic environment. The role of obesity and systemic inflammation in AD pathogenesis is well described, especially in women who have a twofold increased risk compared to men [109]. Increased central adiposity and elevated inflammation are linked to estrogen depletion during perimenopause and menopause elevating women's vulnerability to develop AD [109].

2.8   Implications of the Perimenopausal Transition for Later Life

The perimenopausal transition initiates a targeted, sequential, and orderly disassembly of the reproductive system and the neural substrates that control its function. As a transition state, the perimenopause for women appears to be comparable in its vulnerability as puberty is for both males and females. In this regard, the perimenopause fulfills criteria for a "critical period" in the neuro-adaptive landscape of aging in the female brain. Most women transition through this critical period without complications and are likely to remain relatively healthy without long-term adverse effects. In contrast, a significant proportion of women are vulnerable to the neurological shifts that occur during this transition and emerge from the perimenopause at risk for continued neurological decline. For some, this critical transition period can be a tipping point for the emergence of neurological disease later in life.

It is becoming increasingly clear that complex systems have critical thresholds, often referred to as tipping points, when a system shifts from one state to the other [110]. Analyses of transition state dynamics predict three health states, healthy, pre-disease, and disease [110]. The pre-disease transition state is typically defined as the limit of the normal state that precedes the tipping point into disease. Importantly, the pre-disease state is unstable and is thus potentially reversible. However, the duration of reversibility is limited. The bifurcation point between pre-disease and disease is characterized by a *critical slowing* of the system, in which it becomes increasingly slow to recover from small perturbations to equilibrium [110]. Transition states are inherently unstable, and in the case of neurological transition states, indicators of dysfunction at the limits of normal can be signals of instability and tipping points. The presence, variability, intensity, and duration of perimenopausal symptoms provide potential advance warning signs of impending risk of later health risks, particularly neurodegenerative diseases. Multiple conditions that emerge during the perimenopause, such as insomnia, depression, subjective memory complaints, and cognitive decline, are associated with increased risk of neurodegenerative diseases later in life such as AD. In the same manner, multiple neurodegenerative diseases are characterized by long prodromal periods during which the disease progresses to clinically diagnosed dysfunction. It remains to be determined whether or not the neurological vulnerabilities that can emerge during the perimenopause increase risk for later-life neurological diseases. However, the emergence of hypometabolism during the perimenopause that persists in later years suggests that for some women vulnerability for later-life neurodegenerative disease may have been established. The ability to detect both peripheral and neurological indicators of metabolic dysfunction provides a window of opportunity to prevent late-life neurological disease by sustaining neurological bioenergetic capacity during aging.

2.9 Conclusions

Symptoms of perimenopause are largely neurological and immunological in nature. The experience of this transition can be highly variable, but the outcome, menopause, is inevitable and denotes a transformed neurological system. Determining the best strategy to sustain neurological bioenergetic capacity in women during this critical period in life is crucial to sustain brain function. Identifying women with metabolic or inflammatory at-risk phenotypes for late-onset AD might translate into a target population that is likely to respond to estrogen replacement therapy and adjuvant therapies that serve as metabolic regulators. Transitions of female aging involve a set of sequential, system-level adaptations. Precision hormone therapy during the perimenopausal transition to aid the neuro-adaptations of the aging brain might be the answer to prevent the potential transition into early AD.

References

1. United Nations. Word population prospects: the 2017 revision. Department of Economic and Social Affairs, Population Division. 2017. https://esa.un.org/unpd/wpp/dataquery/. Accessed 17 Jul 2017.
2. Gold EB, Bromberger J, Crawford S, et al. Factors associated with age at natural menopause in a multiethnic sample of midlife women. Am J Epidemiol. 2001;153(9):865–74.
3. Gold EB. The timing of the age at which natural menopause occurs. Obstet Gynecol Clin N Am. 2011;38(3):425–40.
4. Harlow SD, Gass M, Hall JE, et al. Executive summary of the Stages of Reproductive Aging Workshop + 10: addressing the unfinished agenda of staging reproductive aging. Menopause. 2012;19(4):387–95.
5. Brinton RD, Yao J, Yin F, Mack WJ, Cadenas E. Perimenopause as a neurological transition. Nat Rev Endocrinol. 2015;11:393–405.
6. Maki PM, Drogos LL, Rubin LH, Banuvar S, Shulman LP, Geller SE. Objective hot flashes are negatively related to verbal memory performance in midlife women. Menopause. 2008;15(5):848–56.
7. Maki PM, Rubin LH, Cohen M, et al. Depressive symptoms are increased in the early perimenopausal stage in ethnically diverse human immunodeficiency virus-infected and human immunodeficiency virus-uninfected women. Menopause. 2012;19(11):1215–23.
8. Greendale GA, Huang MH, Wight RG, et al. Effects of the menopause transition and hormone use on cognitive performance in midlife women. Neurology. 2009;72(21):1850–7.
9. Greendale GA, Wight RG, Huang MH, et al. Menopause-associated symptoms and cognitive performance: results from the study of women's health across the nation. Am J Epidemiol. 2010;171(11):1214–24.
10. Rasgon N, Shelton S, Halbreich U. Perimenopausal mental disorders: epidemiology and phenomenology. CNS Spectr. 2005;10(6):471–8.

11. Schmidt PJ, Rubinow DR. Reproductive ageing, sex steroids and depression. J Br Menopause Soc. 2006;12(4):178–85.
12. Schmidt PJ, Rubinow DR. Sex hormones and mood in the perimenopause. Ann N Y Acad Sci. 2009;1179:70–85.
13. Weber MT, Rubin LH, Maki PM. Cognition in perimenopause: the effect of transition stage. Menopause. 2013;20(5):511–7.
14. Weber MT, Maki PM, McDermott MP. Cognition and mood in perimenopause: a systematic review and meta-analysis. J Steroid Biochem Mol Biol. 2014;142:90–8.
15. Freeman EW, Sammel MD, Lin H. Temporal associations of hot flashes and depression in the transition to menopause. Menopause. 2009;16(4):728–34.
16. Bromberger JT, Schott LL, Kravitz HM, et al. Longitudinal change in reproductive hormones and depressive symptoms across the menopausal transition: results from the Study of Women's Health Across the Nation (SWAN). Arch Gen Psychiatry. 2010;67(6):598–607.
17. Thurston RC, Santoro N, Matthews KA. Adiposity and hot flashes in midlife women: a modifying role of age. J Clin Endocrinol Metab. 2011;96(10):E1588–95.
18. Nelson HD. Menopause. Lancet. 2008;371(9614):760–70.
19. Usall J, Pinto-Meza A, Fernandez A, et al. Suicide ideation across reproductive life cycle of women. Results from a European epidemiological study. J Affect Disord. 2009;116(1–2):144–7.
20. Genazzani AR, Bernardi F, Pluchino N, et al. Endocrinology of menopausal transition and its brain implications. CNS Spectr. 2005;10(6):449–57.
21. Genazzani AR, Gambacciani M, Simoncini T. Menopause and aging, quality of life and sexuality. Climacteric. 2007;10(2):88–96.
22. Genazzani AR, Pluchino N, Luisi S, Luisi M. Estrogen, cognition and female ageing. Hum Reprod Update. 2007;13(2):175–87.
23. Cray LA, Woods NF, Mitchell ES. Identifying symptom clusters during the menopausal transition: observations from the Seattle Midlife Women's Health Study. Climacteric. 2013;16(5):539–49.
24. Makara-Studzinska MT, Krys-Noszczyk KM, Jakiel G. Epidemiology of the symptoms of menopause - an intercontinental review. Przeglad Menopauzalny. 2014;13(3):203–11.
25. Cray LA, Woods NF, Herting JR, Mitchell ES. Symptom clusters during the late reproductive stage through the early postmenopause: observations from the Seattle Midlife Women's Health Study. Menopause. 2012;19(8):864–9.
26. Brinton RD, Gore AC, Schmidt PJ, Morrison JH. Reproductive aging of females: neural systems. Horm Brain Behav. 2009;4:2199–222.
27. Santoro N, Sutton-Tyrrell K. The SWAN song: Study of Women's Health Across the Nation's recurring themes. Obstet Gynecol Clin N Am. 2011;38(3):417–23.
28. Butler L, Santoro N. The reproductive endocrinology of the menopausal transition. Steroids. 2011;76(7):627–35.
29. Burger H, Woods NF, Dennerstein L, Alexander JL, Kotz K, Richardson G. Nomenclature and endocrinology of menopause and perimenopause. Expert Rev Neurother. 2007;7(11 Suppl):S35–43.
30. Tepper PG, Randolph JF Jr, McConnell DS, et al. Trajectory clustering of estradiol and follicle-stimulating hormone during the menopausal transition among women in the Study of Women's Health across the Nation (SWAN). J Clin Endocrinol Metab. 2012;97(8):2872–80.
31. Bastian LA, Smith CM, Nanda K. Is this woman perimenopausal? JAMA. 2003;289(7):895–902.
32. Avis NE, Stellato R, Crawford S, et al. Is there a menopausal syndrome? Menopausal status and symptoms across racial/ethnic groups. Soc Sci Med. 2001;52(3):345–56.
33. Finch CE, Felicio LS, Mobbs CV, Nelson JF. Ovarian and steroidal influences on neuroendocrine aging processes in female rodents. Endocr Rev. 1984;5(4):467–97.
34. Chen S, Nilsen J, Brinton RD. Dose and temporal pattern of estrogen exposure determines neuroprotective outcome in hippocampal neurons: therapeutic implications. Endocrinology. 2006;147(11):5303–13.

35. Mobbs CV, Gee DM, Finch CE. Reproductive senescence in female C57BL/6J mice: ovarian impairments and neuroendocrine impairments that are partially reversible and delayable by ovariectomy. Endocrinology. 1984;115(5):1653–62.
36. Shughrue PJ, Lane MV, Merchenthaler I. Comparative distribution of estrogen receptor-alpha and -beta mRNA in the rat central nervous system. J Comp Neurol. 1997;388(4):507–25.
37. O'Dowd BF, Nguyen T, Marchese A, et al. Discovery of three novel G-protein-coupled receptor genes. Genomics. 1998;47(2):310–3.
38. Brinton RD. Estrogen-induced plasticity from cells to circuits: predictions for cognitive function. Trends Pharmacol Sci. 2009;30(4):212–22.
39. Nilsson S, Koehler KF, Gustafsson JA. Development of subtype-selective oestrogen receptor-based therapeutics. Nat Rev Drug Discov. 2011;10(10):778–92.
40. Prossnitz ER, Barton M. The G-protein-coupled estrogen receptor GPER in health and disease. Nat Rev Endocrinol. 2011;7(12):715–26.
41. Suzuki H, Barros RP, Sugiyama N, et al. Involvement of estrogen receptor beta in maintenance of serotonergic neurons of the dorsal raphe. Mol Psychiatry. 2013;18(6):674–80.
42. Brailoiu E, Dun SL, Brailoiu GC, et al. Distribution and characterization of estrogen receptor G protein-coupled receptor 30 in the rat central nervous system. J Endocrinol. 2007;193(2):311–21.
43. Naugle MM, Nguyen LT, Merceron TK, et al. G-protein coupled estrogen receptor, estrogen receptor alpha, and progesterone receptor immunohistochemistry in the hypothalamus of aging female rhesus macaques given long-term estradiol treatment. J Exp Zool A Ecol Genet Physiol. 2014;321(7):399–414.
44. Rainbow TC, Parsons B, MacLusky NJ, McEwen BS. Estradiol receptor levels in rat hypothalamic and limbic nuclei. J Neurosci. 1982;2(10):1439–45.
45. Bethea CL, Mirkes SJ, Su A, Michelson D. Effects of oral estrogen, raloxifene and arzoxifene on gene expression in serotonin neurons of macaques. Psychoneuroendocrinology. 2002;27(4):431–45.
46. Maki PM. The timing of estrogen therapy after ovariectomy--implications for neurocognitive function. Nat Clin Pract Endocrinol Metab. 2008;4(9):494–5.
47. Brinton RD. The healthy cell bias of estrogen action: mitochondrial bioenergetics and neurological implications. Trends Neurosci. 2008;31(10):529–37.
48. Rocca WA, Grossardt BR, Shuster LT. Oophorectomy, estrogen, and dementia: a 2014 update. Mol Cell Endocrinol. 2014;389(1–2):7–12.
49. Brinton RD, Thompson RF, Foy MR, et al. Progesterone receptors: form and function in brain. Front Neuroendocrinol. 2008;29(2):313–39.
50. Zhao L, Morgan TE, Mao Z, et al. Continuous versus cyclic progesterone exposure differentially regulates hippocampal gene expression and functional profiles. PLoS One. 2012;7(2):e31267.
51. Rasgon NL, Geist CL, Kenna HA, Wroolie TE, Williams KE, Silverman DH. Prospective randomized trial to assess effects of continuing hormone therapy on cerebral function in postmenopausal women at risk for dementia. PLoS One. 2014;9(3):e89095.
52. Irwin RW, Yao J, To J, Hamilton RT, Cadenas E, Brinton RD. Selective oestrogen receptor modulators differentially potentiate brain mitochondrial function. J Neuroendocrinol. 2012;24(1):236–48.
53. Arnold S, Victor MB, Beyer C. Estrogen and the regulation of mitochondrial structure and function in the brain. J Steroid Biochem Mol Biol. 2012;131(1–2):2–9.
54. Milner TA, Ayoola K, Drake CT, et al. Ultrastructural localization of estrogen receptor beta immunoreactivity in the rat hippocampal formation. J Comp Neurol. 2005;491(2):81–95.
55. Nilsen J, Irwin RW, Gallaher TK, Brinton RD. Estradiol in vivo regulation of brain mitochondrial proteome. J Neurosci. 2007;27(51):14069–77.
56. Heldring N, Pike A, Andersson S, et al. Estrogen receptors: how do they signal and what are their targets. Physiol Rev. 2007;87(3):905–31.
57. NCBI. Homo sapiens gene ESR1, encoding estrogen receptor 1. 2010. http://www.ncbi.nlm.nih.gov/IEB/Research/Acembly/av.cgi?db=human&term=ESR1&submit=Go.
58. NCBI. Homo sapiens complex locus ESR2, encoding estrogen receptor 2 (ER beta). 2010.

59. Ishunina TA, Swaab DF. Age-dependent ERalpha MB1 splice variant expression in discrete areas of the human brain. Neurobiol Aging. 2008;29(8):1177–89.
60. Chung WC, Pak TR, Suzuki S, Pouliot WA, Andersen ME, Handa RJ. Detection and localization of an estrogen receptor beta splice variant protein (ERbeta2) in the adult female rat forebrain and midbrain regions. J Comp Neurol. 2007;505(3):249–67.
61. Wang JM, Hou X, Adeosun S, et al. A dominant negative ERbeta splice variant determines the effectiveness of early or late estrogen therapy after ovariectomy in rats. PLoS One. 2012;7(3):e33493.
62. Weiss G, Skurnick JH, Goldsmith LT, Santoro NF, Park SJ. Menopause and hypothalamic-pituitary sensitivity to estrogen. JAMA. 2004;292(24):2991–6.
63. Rettberg JR, Yao J, Brinton RD. Estrogen: a master regulator of bioenergetic systems in the brain and body. Front Neuroendocrinol. 2014;35(1):8–30.
64. Ding F, Yao J, Rettberg JR, Chen S, Brinton RD. Early decline in glucose transport and metabolism precedes shift to ketogenic system in female aging and Alzheimer's mouse brain: implication for bioenergetic intervention. PLoS One. 2013;8(11):e79977.
65. Yao J, Hamilton RT, Cadenas E, Brinton RD. Decline in mitochondrial bioenergetics and shift to ketogenic profile in brain during reproductive senescence. Biochim Biophys Acta. 2010;1800(10):1121–6.
66. Simpkins JW, Yi KD, Yang SH, Dykens JA. Mitochondrial mechanisms of estrogen neuroprotection. Biochim Biophys Acta. 2010;1800(10):1113–20.
67. Yao J, Irwin R, Chen S, Hamilton R, Cadenas E, Brinton RD. Ovarian hormone loss induces bioenergetic deficits and mitochondrial beta-amyloid. Neurobiol Aging. 2012;33(8):1507–21.
68. Ding F, Yao J, Zhao L, Mao Z, Chen S, Brinton RD. Ovariectomy induces a shift in fuel availability and metabolism in the hippocampus of the female transgenic model of familial Alzheimer's. PLoS One. 2013;8(3):e59825.
69. Mendez P, Wandosell F, Garcia-Segura LM. Cross-talk between estrogen receptors and insulin-like growth factor-I receptor in the brain: cellular and molecular mechanisms. Front Neuroendocrinol. 2006;27(4):391–403.
70. Zhao L, Mao Z, Chen S, Schneider LS, Brinton RD. Early intervention with an estrogen receptor beta-selective phytoestrogenic formulation prolongs survival, improves spatial recognition memory, and slows progression of amyloid pathology in a female mouse model of Alzheimer's disease. J Alzheimers Dis. 2013;37(2):403–19.
71. Cahill GF Jr. Fuel metabolism in starvation. Annu Rev Nutr. 2006;26:1–22.
72. Yao J, Rettberg JR, Klosinski LP, Cadenas E, Brinton RD. Shift in brain metabolism in late onset Alzheimer's disease: implications for biomarkers and therapeutic interventions. Mol Asp Med. 2011;32(4–6):247–57.
73. Yao J, Irwin RW, Zhao L, Nilsen J, Hamilton RT, Brinton RD. Mitochondrial bioenergetic deficit precedes Alzheimer's pathology in female mouse model of Alzheimer's disease. Proc Natl Acad Sci U S A. 2009;106(34):14670–5.
74. Santoro N. Symptoms of menopause: hot flushes. Clin Obstet Gynecol. 2008;51(3):539–48.
75. Freedman RR. Menopausal hot flashes: mechanisms, endocrinology, treatment. J Steroid Biochem Mol Biol. 2014;142:115–20.
76. Maki PM. Minireview: effects of different HT formulations on cognition. Endocrinology. 2012;153(8):3564–70.
77. Avis NE, Colvin A, Bromberger JT, et al. Change in health-related quality of life over the menopausal transition in a multiethnic cohort of middle-aged women: Study of Women's Health Across the Nation. Menopause. 2009;16(5):860–9.
78. Freedman RR, Benton MD, Genik RJ II, Graydon FX. Cortical activation during menopausal hot flashes. Fertil Steril. 2006;85(3):674–8.
79. Simpkins JW, Katovich MJ, Millard WJ. Glucose modulation of skin temperature responses during morphine withdrawal in the rat. Psychopharmacology. 1990;102(2):213–20.
80. Thurston RC, El Khoudary SR, Sutton-Tyrrell K, et al. Vasomotor symptoms and insulin resistance in the study of women's health across the nation. J Clin Endocrinol Metab. 2012;97(10):3487–94.

81. Rasgon NL, Silverman D, Siddarth P, et al. Estrogen use and brain metabolic change in post-menopausal women. Neurobiol Aging. 2005;26(2):229–35.
82. Thurston RC, Chang Y, Mancuso P, Matthews KA. Adipokines, adiposity, and vasomotor symptoms during the menopause transition: findings from the Study of Women's Health Across the Nation. Fertil Steril. 2013;100(3):793–800.
83. Campbell IG, Bromberger JT, Buysse DJ, et al. Evaluation of the association of menopausal status with delta and beta EEG activity during sleep. Sleep. 2011;34(11):1561–8.
84. Kravitz HM, Joffe H. Sleep during the perimenopause: a SWAN story. Obstet Gynecol Clin N Am. 2011;38(3):567–86.
85. Wilson ME, Rosewell KL, Kashon ML, Shughrue PJ, Merchenthaler I, Wise PM. Age differentially influences estrogen receptor-alpha (ERalpha) and estrogen receptor-beta (ERbeta) gene expression in specific regions of the rat brain. Mech Ageing Dev. 2002;123(6):593–601.
86. Yaffe K, Falvey CM, Hoang T. Connections between sleep and cognition in older adults. Lancet Neurol. 2014;13(10):1017–28.
87. Ju YE, Lucey BP, Holtzman DM. Sleep and Alzheimer disease pathology--a bidirectional relationship. Nat Rev Neurol. 2014;10(2):115–9.
88. Maki PM, Resnick SM. Longitudinal effects of estrogen replacement therapy on PET cerebral blood flow and cognition. Neurobiol Aging. 2000;21(2):373–83.
89. Yee LT, Roe K, Courtney SM. Selective involvement of superior frontal cortex during working memory for shapes. J Neurophysiol. 2010;103(1):557–63.
90. Maki PM, Dennerstein L, Clark M, et al. Perimenopausal use of hormone therapy is associated with enhanced memory and hippocampal function later in life. Brain Res. 2011;1379:232–43.
91. Kenna H, Hoeft F, Kelley R, et al. Fasting plasma insulin and the default mode network in women at risk for Alzheimer's disease. Neurobiol Aging. 2013;34(3):641–9.
92. Rasgon NL, Kenna HA, Wroolie TE, Williams KE, DeMuth BN, Silverman DH. Insulin resistance and medial prefrontal gyrus metabolism in women receiving hormone therapy. Psychiatry Res. 2014;223(1):28–36.
93. Mosconi L, Mistur R, Switalski R, et al. Declining brain glucose metabolism in normal individuals with a maternal history of Alzheimer disease. Neurology. 2009;72(6):513–20.
94. Rasgon NL, Kenna HA, Wroolie TE, et al. Insulin resistance and hippocampal volume in women at risk for Alzheimer's disease. Neurobiol Aging. 2011;32(11):1942–8.
95. Mosconi L, Murray J, Tsui WH, et al. Brain imaging of cognitively normal individuals with 2 parents affected by late-onset AD. Neurology. 2014;82(9):752–60.
96. Ryan J, Scali J, Carriere I, et al. Estrogen receptor alpha gene variants and major depressive episodes. J Affect Disord. 2012;136(3):1222–6.
97. Rasgon NL, Kenna HA, Geist C, Small G, Silverman D. Cerebral metabolic patterns in untreated postmenopausal women with major depressive disorder. Psychiatry Res. 2008;164(1):77–80.
98. Yaffe K, Tocco M, Petersen RC, et al. The epidemiology of Alzheimer's disease: laying the foundation for drug design, conduct, and analysis of clinical trials. Alzheimers Dement. 2012;8(3):237–42.
99. Norton S, Matthews FE, Barnes DE, Yaffe K, Brayne C. Potential for primary prevention of Alzheimer's disease: an analysis of population-based data. Lancet Neurol. 2014;13(8):788–94.
100. Hebert LE, Weuve J, Scherr PA, Evans DA. Alzheimer disease in the United States (2010–2050) estimated using the 2010 census. Neurology. 2013;80(19):1778–83.
101. Altmann A, Tian L, Henderson VW, Greicius MD. Sex modifies the APOE-related risk of developing Alzheimer disease. Ann Neurol. 2014;75(4):563–73.
102. Brookmeyer R, Gray S, Kawas C. Projections of Alzheimer's disease in the United States and the public health impact of delaying disease onset. Am J Public Health. 1998;88(9):1337–42.
103. Brookmeyer R, Johnson E, Ziegler-Graham K, Arrighi HM. Forecasting the global burden of Alzheimer's disease. Alzheimers Dement. 2007;3(3):186–91.
104. Morrison JH, Brinton RD, Schmidt PJ, Gore AC. Estrogen, menopause, and the aging brain: how basic neuroscience can inform hormone therapy in women. J Neurosci. 2006;26(41):10332–48.

105. Farrer LA, Cupples LA, van Duijn CM, et al. Apolipoprotein E genotype in patients with Alzheimer's disease: implications for the risk of dementia among relatives. Ann Neurol. 1995;38(5):797–808.
106. Payami H, Zareparsi S, Montee KR, et al. Gender difference in apolipoprotein E-associated risk for familial Alzheimer disease: a possible clue to the higher incidence of Alzheimer disease in women. Am J Hum Genet. 1996;58(4):803–11.
107. Barnes LL, Wilson RS, Bienias JL, Schneider JA, Evans DA, Bennett DA. Sex differences in the clinical manifestations of Alzheimer disease pathology. Arch Gen Psychiatry. 2005;62(6):685–91.
108. Alzheimer's Association. 2014. Alzheimer's Assoc facts_figures_2014.pdf. Chicago.
109. Christensen A, Pike CJ. Menopause, obesity and inflammation: interactive risk factors for Alzheimer's disease. Front Aging Neurosci. 2015;7:130.
110. Chen L, Liu R, Liu ZP, Li M, Aihara K. Detecting early-warning signals for sudden deterioration of complex diseases by dynamical network biomarkers. Sci Rep. 2012;2:342.

Estrogenic Regulation of Neuroprotective and Neuroinflammatory Mechanisms: Implications for Depression and Cognition

3

Natalia Yanguas-Casás, Maria Elvira Brocca, Iñigo Azcoitia, Maria Angeles Arevalo, and Luis M. Garcia-Segura

3.1   Introduction

Hormones are molecules that participate in the communication of different organs to maintain body homeostasis. According to this role, hormones are involved in the maintenance of an adequate physiological function of different body systems, including the peripheral (PNS) and central (CNS) nervous system. Therefore, several hormones exert neuroprotective actions, maintaining the homeostatic function of neurons and glial cells. One of such hormones is estradiol. Estradiol is not only involved in the central control of reproduction but also acts as a protective factor in the brain. Under physiological conditions estradiol regulates synaptic activity, synaptic plasticity, neuroglia communication, and brain metabolism [1–4]. Under pathological conditions, estradiol promotes neuron survival, reducing brain inflammation and facilitating the repair of the damaged neural tissue. Estradiol neuroprotective effects have been described in different animal experimental models of multiple

N. Yanguas-Casás · M. A. Arevalo · L. M. Garcia-Segura (✉)
Instituto Cajal, CSIC, Madrid, Spain

Centro de Investigación Biomédica en Red de Fragilidad y Envejecimiento Saludable (CIBERFES), Instituto de Salud Carlos III, Madrid, Spain
e-mail: nyanguas@cajal.csic.es; arevalo@cajal.csic.es; lmgs@cajal.csic.es

M. E. Brocca
Instituto Cajal, CSIC, Madrid, Spain

I. Azcoitia
Centro de Investigación Biomédica en Red de Fragilidad y Envejecimiento Saludable (CIBERFES), Instituto de Salud Carlos III, Madrid, Spain

Department of Cell Biology, Faculty of Biology, Universidad Complutense, Madrid, Spain
e-mail: azcoitia@bio.ucm.es

© International Society of Gynecological Endocrinology 2019
R. D. Brinton et al. (eds.), *Sex Steroids' Effects on Brain, Heart and Vessels*,
ISGE Series, https://doi.org/10.1007/978-3-030-11355-1_3

sclerosis, stroke, Parkinson's disease, Alzheimer's disease, cognitive decline, affective disorders, and traumatic CNS and PNS injuries [5, 6].

Aging and brain pathology are associated with increased neuroinflammation [6, 7]. Acute neuroinflammation is a physiological response aimed to reduce neural tissue damage. However, under chronic neurodegenerative conditions and with aging, neuroinflammation is a chronic situation that may contribute to increase neural damage [8–11]. Two main cell types are involved in the control of brain inflammation: astrocytes and microglia. Astrocytes exert numerous actions to maintain proper neuronal function. These include the regulation of neuronal metabolism, synaptic function, and neuronal communication. In addition, astrocytes maintain brain tissue homeostasis by the control of neuroinflammation [12]. Microglia are the macrophages of the brain and are the main regulators of the brain immune response. These cells participate in the phagocytosis of neuronal debris and the plastic remodeling of neuronal processes and synapses [13]. Under pathological conditions, both astrocytes and microglia become activated, changing their transcriptomic activity and their phenotype, a phenomenon known as reactive gliosis [14]. One of the characteristics of reactive glial cells is the activation of nuclear factor kappa-light-chain enhancer of activated B cells (NF-κB), which promotes the synthesis and release of pro-inflammatory molecules by astrocytes and microglia [15].

It has been described that in the aged brain, microglia cells present a senescent phenotype and are unable to properly respond with an adequate homeostatic response to tissue damage [7]. Thus, their phagocytic and migratory activity, their activation of NF-κB, and their inflammatory response are dysregulated, contributing to further increase the inflammatory response of other cell types, including astrocytes and neurons. Thus, senescent microglia not only are unable to decrease tissue damage but even contribute to amplify neurodegeneration [16]. A similar situation occurs in chronic neurodegenerative conditions, such as Alzheimer's and Parkinson's diseases [17, 18].

Uncontrolled neuroinflammation not only contributes to neuronal death but also affects the normal functioning and metabolism of surviving neurons and glial cells, altering the processing of information in the brain [19]. Evidence is accumulating on the implication of neuroinflammation in cognitive dysfunction and depression. Clinical studies have revealed that elevated levels of peripheral cytokines correlate with deficits in cognitive performance [20–24]. Changes in peripheral cytokine levels are also associated with depressive disorders in humans [25–30]. Experimental studies in animals have also revealed an association of peripheral inflammation and neuroinflammation with cognitive deficits [31–37] and depressive-like behaviors [38]. The effects of cytokines on cognition [39–44] and depression [45–47] are probably mediated by alterations in the mechanisms of synaptic plasticity and synaptic function (Fig. 3.1) and may involve decreased brain levels of brain-derived neurotrophic factor (BDNF) and other protective molecules [45, 48]. As we will see in the next sections of this chapter, the pro-cognitive effects of estradiol are not only a consequence of direct actions of the hormone on neurons (for instance, regulating synaptic function and plasticity and promoting neuronal survival) but are also mediated by actions on glial cells, regulating reactive gliosis and neuroinflammation.

Fig. 3.1 Brain aging is associated with increased neuroinflammation and gliosis. Inflammation and glial dysfunction impair synaptic plasticity and synaptic function, which contributes to the development of cognitive decline and mood disorders

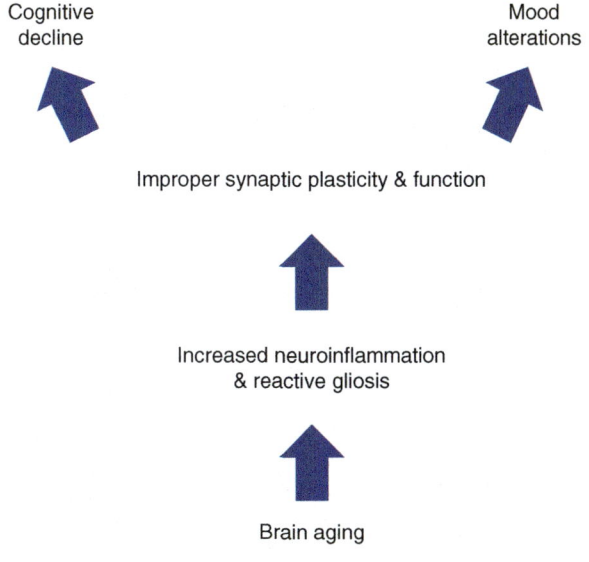

3.2   Role of Estrogen Receptors in Neuroinflammation and Neuroprotection

Estradiol protects the nervous system by decreasing inflammation and reducing apoptosis [49]. In addition, the hormone promotes tissue repair by enhancing dendritic and axonal regeneration, decreasing gliosis and increasing myelination and neurogenesis. These actions of estradiol are exerted directly or indirectly on neurons, astrocytes, microglia, oligodendrocytes, blood vessels, stem cells, and progenitors [5, 50]. All these cells are direct targets for the hormone and are also responsive to signals released by other estradiol target cells. Thus, direct actions of estradiol on glial cells or brain endothelial cells affect the neurons, and direct actions of estradiol on neurons have an impact on the other cell types of the brain. Acting on brain blood vessels, estradiol regulates blood flow, vascular unit metabolism, endothelial cell survival, leukocyte adhesion, and blood-brain barrier function [51, 52]. In neurons, estradiol regulates synaptic transmission and plasticity, neuritogenesis, and cell survival [3, 53, 54]. Acting on astrocytes and microglia, estradiol regulates local inflammation, gliosis, and the release of trophic factors for neurons [55, 56]. Estradiol also regulates cell survival, myelination, and re-myelination, acting on oligodendrocytes, and modulates developmental and adult neurogenesis, acting on stem cells and progenitors [5].

As in other tissues, estradiol acts in brain cells by binding to a variety of estrogen receptors (ERs). The best characterized are ERα, ERβ, and G-protein-coupled ER 1 (GPER) [57–59] (Fig. 3.2). ERα and ERβ are nuclear transcription factors that, among other protein domains, have a binding domain for estradiol (ligand binding domain, LBD) and a DNA binding domain (DBD). Through the DBD, ERα and ERβ

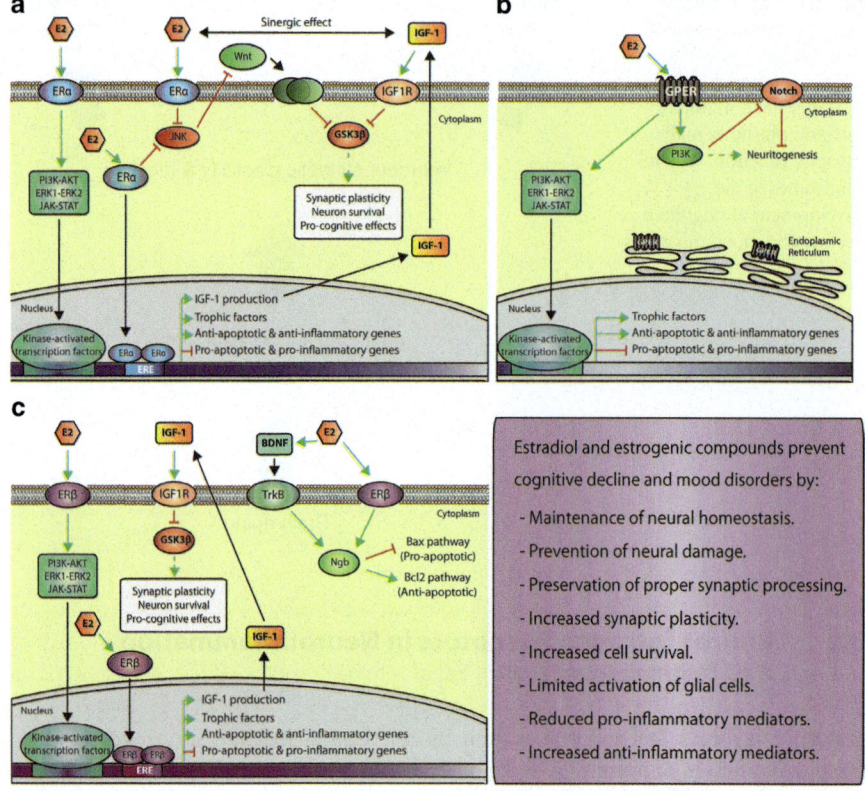

Fig. 3.2 Estradiol (E2) roles in the prevention of cognitive decline and mood disorders. E2 or estrogenic compound binding to (**a**) estrogen receptor alpha (ERα), (**b**) G-protein-coupled estrogen receptor 1 (GPER), and/or (**c**) estrogen receptor beta (ERβ) induces the expression of molecules that promote neuronal survival and represses the expression of molecules that promote neuronal cell death and neuroinflammation. In addition, E2 signaling interacts with the signaling of other neuroprotective factors, such as insulin-like growth factor 1 (IGF-1), brain-derived neurotrophic factor (BDNF), and neuroglobin (Ngb). *PI3K-Akt* phosphoinositide 3-kinase-Akt signaling pathway, *ERK1-ERK2* extracellular signal-regulated kinases signaling pathway, *JAK-STAT* Janus kinases-signal transducers and activators of transcription signaling pathway, *EREs* estrogen-responsive elements, *JNK* c-Jun-N-terminal kinase, *GSK3β* glycogen synthase kinase-3β, *IGF1R* insulin-like growth factor 1 receptor, *TrkB* tyrosine receptor kinase B

bind to estrogen-responsive elements (EREs) in target genes to regulate their transcription. In addition, ERα and ERβ have a hinge region domain, located between the LBD and the DBD, which participates in the subcellular distribution of the receptors. Indeed, ERα and ERβ are not only located in the cell nucleus, to act as transcription factors, but are also localized in the cytoplasm and the plasma membrane, where they interact with the signaling pathways of other factors and regulate the activity of different kinases, such as phosphoinositide 3-kinase (PI3K), c-Jun N-terminal kinase (JNK), and extracellular signal-regulated kinases (ERKs) [60]. Furthermore, GPER, a G-protein-coupled receptor that is located in the plasma membrane or in the endoplasmic reticulum, also regulates the activity of these kinases [60]. The regulation of kinases by ERs results in modifications in the transcriptional activity of different genes mediated by kinase-activated transcription factors. The direct regulation of transcriptional activity by ERα and ERβ and the indirect regulation of transcriptional activity by ERα, ERβ, and GPER, mediated by kinase-activated transcription factors, result in the upregulation of anti-apoptotic and neuroprotective genes and the downregulation of pro-apoptotic and pro-inflammatory molecules. Thus, estradiol, through ERα, ERβ, and GPER, increases the expression of molecules that promote neuronal survival and represses the expression of molecules that promote neuronal cell death and neuroinflammation [60].

3.3   Interaction of Estrogen Receptor Signaling in the Brain with the Signaling of Other Neuroprotective and Anti-inflammatory Factors

The neuroprotective and anti-inflammatory molecular mechanisms of estradiol include the interaction with the signaling of other neuroprotective and anti-inflammatory factors. Recent studies have shown that estradiol, via ERβ (Fig. 3.2c), upregulates the expression of neuroglobin, a member of the globin family of proteins, which also include hemoglobin and myoglobin, among others [61–63]. Neuroglobin is a neuroprotective factor that reduces apoptosis in neurons and glial cells and decreases the inflammatory response of astrocytes [61–63]. Neuroglobin signaling involves the activation of Akt, the downregulation of the pro-apoptotic protein Bax, and the upregulation of the anti-apoptotic protein Bcl-2. The association of neuroglobin with huntingtin is necessary for the neuroprotective action of this protein. Estradiol requires huntingtin to upregulate neuroglobin levels. In addition, huntingtin facilitates the translocation of neuroglobin to the mitochondria, and mutated forms of huntingtin, characteristic of Huntington disease, prevent the neuroprotective actions of estradiol mediated by the upregulation of neuroglobin [64].

Another molecule that upregulates neuroglobin expression in neural cells is BDNF (Fig. 3.2c). As it has been observed for estradiol, BDNF also requires huntingtin to upregulate neuroglobin expression [64]. In turn, BDNF is upregulated by estradiol in the brain [65]. This neurotrophic factor activates the PI3K signaling pathway acting on the neurotrophin receptor tyrosine receptor kinase B (TrkB). The BDNF/TrkB/PI3K signaling pathway promotes neuritogenesis, synaptic plasticity, neuron survival, and neurogenesis, reduces neuroinflammation, is involved in memory processes, and reduces depressive symptoms [2, 53, 66–68]. BDNF is therefore implicated in the affective and cognitive effects of estradiol in the brain. It is important to note that brain BDNF levels increase with physical exercise [69], pointing to the possibility that lifestyle in postmenopausal women may affect the outcome of estrogen therapy for cognition and depression.

Acting on GPER (Fig. 3.2b), estradiol also activates PI3K, which inhibits Notch signaling, causing an increase in neuritogenesis. Acting on membrane-associated ERα (Fig. 3.2a), estradiol inhibits JNK. JNK induces the expression of dickkopf

(DKK1), a negative regulator of the Wnt signaling pathway. Thus, by inhibiting JNK, estradiol increases Wnt signaling, causing the inhibition of glycogen synthase kinase-3β (GSK3β) [60]. Inhibition of GSK3β promotes synaptic plasticity and neuron survival, reduces inflammation, and has pro-cognitive effects [70–73]. Furthermore, GSK3β activation may be associated with depressive disorders [73], and GSK3β inhibition with lithium is a classical intervention for the treatment of depression and other mental disorders.

Estradiol also interacts with insulin-like growth factor-1 (IGF-1) signaling [74–76] (Fig. 3.2a, c). Acting on nuclear ERs, estradiol promotes IGF-1 synthesis in the brain. In turn, IGF-1 exerts a ligand-independent activation of ERα in the brain [77]. IGF-1 acts on IGF-1 receptor, a tyrosine kinase receptor that activates ERK and PI3K. PI3K inhibits GSK3β, which, as mentioned before, promotes neural function and cognition. In addition, estradiol induces the interaction of ERα with the PI3K/ GSK3β signaling pathway. Indeed, estradiol and IGF-1 exert a synergic activation of this neuroprotective and anti-inflammatory signaling pathway in the brain, and the neuroprotective actions of each of these two factors depend on the presence of the other. Thus estradiol neuroprotective actions are lost when IGF-1 receptor is inhibited in the brain, and IGF-1 neuroprotective actions are lost when ERs are inhibited in the brain [74–76, 78]. Since IGF-1 plasma levels decrease with aging in humans and in other species, the interdependence of estradiol and IGF-1 signaling for neuroprotection is highly relevant to understand the actions of estrogen therapy in the brain of postmenopausal women. Thus, it has been shown that estradiol neuroprotective effects in a stroke model are lost in older female mice, in which IGF-1 levels are decreased. However, estradiol recovers its protective action after IGF-1 administration [76]. This suggests that the effect of estradiol in older women may be different, depending on the available levels of IGF-1 in the brain or on the brain expression of IGF-1 receptor. As mentioned before for BDNF, physical exercise also increases brain IGF-1 levels [79], suggesting that it may benefit the actions of estrogen therapy on brain function.

3.4 Neuroprotective and Anti-inflammatory Actions of Synthetic Estrogenic Compounds

In addition to estradiol, the neuroprotective and anti-inflammatory actions of synthetic estrogenic compounds used in clinical practice have been tested in animal models. These studies have shown that some selective estrogen receptor modulators (SERMs), used for the treatment of osteoporosis or climacteric symptoms or for the treatment of ER positive cancers, also exert neuroprotective and anti-inflammatory actions in different experimental models of neurodegenerative, cognitive, and affective disorders. SERMs, such as tamoxifen, raloxifene, ospemifene, and bazedoxifene, reduce excitotoxic neuronal damage, decrease the expression of neuroinflammatory molecules, and reduce the activation of astrocytes and microglia [80–88]. Tamoxifen has been also shown to promote neuronal regeneration after spinal cord lesions [89]. In addition, in ovariectomized rats, tamoxifen and raloxifene increase the number of dendritic spines in cognitive brain regions, such as the hippocampus and the medial prefrontal cortex, and promote memory performance [90–92]. Furthermore, tamoxifen and raloxifene exert anxiolytic and antidepressive actions in ovariectomized mice subjected to chronic stress [93].

Tibolone is another synthetic steroid used in numerous countries for the treatment of menopause-associated symptoms. The actions of tibolone are mediated by its metabolites, which have estrogenic, progestagenic, and androgenic activity. Tibolone is considered to be a selective tissue estrogenic activity regulator (STEAR). Local differences in tibolone metabolism and in the expression of steroid receptors confer selective tissue actions to this drug. Pro-cognitive effects of tibolone treatment and positive effects on mood and well-being have been reported in postmenopausal women [94–96]. Experimental studies in vitro and in animal models indicate that tibolone reduces reactive gliosis and protects glial cells from different metabolic insults, preserving mitochondrial function and reducing oxidative stress [97, 98]. The protective actions of tibolone on glial cells are mediated, at least in part, by the upregulation of neuroglobin [98]. In addition, tibolone increases β-endorphin levels in the brain of ovariectomized rats [99] and in the plasma of postmenopausal women [100]. Pro-cognitive actions of tibolone could also be mediated by promoting cholinergic activity [101]. Furthermore, tibolone increases the number of dendritic spines in brain cognitive regions, such as the hippocampus [102].

3.5   Interactions Between Brain Estradiol Synthesis, Neuroinflammation, and Neuroprotection

The nervous system is not only a target of estradiol but also a source of this steroid. The enzyme aromatase, which converts testosterone in estradiol, is expressed by different neuronal populations in the human brain, including those in cognitive regions such as the hippocampus and the cerebral cortex [103, 104]. Aromatase has been localized in the presynaptic terminals. In addition, ERs have been localized in the pre- and postsynaptic terminals, suggesting that estradiol may act as a neuro-modulator, being released by presynaptic terminals, where aromatase is located, and acting on ERs in the pre- and postsynaptic terminals [105–107]. Neuronal-derived estradiol also participates in the regulation of the synthesis of synaptic proteins and in the structural and functional plasticity of synapses [108–113]. These actions of brain endogenous estradiol may affect behavior, mood, and cognition [114]. In addition, it has been described that brain injury in different animal models induces the expression of aromatase and ERs by astrocytes. Furthermore, the inhibition of brain aromatase after brain injury increases neurodegeneration and gliosis, indicating that brain estradiol production exerts neuroprotective actions [60]. Therefore, estradiol not only acts in the brain as a hormone but also as a local paracrine or autocrine factor to regulate the function of neurons and glial cells under physiological and pathological conditions.

The local production of estradiol by the nervous system may explain cognitive and depressive effects of aromatase inhibitors observed in animal studies. For instance, in ovariectomized rodents, the aromatase inhibitor letrozole increases anxiety and depressive behaviors and impairs cognition. Since animals were ovariectomized, these effects are evidently mediated by extragonadal aromatase inhibition and may be mediated by the inhibition of brain estradiol synthesis [115–117]. Aromatase-deficient female mice also exhibit depressive behaviors [118]. The effects of aromatase inhibition on cognition in female mice is associated with a decrease in Wnt signaling in the hippocampus [117]. Some studies in breast cancer patients treated with aromatase inhibitors also suggest effects of the inhibition of estradiol synthesis on cognition and depression, although numerous confounding factors do not allow to attain definitive conclusions [119–121]. In addition, an increased risk for Alzheimer's disease has been associated with some polymorphisms of the CYP19A1 gene, which encodes for the enzyme aromatase [122–128].

The production of estradiol by brain cells raises the question on the possible interactions between systemic estradiol and intracerebral estradiol. Interestingly, it has been described that brain-derived estradiol mediates the effect of systemic estradiol on cognition in rats [129]. In addition, brain-derived estradiol may determine the neuroprotective actions of exogenous estradiol, as it has been observed in a mouse model of Alzheimer's disease [130]. On the other hand, systemic estradiol enhances the synthesis of brain-derived estradiol by acting on gonadotropin-releasing hormone receptors in the hippocampus [129, 131]. Then, brain-derived estradiol may reach high local concentration levels necessary for the activation on membrane-associated neuroprotective and anti-inflammatory signaling pathways. Further research is needed to fully understand the significance and implications of brain estradiol synthesis in postmenopausal women.

3.6   Concluding Remarks

As we have seen in this chapter, estradiol, either from ovarian or central origin, and some estrogenic compounds, such as some SERMs and tibolone, exert neuroprotective and anti-inflammatory actions in the brain. These actions of estradiol and estrogenic compounds have implications for cognition and depression. Estrogens prevent cognitive decline and mood disorders by maintaining neuronal homeostasis, preventing neuronal damage, and preserving a proper synaptic processing of information in the brain. One of the brain regions where estrogen actions on neurons and synapses have been studied with more detail is the hippocampus, which is involved in both cognition and mood [132]. Synaptic actions of estrogens in other brain regions, such as the cerebral cortex, may also prevent cognitive decline and depression. Furthermore, glial cells are also involved in information processing in the brain, and alteration of these cells by neuroinflammation may compromise neuronal and synaptic function. Therefore, actions of estrogens in the regulation of neuroinflammation may also contribute to prevent mood disorders and cognitive decline.

In addition to the effects of estrogens on neurons and glial cells, other estrogenic actions in the brain may contribute to maintain cognition and mood. For instance, inflammation and aging alter the function of blood-brain barrier, which may cause affective and cognitive problems. Estradiol may contribute to preserve brain function conserving blood-brain barrier integrity [76, 133] and promoting the transport of peripheral neuroprotective molecules, such as IGF-1 [134], into the brain parenchyma. The role of blood-brain barrier preservation in the neuroprotective, cognitive, and affective actions of estrogens merits therefore to be addressed in future studies.

Acknowledgments Authors acknowledge the support from Ministerio de Economía, Industria y Competitividad (MINECO), Spain (grant number BFU2017-82754-R); Centro de Investigación Biomédica en Red de Fragilidad y Envejecimiento Saludable (CIBERFES); Instituto de Salud Carlos III, Madrid, Spain; and Fondos FEDER.

References

1. Acaz-Fonseca E, Avila-Rodriguez M, Garcia-Segura LM, Barreto GE. Regulation of astroglia by gonadal steroid hormones under physiological and pathological conditions. Prog Neurobiol. 2016;144:5–26.
2. Arevalo MA, Azcoitia I, Gonzalez-Burgos I, Garcia-Segura LM. Signaling mechanisms mediating the regulation of synaptic plasticity and memory by estradiol. Horm Behav. 2015;74:19–27.
3. Frankfurt M, Luine V. The evolving role of dendritic spines and memory: interaction(s) with estradiol. Horm Behav. 2015;74:28–36.
4. Rettberg JR, Yao J, Brinton RD. Estrogen: a master regulator of bioenergetic systems in the brain and body. Front Neuroendocrinol. 2014;35(1):8–30.
5. Azcoitia I, Arevalo MA, De Nicola AF, Garcia-Segura LM. Neuroprotective actions of estradiol revisited. Trends Endocrinol Metab. 2011;22(12):467–73.
6. Villa A, Vegeto E, Poletti A, Maggi A. Estrogens, neuroinflammation, and neurodegeneration. Endocr Rev. 2016;37(4):372–402.
7. Barrientos RM, Frank MG, Watkins LR, Maier SF. Aging-related changes in neuroimmune-endocrine function: implications for hippocampal-dependent cognition. Horm Behav. 2012;62(3):219–27.
8. Sparkman NL, Johnson RW. Neuroinflammation associated with aging sensitizes the brain to the effects of infection or stress. Neuroimmunomodulation. 2008;15(4–6):323–30.
9. DiSabato DJ, Quan N, Godbout JP. Neuroinflammation: the devil is in the details. J Neurochem. 2016;139(Suppl 2):136–53.
10. von Bernhardi R, Eugenin-von Bernhardi L, Eugenin J. Microglial cell dysregulation in brain aging and neurodegeneration. Front Aging Neurosci. 2015;7:124.
11. Niraula A, Sheridan JF, Godbout JP. Microglia priming with aging and stress. Neuropsychopharmacology. 2017;42(1):318–33.
12. Belanger M, Magistretti PJ. The role of astroglia in neuroprotection. Dialogues Clin Neurosci. 2009;11(3):281–95.
13. Chen Z, Trapp BD. Microglia and neuroprotection. J Neurochem. 2016;136(Suppl 1):10–7.
14. Pekny M, Pekna M. Reactive gliosis in the pathogenesis of CNS diseases. Biochim Biophys Acta. 2016;1862(3):483–91.
15. Kaltschmidt B, Kaltschmidt C. NF-kappaB in the nervous system. Cold Spring Harb Perspect Biol. 2009;1(3):a001271.
16. von Bernhardi R, Tichauer JE, Eugenin J. Aging-dependent changes of microglial cells and their relevance for neurodegenerative disorders. J Neurochem. 2010;112(5):1099–114.

17. Blaylock RL. Parkinson's disease: microglial/macrophage-induced immunoexcitotoxicity as a central mechanism of neurodegeneration. Surg Neurol Int. 2017;8:65.
18. Alam Q, Alam MZ, Mushtaq G, Damanhouri GA, Rasool M, Kamal MA, et al. Inflammatory process in Alzheimer's and Parkinson's diseases: central role of cytokines. Curr Pharm Des. 2016;22(5):541–8.
19. Chen WW, Zhang X, Huang WJ. Role of neuroinflammation in neurodegenerative diseases (Review). Mol Med Rep. 2016;13(4):3391–6.
20. Andreotti C, King AA, Macy E, Compas BE, DeBaun MR. The association of cytokine levels with cognitive function in children with sickle cell disease and normal MRI studies of the brain. J Child Neurol. 2015;30(10):1349–53.
21. Ganz PA, Bower JE, Kwan L, Castellon SA, Silverman DH, Geist C, et al. Does tumor necrosis factor-alpha (TNF-alpha) play a role in post-chemotherapy cerebral dysfunction? Brain Behav Immun. 2013;30(Suppl):S99–108.
22. Cvejic E, Lemon J, Hickie IB, Lloyd AR, Vollmer-Conna U. Neurocognitive disturbances associated with acute infectious mononucleosis, Ross River fever and Q fever: a preliminary investigation of inflammatory and genetic correlates. Brain Behav Immun. 2014;36:207–14.
23. Yuan L, Liu A, Qiao L, Sheng B, Xu M, Li W, et al. The relationship of CSF and plasma cytokine levels in HIV infected patients with neurocognitive impairment. Biomed Res Int. 2015;2015:506872.
24. Skvarc DR, Berk M, Byrne LK, Dean OM, Dodd S, Lewis M, et al. Post-operative cognitive dysfunction: an exploration of the inflammatory hypothesis and novel therapies. Neurosci Biobehav Rev. 2018;84:116–33.
25. Dantzer R, O'Connor JC, Freund GG, Johnson RW, Kelley KW. From inflammation to sickness and depression: when the immune system subjugates the brain. Nat Rev Neurosci. 2008;9(1):46–56.
26. Dowlati Y, Herrmann N, Swardfager W, Liu H, Sham L, Reim EK, et al. A meta-analysis of cytokines in major depression. Biol Psychiatry. 2010;67(5):446–57.
27. Roomruangwong C, Anderson G, Berk M, Stoyanov D, Carvalho AF, Maes M. A neuro-immune, neuro-oxidative and neuro-nitrosative model of prenatal and postpartum depression. Prog Neuropsychopharmacol Biol Psychiatry. 2018;81:262–74.
28. Jha MK, Trivedi MH. Personalized antidepressant selection and pathway to novel treatments: clinical utility of targeting inflammation. Int J Mol Sci. 2018;19(1). pii: E233.
29. Miller AH, Raison CL. The role of inflammation in depression: from evolutionary imperative to modern treatment target. Nat Rev Immunol. 2016;16(1):22–34.
30. Shariq AS, Brietzke E, Rosenblat JD, Barendra V, Pan Z, McIntyre RS. Targeting cytokines in reduction of depressive symptoms: a comprehensive review. Prog Neuropsychopharmacol Biol Psychiatry. 2018;83:86–91.
31. Barrientos RM, Higgins EA, Biedenkapp JC, Sprunger DB, Wright-Hardesty KJ, Watkins LR, et al. Peripheral infection and aging interact to impair hippocampal memory consolidation. Neurobiol Aging. 2006;27(5):723–32.
32. Hein AM, Stasko MR, Matousek SB, Scott-McKean JJ, Maier SF, Olschowka JA, et al. Sustained hippocampal IL-1beta overexpression impairs contextual and spatial memory in transgenic mice. Brain Behav Immun. 2010;24(2):243–53.
33. Barrientos RM, Higgins EA, Sprunger DB, Watkins LR, Rudy JW, Maier SF. Memory for context is impaired by a post context exposure injection of interleukin-1 beta into dorsal hippocampus. Behav Brain Res. 2002;134(1–2):291–8.
34. Godbout JP, Johnson RW. Interleukin-6 in the aging brain. J Neuroimmunol. 2004;147(1–2):141–4.
35. Pei B, Sun J. Pinocembrin alleviates cognition deficits by inhibiting inflammation in diabetic mice. J Neuroimmunol. 2018;314:42–9.
36. Vagnozzi AN, Giannopoulos PF, Pratico D. The direct role of 5-lipoxygenase on tau pathology, synaptic integrity and cognition in a mouse model of tauopathy. Transl Psychiatry. 2017;7(12):1288.

37. Au A, Feher A, McPhee L, Jessa A, Oh S, Einstein G. Estrogens, inflammation and cognition. Front Neuroendocrinol. 2016;40:87–100.
38. Wang HT, Huang FL, Hu ZL, Zhang WJ, Qiao XQ, Huang YQ, et al. Early-life social isolation-induced depressive-like behavior in rats results in microglial activation and neuronal histone methylation that are mitigated by minocycline. Neurotox Res. 2017;31(4):505–20.
39. Vereker E, O'Donnell E, Lynch MA. The inhibitory effect of interleukin-1beta on long-term potentiation is coupled with increased activity of stress-activated protein kinases. J Neurosci. 2000;20(18):6811–9.
40. Vereker E, Campbell V, Roche E, McEntee E, Lynch MA. Lipopolysaccharide inhibits long term potentiation in the rat dentate gyrus by activating caspase-1. J Biol Chem. 2000;275(34):26252–8.
41. Hauss-Wegrzyniak B, Lynch MA, Vraniak PD, Wenk GL. Chronic brain inflammation results in cell loss in the entorhinal cortex and impaired LTP in perforant path-granule cell synapses. Exp Neurol. 2002;176(2):336–41.
42. Tancredi V, D'Antuono M, Cafe C, Giovedi S, Bue MC, D'Arcangelo G, et al. The inhibitory effects of interleukin-6 on synaptic plasticity in the rat hippocampus are associated with an inhibition of mitogen-activated protein kinase ERK. J Neurochem. 2000;75(2):634–43.
43. Cumiskey D, Curran BP, Herron CE, O'Connor JJ. A role for inflammatory mediators in the IL-18 mediated attenuation of LTP in the rat dentate gyrus. Neuropharmacology. 2007;52(8):1616–23.
44. Lynch MA. Neuroinflammatory changes negatively impact on LTP: a focus on IL-1beta. Brain Res. 2015;1621:197–204.
45. Zhang XL, Wang L, Xiong L, Huang FH, Xue H. Timosaponin B-III exhibits antidepressive activity in a mouse model of postpartum depression by the regulation of inflammatory cytokines, BNDF signaling and synaptic plasticity. Exp Ther Med. 2017;14(4):3856–61.
46. Wohleb ES, Franklin T, Iwata M, Duman RS. Integrating neuroimmune systems in the neurobiology of depression. Nat Rev Neurosci. 2016;17(8):497–511.
47. Riazi K, Galic MA, Kentner AC, Reid AY, Sharkey KA, Pittman QJ. Microglia-dependent alteration of glutamatergic synaptic transmission and plasticity in the hippocampus during peripheral inflammation. J Neurosci. 2015;35(12):4942–52.
48. Barrientos RM, Frank MG, Crysdale NY, Chapman TR, Ahrendsen JT, Day HE, et al. Little exercise, big effects: reversing aging and infection-induced memory deficits, and underlying processes. J Neurosci. 2011;31(32):11578–86.
49. Gatson JW, Maass DL, Simpkins JW, Idris AH, Minei JP, Wigginton JG. Estrogen treatment following severe burn injury reduces brain inflammation and apoptotic signaling. J Neuroinflammation. 2009;6:30.
50. Johann S, Beyer C. Neuroprotection by gonadal steroid hormones in acute brain damage requires cooperation with astroglia and microglia. J Steroid Biochem Mol Biol. 2013;137: 71–81.
51. Razmara A, Sunday L, Stirone C, Wang XB, Krause DN, Duckles SP, et al. Mitochondrial effects of estrogen are mediated by estrogen receptor alpha in brain endothelial cells. J Pharmacol Exp Ther. 2008;325(3):782–90.
52. Maggioli E, McArthur S, Mauro C, Kieswich J, Kusters DH, Reutelingsperger CP, et al. Estrogen protects the blood-brain barrier from inflammation-induced disruption and increased lymphocyte trafficking. Brain Behav Immun. 2016;51:212–22.
53. Arevalo MA, Ruiz-Palmero I, Scerbo MJ, Acaz-Fonseca E, Cambiasso MJ, Garcia-Segura LM. Molecular mechanisms involved in the regulation of neuritogenesis by estradiol: recent advances. J Steroid Biochem Mol Biol. 2012;131(1–2):52–6.
54. Sellers K, Raval P, Srivastava DP. Molecular signature of rapid estrogen regulation of synaptic connectivity and cognition. Front Neuroendocrinol. 2015;36:72–89.
55. Acaz-Fonseca E, Sanchez-Gonzalez R, Azcoitia I, Arevalo MA, Garcia-Segura LM. Role of astrocytes in the neuroprotective actions of 17beta-estradiol and selective estrogen receptor modulators. Mol Cell Endocrinol. 2014;389(1–2):48–57.

56. Arevalo MA, Santos-Galindo M, Bellini MJ, Azcoitia I, Garcia-Segura LM. Actions of estrogens on glial cells: implications for neuroprotection. Biochim Biophys Acta. 2010;1800(10):1106–12.
57. Toran-Allerand CD. Minireview: A plethora of estrogen receptors in the brain: where will it end? Endocrinology. 2004;145(3):1069–74.
58. Nilsson S, Gustafsson JA. Estrogen receptors: therapies targeted to receptor subtypes. Clin Pharmacol Ther. 2011;89(1):44–55.
59. Tang H, Zhang Q, Yang L, Dong Y, Khan M, Yang F, et al. Reprint of "GPR30 mediates estrogen rapid signaling and neuroprotection". Mol Cell Endocrinol. 2014;389(1–2):92–8.
60. Arevalo MA, Azcoitia I, Garcia-Segura LM. The neuroprotective actions of oestradiol and oestrogen receptors. Nat Rev Neurosci. 2015;16(1):17–29.
61. De Marinis E, Acaz-Fonseca E, Arevalo MA, Ascenzi P, Fiocchetti M, Marino M, et al. 17beta-Oestradiol anti-inflammatory effects in primary astrocytes require oestrogen receptor beta-mediated neuroglobin up-regulation. J Neuroendocrinol. 2013;25(3):260–70.
62. De Marinis E, Ascenzi P, Pellegrini M, Galluzzo P, Bulzomi P, Arevalo MA, et al. 17beta-estradiol--a new modulator of neuroglobin levels in neurons: role in neuroprotection against H(2)O(2)-induced toxicity. Neurosignals. 2010;18(4):223–35.
63. De Marinis E, Marino M, Ascenzi P. Neuroglobin, estrogens, and neuroprotection. IUBMB Life. 2011;63(3):140–5.
64. Nuzzo MT, Fiocchetti M, Totta P, Melone MAB, Cardinale A, Fusco FR, et al. Huntingtin polyQ mutation impairs the 17beta-estradiol/neuroglobin pathway devoted to neuron survival. Mol Neurobiol. 2017;54(8):6634–46.
65. Pietranera L, Brocca ME, Roig P, Lima A, Garcia-Segura LM, De Nicola AF. Estrogens are neuroprotective factors for hypertensive encephalopathy. J Steroid Biochem Mol Biol. 2015;146:15–25.
66. Harte-Hargrove LC, Maclusky NJ, Scharfman HE. Brain-derived neurotrophic factor-estrogen interactions in the hippocampal mossy fiber pathway: implications for normal brain function and disease. Neuroscience. 2013;239:46–66.
67. Srivastava DP, Woolfrey KM, Evans PD. Mechanisms underlying the interactions between rapid estrogenic and BDNF control of synaptic connectivity. Neuroscience. 2013;239:17–33.
68. Luine V, Frankfurt M. Interactions between estradiol, BDNF and dendritic spines in promoting memory. Neuroscience. 2013;239:34–45.
69. Alkadhi KA. Exercise as a positive modulator of brain function. Mol Neurobiol. 2018;55(4):3112–30.
70. King MK, Pardo M, Cheng Y, Downey K, Jope RS, Beurel E. Glycogen synthase kinase-3 inhibitors: rescuers of cognitive impairments. Pharmacol Ther. 2014;141(1):1–12.
71. Datusalia AK, Sharma SS. Amelioration of diabetes-induced cognitive deficits by GSK-3beta inhibition is attributed to modulation of neurotransmitters and neuroinflammation. Mol Neurobiol. 2014;50(2):390–405.
72. Venna VR, Benashski SE, Chauhan A, McCullough LD. Inhibition of glycogen synthase kinase-3beta enhances cognitive recovery after stroke: the role of TAK1. Learn Mem. 2015;22(7):336–43.
73. Pardo M, Abrial E, Jope RS, Beurel E. GSK3beta isoform-selective regulation of depression, memory and hippocampal cell proliferation. Genes Brain Behav. 2016;15(3):348–55.
74. Reshma MV, Saritha SS, Balachandran C, Arumughan C. Lipase catalyzed interesterification of palm stearin and rice bran oil blends for preparation of zero trans shortening with bioactive phytochemicals. Bioresour Technol. 2008;99(11):5011–9.
75. Garcia-Segura LM, Arevalo MA, Azcoitia I. Interactions of estradiol and insulin-like growth factor-I signalling in the nervous system: new advances. Prog Brain Res. 2010;181:251–72.
76. Sohrabji F. Estrogen-IGF-1 interactions in neuroprotection: ischemic stroke as a case study. Front Neuroendocrinol. 2015;36:1–14.
77. Grissom EM, Daniel JM. Evidence for ligand-independent activation of hippocampal estrogen receptor-alpha by IGF-1 in hippocampus of ovariectomized rats. Endocrinology. 2016;157(8):3149–56.

78. Cardona-Gomez GP, Mendez P, DonCarlos LL, Azcoitia I, Garcia-Segura LM. Interactions of estrogens and insulin-like growth factor-I in the brain: implications for neuroprotection. Brain Res Brain Res Rev. 2001;37(1–3):320–34.
79. Trejo JL, Carro E, Torres-Aleman I. Circulating insulin-like growth factor I mediates exercise-induced increases in the number of new neurons in the adult hippocampus. J Neurosci. 2001;21(5):1628–34.
80. Barreto G, Santos-Galindo M, Diz-Chaves Y, Pernia O, Carrero P, Azcoitia I, et al. Selective estrogen receptor modulators decrease reactive astrogliosis in the injured brain: effects of aging and prolonged depletion of ovarian hormones. Endocrinology. 2009;150(11): 5010–5.
81. Arevalo MA, Santos-Galindo M, Lagunas N, Azcoitia I, Garcia-Segura LM. Selective estrogen receptor modulators as brain therapeutic agents. J Mol Endocrinol. 2011;46(1):R1–9.
82. Arevalo MA, Diz-Chaves Y, Santos-Galindo M, Bellini MJ, Garcia-Segura LM. Selective oestrogen receptor modulators decrease the inflammatory response of glial cells. J Neuroendocrinol. 2012;24(1):183–90.
83. Li R, Xu W, Chen Y, Qiu W, Shu Y, Wu A, et al. Raloxifene suppresses experimental autoimmune encephalomyelitis and NF-kappaB-dependent CCL20 expression in reactive astrocytes. PLoS One. 2014;9(4):e94320.
84. Barreto GE, Santos-Galindo M, Garcia-Segura LM. Selective estrogen receptor modulators regulate reactive microglia after penetrating brain injury. Front Aging Neurosci. 2014;6:132.
85. Bourque M, Morissette M, Di Paolo T. Raloxifene activates G protein-coupled estrogen receptor 1/Akt signaling to protect dopamine neurons in 1-methyl-4-phenyl-1,2,3,6-tetrahydropyridine mice. Neurobiol Aging. 2014;35(10):2347–56.
86. Wang X, Zhao L, Zhang Y, Ma W, Gonzalez SR, Fan J, et al. Tamoxifen provides structural and functional rescue in murine models of photoreceptor degeneration. J Neurosci. 2017;37(12):3294–310.
87. Jover-Mengual T, Castello-Ruiz M, Burguete MC, Jorques M, Lopez-Morales MA, Aliena-Valero A, et al. Molecular mechanisms mediating the neuroprotective role of the selective estrogen receptor modulator, bazedoxifene, in acute ischemic stroke: a comparative study with 17beta-estradiol. J Steroid Biochem Mol Biol. 2017;171:296–304.
88. Rzemieniec J, Litwa E, Wnuk A, Lason W, Kajta M. Bazedoxifene and raloxifene protect neocortical neurons undergoing hypoxia via targeting ERalpha and PPAR-gamma. Mol Cell Endocrinol. 2018;461:64–78.
89. Colon JM, Gonzalez PA, Cajigas A, Maldonado WI, Torrado AI, Santiago JM, et al. Continuous tamoxifen delivery improves locomotor recovery 6h after spinal cord injury by neuronal and glial mechanisms in male rats. Exp Neurol. 2018;299(Pt A):109–21.
90. Gonzalez-Burgos I, Rivera-Cervantes MC, Velazquez-Zamora DA, Feria-Velasco A, Garcia-Segura LM. Selective estrogen receptor modulators regulate dendritic spine plasticity in the hippocampus of male rats. Neural Plast. 2012;2012:309494.
91. Velazquez-Zamora DA, Garcia-Segura LM, Gonzalez-Burgos I. Effects of selective estrogen receptor modulators on allocentric working memory performance and on dendritic spines in medial prefrontal cortex pyramidal neurons of ovariectomized rats. Horm Behav. 2012;61(4):512–7.
92. Pandey D, Banerjee S, Basu M, Mishra N. Memory enhancement by Tamoxifen on amyloidosis mouse model. Horm Behav. 2016;79:70–3.
93. Calmarza-Font I, Lagunas N, Garcia-Segura LM. Antidepressive and anxiolytic activity of selective estrogen receptor modulators in ovariectomized mice submitted to chronic unpredictable stress. Behav Brain Res. 2012;227(1):287–90.
94. Genazzani AR, Pluchino N, Bernardi F, Centofanti M, Luisi M. Beneficial effect of tibolone on mood, cognition, well-being, and sexuality in menopausal women. Neuropsychiatr Dis Treat. 2006;2(3):299–307.
95. Gulseren L, Kalafat D, Mandaci H, Gulseren S, Camli L. Effects of tibolone on the quality of life, anxiety-depression levels and cognitive functions in natural menopause: an observational follow-up study. Aust N Z J Obstet Gynaecol. 2005;45(1):71–3.

96. Pinto-Almazan R, Segura-Uribe JJ, Farfan-Garcia ED, Guerra-Araiza C. Effects of Tibolone on the central nervous system: clinical and experimental approaches. Biomed Res Int. 2017;2017:8630764.

97. Avila Rodriguez M, Garcia-Segura LM, Cabezas R, Torrente D, Capani F, Gonzalez J, et al. Tibolone protects T98G cells from glucose deprivation. J Steroid Biochem Mol Biol. 2014;144(Pt B):294–303.

98. Avila-Rodriguez M, Garcia-Segura LM, Hidalgo-Lanussa O, Baez E, Gonzalez J, Barreto GE. Tibolone protects astrocytic cells from glucose deprivation through a mechanism involving estrogen receptor beta and the upregulation of neuroglobin expression. Mol Cell Endocrinol. 2016;433:35–46.

99. Genazzani AR, Bernardi F, Pluchino N, Giretti MS, Begliuomini S, Casarosa E, et al. Effect of tibolone administration on central and peripheral levels of allopregnanolone and beta-endorphin in female rats. Menopause. 2006;13(1):57–64.

100. Genazzani AR, Petraglia F, Facchinetti F, Grasso A, Alessandrini G, Volpe A. Steroid replacement treatment increases beta-endorphin and beta-lipotropin plasma levels in postmenopausal women. Gynecol Obstet Investig. 1988;26(2):153–9.

101. Gibbs RB, Nelson D, Anthony MS, Clarkson TB. Effects of long-term hormone replacement and of tibolone on choline acetyltransferase and acetylcholinesterase activities in the brains of ovariectomized, cynomologus monkeys. Neuroscience. 2002;113(4):907–14.

102. Beltran-Campos V, Diaz-Ruiz A, Padilla-Gomez E, Aguilar Zavala H, Rios C, Diaz Cintra S. Effect of tibolone on dendritic spine density in the rat hippocampus. Neurologia. 2015;30(7):401–6.

103. Azcoitia I, Yague JG, Garcia-Segura LM. Estradiol synthesis within the human brain. Neuroscience. 2011;191:139–47.

104. Biegon A. In vivo visualization of aromatase in animals and humans. Front Neuroendocrinol. 2016;40:42–51.

105. Balthazart J, Ball GF. Is brain estradiol a hormone or a neurotransmitter? Trends Neurosci. 2006;29(5):241–9.

106. Saldanha CJ, Remage-Healey L, Schlinger BA. Synaptocrine signaling: steroid synthesis and action at the synapse. Endocr Rev. 2011;32(4):532–49.

107. Cornil CA, Leung CH, Pletcher ER, Naranjo KC, Blauman SJ, Saldanha CJ. Acute and specific modulation of presynaptic aromatization in the vertebrate brain. Endocrinology. 2012;153(6):2562–7.

108. Kretz O, Fester L, Wehrenberg U, Zhou L, Brauckmann S, Zhao S, et al. Hippocampal synapses depend on hippocampal estrogen synthesis. J Neurosci. 2004;24(26):5913–21.

109. Prange-Kiel J, Fester L, Zhou L, Lauke H, Carretero J, Rune GM. Inhibition of hippocampal estrogen synthesis causes region-specific downregulation of synaptic protein expression in hippocampal neurons. Hippocampus. 2006;16(5):464–71.

110. Srivastava DP, Woolfrey KM, Liu F, Brandon NJ, Penzes P. Estrogen receptor ss activity modulates synaptic signaling and structure. J Neurosci. 2010;30(40):13454–60.

111. Vierk R, Glassmeier G, Zhou L, Brandt N, Fester L, Dudzinski D, et al. Aromatase inhibition abolishes LTP generation in female but not in male mice. J Neurosci. 2012;32(24):8116–26.

112. Bender RA, Zhou L, Vierk R, Brandt N, Keller A, Gee CE, et al. Sex-dependent regulation of aromatase-mediated synaptic plasticity in the basolateral amygdala. J Neurosci. 2017;37(6):1532–45.

113. Liu M, Huangfu X, Zhao Y, Zhang D, Zhang J. Steroid receptor coactivator-1 mediates letrozole induced downregulation of postsynaptic protein PSD-95 in the hippocampus of adult female rats. J Steroid Biochem Mol Biol. 2015;154:168–75.

114. Bailey DJ, Ma C, Soma KK, Saldanha CJ. Inhibition of hippocampal aromatization impairs spatial memory performance in a male songbird. Endocrinology. 2013;154(12):4707–14.

115. Meng FT, Ni RJ, Zhang Z, Zhao J, Liu YJ, Zhou JN. Inhibition of oestrogen biosynthesis induces mild anxiety in C57BL/6J ovariectomized female mice. Neurosci Bull. 2011;27(4):241–50.

116. Taylor GT, Manzella FM, Huffman J, Cabrera OH, Hoffman J. Cognition in female rats after blocking conversion of androgens to estrogens. Horm Behav. 2017;90:84–9.
117. Zameer S, Vohora D. Effect of aromatase inhibitors on learning and memory and modulation of hippocampal dickkopf-1 and sclerostin in female mice. Pharmacol Rep. 2017;69(6):1300–7.
118. Dalla C, Antoniou K, Papadopoulou-Daifoti Z, Balthazart J, Bakker J. Oestrogen-deficient female aromatase knockout (ArKO) mice exhibit depressive-like symptomatology. Eur J Neurosci. 2004;20(1):217–28.
119. Phillips KA, Aldridge J, Ribi K, Sun Z, Thompson A, Harvey V, et al. Cognitive function in postmenopausal breast cancer patients one year after completing adjuvant endocrine therapy with letrozole and/or tamoxifen in the BIG 1-98 trial. Breast Cancer Res Treat. 2011;126(1):221–6.
120. Li C, Zhou C, Li R. Can exercise ameliorate aromatase inhibitor-induced cognitive decline in breast cancer patients? Mol Neurobiol. 2016;53(6):4238–46.
121. Seliktar N, Polek C, Brooks A, Hardie T. Cognition in breast cancer survivors: hormones versus depression. Psychooncology. 2015;24(4):402–7.
122. Iivonen S, Corder E, Lehtovirta M, Helisalmi S, Mannermaa A, Vepsalainen S, et al. Polymorphisms in the CYP19 gene confer increased risk for Alzheimer disease. Neurology. 2004;62(7):1170–6.
123. Huang R, Poduslo SE. CYP19 haplotypes increase risk for Alzheimer's disease. J Med Genet. 2006;43(8):e42.
124. Combarros O, Sanchez-Juan P, Riancho JA, Mateo I, Rodriguez-Rodriguez E, Infante J, et al. Aromatase and interleukin-10 genetic variants interactively modulate Alzheimer's disease risk. J Neural Transm (Vienna). 2008;115(6):863–7.
125. Corbo RM, Gambina G, Ulizzi L, Moretto G, Scacchi R. Genetic variation of CYP19 (aromatase) gene influences age at onset of Alzheimer's disease in women. Dement Geriatr Cogn Disord. 2009;27(6):513–8.
126. Chace C, Pang D, Weng C, Temkin A, Lax S, Silverman W, et al. Variants in CYP17 and CYP19 cytochrome P450 genes are associated with onset of Alzheimer's disease in women with down syndrome. J Alzheimers Dis. 2012;28(3):601–12.
127. Janicki SC, Park N, Cheng R, Schupf N, Clark LN, Lee JH. Aromatase variants modify risk for Alzheimer's disease in a multiethnic female cohort. Dement Geriatr Cogn Disord. 2013;35(5–6):340–6.
128. Zheng J, Yan H, Shi L, Kong Y, Zhao Y, Xie L, et al. The CYP19A1 rs3751592 variant confers susceptibility to Alzheimer disease in the Chinese Han population. Medicine (Baltimore). 2016;95(35):e4742.
129. Nelson BS, Black KL, Daniel JM. Circulating estradiol regulates brain-derived estradiol via actions at GnRH receptors to impact memory in ovariectomized rats. eNeuro. 2016;3(6). https://doi.org/10.1523/ENEURO.0321-16.2016
130. Li R, He P, Cui J, Staufenbiel M, Harada N, Shen Y. Brain endogenous estrogen levels determine responses to estrogen replacement therapy via regulation of BACE1 and NEP in female Alzheimer's transgenic mice. Mol Neurobiol. 2013;47(3):857–67.
131. Fester L, Rune GM. Sexual neurosteroids and synaptic plasticity in the hippocampus. Brain Res. 1621;2015:162–9.
132. Anacker C, Hen R. Adult hippocampal neurogenesis and cognitive flexibility - linking memory and mood. Nat Rev Neurosci. 2017;18(6):335–46.
133. Sohrabji F, Bake S. Age-related changes in neuroprotection: is estrogen pro-inflammatory for the reproductive senescent brain? Endocrine. 2006;29(2):191–7.
134. Munive V, Santi A, Torres-Aleman I. A concerted action of estradiol and insulin like growth factor I underlies sex differences in mood regulation by exercise. Sci Rep. 2016;6:25969.

Estetrol and Its Effects on the Damaged Brain

4

Ekaterine Tskitishvili and Jean Michel Foidart

4.1 Development of the Nervous System

Development of the nervous system in humans during pregnancy is passing through critical and complex periods of morphological and functional differentiation. During ontogenesis newly developed structures of the nervous system, which differ by function and localization, are unified in one complete functional system.

Main steps in human organogenesis are taking place before the eighth week of fertilization. Development of the brain by itself includes several major stages and lasts during the whole pregnancy. Major events in human brain development include primary neurulation, prosencephalic development, neuronal proliferation and migration, organization, and myelination [1]. The neuronal tube formation is already finished by the 20th day of fertilization [2], and the formation of the cortical plate takes place between 7 and 16 weeks of gestation though the cortex increases in thickness until neurogenesis is completed after midgestation. The total number of neurons in the central nervous system (CNS) reaches a maximum in the first 20–24 weeks of the antenatal period and remains relatively constant up to adulthood, only slightly decreasing in early postnatal period.

By the 9th week of gestation, ERα is detected in the proliferating zones and the cortical plate [2, 3]. In contrast to the expression patterns of ERα, ERβ is detected at 15 weeks of gestation in proliferating zones and at 16–17 weeks of gestation in the

E. Tskitishvili (✉)
Laboratory of Tumor Biology and Development, GIGA-Cancer, University of Liege, Liege, Belgium

J. M. Foidart (✉)
Laboratory of Tumor Biology and Development, GIGA-Cancer, University of Liege, Liege, Belgium

Department of Obstetrics and Gynecology, Faculty of Medicine, University of Liege, Liege, Belgium

Department of Clinical Sciences, Faculty of Medicine, University of Liege, Liege, Belgium

© International Society of Gynecological Endocrinology 2019
R. D. Brinton et al. (eds.), *Sex Steroids' Effects on Brain, Heart and Vessels*,
ISGE Series, https://doi.org/10.1007/978-3-030-11355-1_4

cortical plate. From the same period of time, both receptors are expressed in different subregions of the hippocampus [3]. In the rat pups, ERs are present in the developing as well as adult hippocampus [4, 5] with a peak in binding at postnatal day 4 declining to adult levels already by postnatal day 15 [6, 7]. Thus, ERα plays a role in early developmental processes, whereas ERβ might be more important for later events of corticogenesis [8]. Two pairs of internal carotid and vertebral arteries, connected by the circle of Willis, supply the brain with blood [2]. The internal carotid arteries develop quite early, by the 4th week of gestation, whereas by the 5th week of gestation, most of arteries are developed by forming a specific pattern [2]. At 16 weeks of gestation, the anterior, middle, and posterior cerebral arteries are already well established. In premature newborns between 22 and 30 weeks of gestation, the blood vessels of the germinal and periventricular zone and the perforating ventriculopetal vessels are particularly vulnerable to perinatal asphyxia [2], whereas between 30 and 34 weeks of gestation, the fetal white matter is vulnerable to hypoxic ischemic injury, and the injury leads to the formation of focal hemorrhagic lesions and periventricular leukomalacia (PVL) [often resulting in infarction (necrosis) and cavitation], respectively [2].

Myelination in the CNS is performed by oligodendrocytes and is a slow process which is a significant mark of the maturity of the CNS. Notably, in the brain stem, myelination starts at the 8th week of gestation though not completed until after birth, and the rate of myelin deposition is greatest during the first 2 postnatal years [9].

4.2   Estrogens, Estrogen Receptors (ERs), and the Brain

4.2.1   Estrogens

Successful maintenance of pregnancy requires the coordinated secretion of hormones. Indeed, placenta, feto-placental unit, and fetus become the main sources of estrogens: estrone (E1), estradiol (E2), estriol (E3), and estetrol (E4). Appearance of each estrogen in maternal plasma after 9 weeks of gestation coincides with main events of the brain development, pointing out the importance of estrogens in formation of brain morphology and its functionality. For example, we can easily follow the manifestation of unconjugated estradiol (E2) in maternal plasma by the 9th week of gestation and the detection of ERα in the proliferating zones and the cortical plate [2, 3], like that showing the importance of E2 in early corticogenesis. Plasma concentrations of E1, E2, E3, and E4 increase as human pregnancy progresses [10, 11] implicating importance of estrogens in fetal development during pregnancy in general as well as in parturition.

Some recent studies already have shown role of estrogens in (1) fetal neurogenesis, (2) prevention of neuronal cell death, (3) axonal sprouting, and (4) synaptic transmission [12, 13]. Others implicated estrogens as major players for fetal cerebral angiogenesis and cerebral blood flow maintenance due to (1) neurovascular sharing of major signaling pathways and the development of blood-brain barrier, (2) interaction between neurons and vessels mediated by Ca^{2+} ions released from astrocytes, (3) direct effects of estrogens on cerebral vessels [14–18], (4) decrease in water permeability of the blood-brain barrier (BBB) [19], and (5) upregulation of vascular endothelial growth factor (VEGF) expression from neuronal cells [20].

VEGF is an angiogenic protein with neurotrophic and neuroprotective effects which stimulate neurogenesis in vitro and in vivo in the subventricular zone (SVZ) and the subgranular zone (SGZ) of the hippocampal dentate gyrus (DG) [21] and promotes proliferation of cortical neuron precursors by regulating E2F expression (the family of transcription factors, a key regulator of the cell cycle machinery) [22]. Usually neuronal VEGF expression correlates with angiogenesis in postnatal developing rat brain and might be upregulated by hypoxia [23], but it has importance in the developing brain as well. As it was already evidenced, loss of VEGF expression by CNS neurons impairs vascularization, curbs neuronal expansion, and results in neuronal apoptosis in the developing brain, pointing out that VEGF-induced blood vessel growth is essential for nervous tissue growth during embryonic development [24, 25].

According to different studies, general impact of estrogens on the CNS includes (1) neuromodulatory effect by affecting neuron excitability, synaptic plasticity, and neurotransmitter system; (2) neurotrophic effect by influencing glial morphology and functions, neurite outgrowth and sprouting, and cell viability; and (3) neuroprotective effect by exerting proneurogenic, antiexcitatory, antioxidative, antiapoptotic, and anti-inflammatory profile [26, 27].

Estrogen administration in animal models and clinical studies of Parkinson's and Alzheimer's diseases, ischemic stroke, spinal cord injury, and multiple sclerosis has already demonstrated neuroprotective effect [12, 28–32], suggesting the early protective effect of estrogens administered particularly in younger patients (50–62 years) [33] or in women soon after menopause [34]. Even short-term estrogen treatment increases dopamine transporters in the caudate putamen [35] and amyloid beta-protein (Aβ) uptake by microglia. It also prevents Aβ peptide formation by neurons [36, 37] and protects against loss of DA neurons [38, 39]. According to the "healthy cell bias of estrogen action hypothesis," if estrogens are administered too late in the disease, they are not protective [40, 41].

At cellular and molecular levels, estrogens might have different important actions: (1) increase of astrocyte ability to uptake glutamate and like that preventing neuronal loss due to glutamate toxicity [42, 43], (2) direct neuroprotective effect on mitochondria [44–48], (3) induction of expression of genes regulating cytoskeleton of neuron cells (e.g., neurofilaments, microtubule-associated proteins), and (4) increase of aerobic glycolysis, respiratory efficiency, ATP generation, and Ca^{2+} load tolerance leading to antioxidant defense [49].

4.2.2 Estrogen Receptors (ERs)

Estrogen actions are realized through specific estrogen receptors (ERs).

GPER is a membrane-bound receptor, though some research groups found it in the Golgi complex [50] or at the endoplasmic reticulum [51] or even intracellularly in some transfection experiments [52]. Estrogens may affect serotonin signaling in the hypothalamus [53] and dopamine efflux in PC-12 cells [54] or mechanical hyperalgesia in nociceptive neurons of rat dorsal root ganglia [55] and control the energy homeostasis in the hypothalamus [56] by employing GPER.

ERs have specific regions, activation function 1 and 2 (AF1 and AF2), which are responsible for formation of initial transcriptional complexes. AF1 and AF2 are situated in the amino-terminal and carboxyl-terminal domains of the receptors, respectively [57]. These functions characterize most of nuclear receptors and correspond to two active domains which are responsible for recruitment of specific co-regulator proteins, and these proteins in turn might modulate transcriptional activity of ERα. The level of AF1 activity does not depend on the presence of ligand, whereas the activity of AF2 is ligand-dependent [57]. Inactive receptors are linked to the heat shock proteins, and binding of ligand to the ERs leads to dissociation of heat shock proteins from ERs followed by dimerization of ERs. ERs are forming homo- and heterodimers [58]. Zinc (Zn^{2+}) fingers of ligand-ERs complex bind to DNA at specific ERs elements (EREs) which are located in the regulatory regions of target genes and where they act as a hub for a large transcriptional complex including coactivators and corepressors resulting in gene transcription. EREs can alter transcription indirectly by interacting with other transcription factors (AP1, C/EBPβ, and SP1) [57, 58].

According to different studies, estrogen receptors (ERs), ERα, ERβ, and G protein-coupled estrogen receptor 1 (*GPER*, also known as G protein-coupled receptor 30 (GPR30)), may coexist in many brain areas, although their expression levels and distribution patterns are different and sometimes gender specific [59–63]. Like that in adult human brain, ERα, ERβ, and GPER coexist in the basal forebrain, hypothalamus, and hippocampus; ERα and ERβ are expressed in the prefrontal cortex, amygdala, locus coeruleus, and raphe nucleus; ERβ and GPER coexist in the thalamus, whereas only ERβ is expressed in the posterior cingulate [63]. During development ERα and ERβ display distinct chronology and distribution patterns that undergo dynamic changes in the course of corticogenesis as already discussed above.

In terms of subcellular localization, there is a difference between ER localization during development and in adults. During development ERα and ERβ are located in the cell nuclei, whereas in the adult human brain, the ERα staining is localized in both cell compartments (cytoplasm and nucleus), and ERβ has exclusively cytoplasmic localization [64, 65]. The ERα staining is clearly cytoplasmic in the pyramidal cells of Ammon's horn (CA) and in layer II of the entorhinal cortex, whereas it is more nuclear in the dentate gyrus (DG) and in layer V of the entorhinal cortex and temporal cortex [59, 64, 65]. Some recent investigations already have shown localization patterns of ERα, ERβ, and GPER in different neuronal cells pointing out involvement of these receptors in neurogenesis and myelination. In astrocytes and microglia, expression of ERα and ERβ is observed in the nuclei, whereas ERβ is expressed in the cytoplasm; nuclei of the axonal bodies express ERα and ERβ, whereas ERα, ERβ, and GPER are manifested in the cytoplasm; basal dendrites, axonal (initial) segments, and myelin sheaths are rich with ERβ [63]. Another question that became the main direction of research is subcellular localization of ERs in the dentate gyrus (DG) region of the hippocampus which is important for neurogenesis and synaptic remodeling as well as neuroprotection and realization of cognitive function. In DG, a subset of GABAergic interneurons contains nuclear ERα, whereas granule cells, newly born cells, and some GABAergic interneurons contain cytosolic and plasma membrane-associated ERβ [64]. Dendritic spines, mostly originating from granule cells, contain ERα and ERβ. A few dendritic spines in the hilus of DG, originating from mossy cells, contain ERα and ERβ. Interestingly, some ERα-containing axon terminals are cholinergic, whereas some ERβ-containing terminals are monoaminergic. Astrocytes, mostly in the molecular layer, also contain ERα and ERβ [64].

In general, expression of ERα mRNA in the neonatal cortex, olfactory bulb and cerebellum suggests its role in the regulation of early postnatal differentiation and development of these brain areas by estrogens, since ERα is supposed closely related to cellular differentiation and sexual differentiation of developing brain [6].

Different studies already have demonstrated the presence of ERs in rat pial arteries and intracerebral blood vessels [65] and also proved expression of ERα in nuclei, membranes, and mitochondria of endothelial and vascular smooth muscles of cerebral arteries [19, 65]. Although ERβ was detected in immunoblots of cerebral artery lysates, the definitive role of ERβ is not fully understood [65], though ERα and ERβ may modulate each other's activity [66].

According to some studies, ER activation might offer neuroprotection, in part, through transcriptional mechanisms affecting the apoptotic cascade including BCl2, caspases, and Apaf-1 like that limiting cell death [67–70]. ERs can also directly activate signal transduction pathways involving MAP kinase resulting in neuroprotection that is receptor-mediated [71]. As it was shown in Parkinson's disease animal model of 6-hydroxydopamine (6-OHDA), estradiol can also act indirectly by activating the insulin-like growth factor-1 (IGF-1) receptor to protect against 6-OHDA-induced neuronal loss [72].

If the abovementioned effects of estrogens and ERs in the CNS were prominent mainly for E2, information on how E4 affects the CNS became available only few years ago based on studies performed by our research group.

4.2.3   Estetrol

Estetrol (E4) is a steroid hormone, discovered in 1965 by Egon Diczfalusy and co-workers [73]. Structurally, estetrol is an estrogenic steroid with four hydroxyl groups, explaining the acronym E4. Estetrol is produced in nature by the human fetal liver, since its synthesis requires two hydroxylases (15α- and 16α-hydroxylase) only expressed by the fetal liver during pregnancy. Substrates for E4 are estradiol (E2), requiring both 15- and 16-hydroxylation, and estriol (E3), requiring 15-hydroxylation only. Estetrol is an end product of steroid metabolism. There is no metabolism backward to E3, E2, or E1, and there are no active metabolites [74]. The chemical name of estetrol is estra-1,3,5(10)-trien-3,15a,16a,17b-tetrol, and it is known under CAS No. 15183-37-6. The molecular formula of E4 is

$C_{18}H_{24}O_4$, and it has a molecular weight of 304.38. Its physical appearance is that of a white to off-white solid. Estetrol has a melting point in the range of 240–245 °C [73]. Experience so far indicates that E4 is very stable, even under nonoptimal storage conditions. E4 might be slightly hygroscopic. Storage conditions of E4 should therefore be optimized to prevent moisture and water uptake. Both in pure water and in phosphate buffers, E4 is highly soluble. In water, the solubility amounted to 1.0 mg/ml. The octanol-water partition coefficient (Pow) is a measure of the lipophilic or hydrophilic properties of a compound and is expressed as the logarithm of Pow. The lipophilic and hydrophilic properties largely determine the passive gastrointestinal absorption, the distribution through the body, and the passive passage of the blood-brain barrier. In two sets of experiments, using different methods to determine the partition coefficient of E4, the observed log Pow values were 1.470 and 1.695 [73, 74]. This means that concentrations in the octanol phase were about 30–50 times higher compared to those in the water phase. A log Pow of about 2.0 is considered optimal to allow passage through the blood-brain barrier [74].

E4 is found in maternal urine as early as 9 weeks of gestation, increasing substantially as pregnancy progresses [74, 75]. Estetrol produces a number of biological changes in the rodent uterus, such as weight increase, progesterone receptor stimulation, enzyme induction, and histological and ultrastructural changes. From a teleological viewpoint, it seems likely that an estrogenic steroid produced in such significant quantities by the male and female human fetal liver during pregnancy is safe and has physiological significance. As it was concluded, genomic clinical effects of E4 will most likely occur through the estrogen receptors. E4 has a moderate affinity for human ERα and ERβ, with Ki values of 4.9 + 0.567 nmol/l and 19 + 1 nmol/l, respectively, demonstrating a four- to fivefold preference for the ERα (lower Ki value) [76]. Estetrol has high selectivity for the estrogen receptors. Binding to the glucocorticoid, progesterone, and testosterone receptors was only 11–15% at a concentration of 10 mmol/l, and further profiling of E4 in a set of 124 receptors and enzymes demonstrated inactivity toward 123 molecular targets. The single target showing interaction with E4 was the adrenergic α1β receptor (weak binding) [76]. It is concluded that genomic clinical effects of E4 will most likely occur through the estrogen receptors. The high selectivity of E4 suggests a low risk of unexpected side effects [77, 78]. E4 could be a safe and efficacious candidate for the treatment of early brain damage in newborn. The use of E2 unlike the use of E4 might have diverse effects on inflammation and immune responses [79], cardiovascular complications, venous thrombosis, and stroke [80–82], even the initiation/progression of several endocrine-related cancers (e.g., breast, prostate, ovarian, and endometrial cancer) [83].

Main properties of E4 are as follows: (1) slow metabolism and the long half-life; (2) strong antioxidant properties; (3) no binding to sex hormone-binding globulins (SHBG), suggesting that E4 may not influence the plasma levels of SHBG; and (4) log Pow index about 1.470–1.695 which is enough for any compound to pass the blood-brain barrier [75–77]. These properties of E4 might be important to assume the possible neuroprotective actions of E4.

4.3   Neonatal Hypoxic-Ischemic Encephalopathy

Neonatal encephalopathy (NE) is a clinically defined syndrome of disturbed neurologic function in the earliest days of life in an infant born at or beyond 35 weeks of gestation, manifested by a subnormal level of consciousness or seizures and often accompanied by difficulty with initiating and maintaining respiration and depression of tone and reflexes [84]. Neonatal hypoxic-ischemic encephalopathy is associated with increased lethality and long-term morbidity. Mortality and the neurodevelopmental outcomes in infants with moderate and severe HIE are as follows: 23–27% of infants die prior to discharge from the neonatal IC unit (NICU), whereas 37–38% die at follow-up 18–22 months later. The neurodevelopmental outcome at 18 months includes mental and psychomotor development retardation, cerebral palsy, epilepsy, blindness, and hearing impairment [85, 86]. Usually neonates with HIE have different complications manifested with the different degree of severity as follows: mental development index (MDI) <70 (39%), psychomotor development index (PDI) <70 (35–41%), disabling cerebral palsy (30%), epilepsy (16%), blindness (14–17%), and severe hearing impairment (6%) [85, 86], and HIE is the fifth largest cause of death of children before age 5 [87–89].

Perinatal asphyxia or birth asphyxia, more appropriately known as neonatal hypoxic-ischemic encephalopathy (HIE) or hypoxic and ischemic brain injury in the newborn, is characterized by clinical and laboratory evidence of acute or subacute brain injury (encephalopathy) due to intrapartum or late antepartum brain hypoxia and ischemia [90, 91]. A common but crucial problem is the inability to time the onset, duration, magnitude, and single or repetitive nature of the exact insult that causes brain injury resulting in neonatal encephalopathy. The uncertain timing and etiology of brain injury in most cases of neonatal encephalopathy also fuel birth injury malpractice litigation. It is usually unknown whether the ultimate brain injury is caused by the events only around delivery or by cumulative insults throughout pregnancy [84].

Health factors that influence the risk of neonatal encephalopathy include maternal diseases, multiple pregnancy, gestational age at delivery, malformations within or outside the nervous system, intrauterine growth restriction, congenital infections, intrapartum hypoxic-ischemic events, metabolic problems, and stroke [84–86]. Type and timing of contributing factors that are consistent with an acute peripartum or intrapartum events include sentinel hypoxic or ischemic event occurring immediately before or during labor and delivery (a ruptured uterus, severe abruption placentae, umbilical cord prolapsed, amniotic fluid embolus with coincident severe and prolonged maternal hypotension and hypoxemia, maternal cardiovascular collapse, fetal exsanguinations from either vasa previa or massive feto-maternal hemorrhage) [84]. More precisely, there are several risk factors associated with the development of perinatal HIE: preconceptual (e.g., diabetes mellitus type 1, thyroid disease, fertility treatment, nulliparity, advanced maternal age), antepartum (severe preeclampsia, placental abruption, multiple pregnancy, antepartum hemorrhage, fetal growth restriction), and intrapartum (e.g., breech and malpresentation, cord prolapse, caesarean section, maternal pyrexia, induction) [84, 91, 92]. Given the history of the understanding of NE and HIE, it's not surprising that HIE has been most commonly studied in vitro and in vivo. Consequently we will focus on the understanding of the cellular mechanisms of HIE because this is the pathway to NE that has been best studied [84].

The principal pathogenetic mechanism underlying most of the neuropathological conditions leading to hypoxia-ischemia is a failure of compensatory mechanisms and impaired cerebral blood flow (CBF). At the cellular level, hypoxia-ischemia initially causes energy failure, reperfusion and oxidative and nitrosative stress (immediate phase), and then the loss of mitochondrial function and caspase activation (delayed phase) [88, 93]. Step by step, the primary energy failure is accompanied by glutamate-mediated excitotoxicity. Excitotoxic cellular injury occurs via excess activation of glutamate receptors, which leads to necrotic cell death within 6 h after insult and is more prominent within 1.5 h after insult. There are four receptor types for glutamate, but the N-methyl-D-aspartate (NMDA) receptors are the most avid and physiologically active. The channels activated by NMDA receptors are voltage-dependent and calcium-permeable. Their activation causes neuron depolarization. Repeated depolarization of a neuron by unregulated glutamate release results in accumulation of intracellular calcium. Consequently, an increase of intracellular calcium sets off additional pathologic cascades [88, 93] including oxidative stress and interaction with nitric oxide pathway to produce reactive nitrogen species—peroxynitrites leading to peroxynitrite-induced neurotoxicity, lipid peroxidation, mitochondrial damage and remodeling, depletion of antioxidant reserve, and DNA damage [94]. Between 6 and 72 h after insult, development of mitochondrial dysfunction leads to caspase activation and to the apoptotic cell death which is more prominent during the first 6–8 h after insult [88]. This is the point of "no return." Inflammatory mediators (cytokines and chemokines) have been implicated in the pathogenesis of hypoxic-ischemic encephalopathy and may represent a final common pathway of brain injury. As it was shown, NF-kB activation in neurons could provide survival, whereas activation in glial cells enhances neuronal cell death [95].

Assuming that hypoxic-ischemic encephalopathy represents the clinical condition affecting mostly the brain, brain lesions have been reported in many studies. Pial arteriolar vasodilatation is a constant finding in the brain of asphyxiated newborns. It is simply evidenced at panoramic view, and it is mainly related to the loss of microvascular reactivity in cerebral vessels [95, 96]. Endothelial damage represents probably the most important change in the brain of asphyxiated newborns. All the endothelial lesions previously reported may be encountered at the histological examination of brain samples [97]. Endothelial swelling represents a peculiar feature in the small intracerebral vessels. Given the narrow lumen of the intravascular capillaries, endothelial swelling may lead to the occlusion of the vascular lumen, leading to the block of the intracerebral circulation, aggravating brain hypoxia. The endothelial damage is followed by the dysfunction of the neurovascular unit that contributes to subsequent neuronal cell death [97, 98]. Neuronal cell death represents a major pathological finding in the interpretation of the severity of the hypoxic encephalopathy. Apoptosis is the most frequent type of cell death occurring in the brain of asphyxiated newborns. At histology, affected neurons show shrinkage, increased eosinophilia of the cytoplasm, nuclear pyknosis, and karyorrhexis, ending with the formation of roundish eosinophilic globules that appear intermingled with preserved neurons [97]. Neuronal apoptosis may be encountered, in the clinical setting of asphyxia, in all the cerebral regions. In our experience, neurons of the brain stem, basal nuclei, and cerebellum appear as the most frequently affected by apoptosis, often in association with apoptosis of the cerebral cortical neurons. Recently, the increased expression of pro-apoptotic proteins—including BAX, cytoplasmic cytochrome C and caspase-3—has been reported in the cortex and thalamus of the brain of mice affected by birth hypoxia [97, 99], suggesting the use of these antibodies in cases in which histology could not clearly evidence the typical features of neuronal cell death. The hippocampus should be always sampled for histological studies, given the frequent functional compromise of this brain region in newborns affected by asphyxia, particularly in female infants [96, 100]. In a recent study, all 16 full-term asphyxiated infants displayed neuronal cell damage and glial reactivity in the hippocampus [96, 101]. If we are talking about the patterns of neonatal HIE at term, there are five patterns of brain injury identified by imaging studies in neonates with this pathological condition: pattern I, basal ganglia and thalami lesions associated with severe white matter damage; pattern II, basal ganglia and thalami lesions with mild or moderate white matter changes; pattern III, isolated thalamic injury; pattern IV, moderate white matter damage only; and pattern V, mild white matter changes or normal findings. Usually infants with patterns III and IV had developmental delay and diplegic cerebral palsy, respectively, and pattern V is associated with normal outcomes [102]. Thus, the basal ganglia and thalami lesions are the imaging signature in term neonates exposed to hypoxic-ischemic sentinel events, and in general, patterns of central gray matter and secondary white matter injury are associated with higher risks of severe morbidity and death [102].

Clinical manifestation of neonatal encephalopathy varies depending on encephalopathy severity.

Neonates with suspected encephalopathy are classified according to the Sarnat staging system, which evaluates the level of consciousness, muscle tone, tendon reflexes, complex reflexes, and autonomic function and classifies HIE into the following three categories: stage I (mild), stage II (moderate), and stage III (severe) [103, 104].

*Stage I: Mild Encephalopathy*Muscle tone may be slightly increased, and deep tendon reflexes may be brisk during the first few days. Transient behavioral abnormalities, such as poor feeding, irritability, or excessive crying or sleepiness (typically in an alternating pattern), may be observed [88, 103, 104].

*Stage II: Moderate Encephalopathy*The infant is lethargic, with significant hypotonia and diminished deep tendon reflexes. The grasping, Moro, and sucking reflexes may be sluggish or absent. The infant may experience occasional periods of apnea. Seizures typically occur early within the first 24 h after birth [103]. Full recovery within 1–2 weeks is possible and is associated with a better long-term outcome. An initial period of well-being of mild encephalopathy may be followed by sudden deterioration, suggesting ongoing brain cell dysfunction, injury, and death; during this period, seizure intensity might increase [88, 103, 104].

*Stage III: Severe Encephalopathy*Stupor or coma is typical. The infant may not respond to any physical stimulus. Breathing may be irregular, and the infant often requires ventilatory support. Generalized hypotonia and depressed deep tendon reflexes are common. Neonatal reflexes (e.g., sucking, swallowing, grasping, Moro) are absent [88, 103, 104]. Disturbances of ocular motion, such as a skewed deviation of the eyes, nystagmus, bobbing, and loss of "doll's eye" (i.e., conjugate) movements may be revealed by cranial nerve examination [88]. Pupils may be dilated, fixed, or poorly reactive to light. Seizures are delayed, can be severe, and may be initially resistant to conventional treatments. The seizures are usually generalized, and their frequency may increase during the 24–48 h after onset, correlating with the phase of reperfusion injury. As the injury progresses, seizures subside, and the EEG becomes isoelectric or shows a burst suppression pattern. At that time, wakefulness may deteriorate further, and the fontanelle may bulge, suggesting increasing cerebral edema [88].

Irregularities of heart rate and blood pressure (BP) are common during the period of reperfusion injury, as is death from cardiorespiratory failure. Multiple organ dysfunction also presents [88]. Multi-organ systems involvement is a hallmark of NE associated with perinatal asphyxia [88]. Organs involved following a hypoxic-ischemic events include the heart (43–78%) with reduced myocardial contractility, severe hypotension, passive cardiac dilatation, and tricuspid regurgitation; lungs (71–86%) with severe pulmonary hypertension requiring assisted ventilation; kidneys (46–72%) with renal failure presenting as oliguria and, during recovery, as high-output tubular failure, leading to significant water and electrolyte imbalances; liver (80–85%) with elevated liver function test results, hyperammonemia, and coagulopathy; and gastrointestinal system with poor peristalsis and delayed gastric emptying, and necrotizing enterocolitis is rare, and intestinal injuries may not be apparent in the first few days of life or until feeds are initiated; hematologic disturbances (32–54%) include increased nucleated red blood cells (RBCs), neutropenia or neutrophilia, thrombocytopenia, and coagulopathy [88]. Severely depressed respiratory and cardiac functions and signs of brain stem compression suggest a life-threatening rupture of the vein of Galen (i.e., great cerebral vein) with a hematoma in the posterior cranial fossa.

NE is often reported to be the most frequent cause of neonatal seizures [88]. Large, unilateral infarcts occur with neonatal seizures in as many as 80% of patients. Infants with multiple or diffuse lesions and cerebral venous infarcts often have multifocal or migratory seizures observed even during physical examination [88].

A single valuable test for the diagnosis of HIE does not exist. It is important to assess the neonate at birth for detection of signs consistent with an acute peripartum or intrapartum event and the designation of perinatal asphyxia severe enough to result in acute neurologic injury [84]. The following parameters should be taken into consideration: (1) Apgar score of less than 5 at 5 and 10 min after birth; (2) umbilical artery pH less than 7.0, or base deficit greater than or equal to 12 mmol/l, or both; (3) neonatal neurologic sequelae (e.g., seizures, coma, hypotonia); and (4) multiple organ involvement (e.g., renal injury, hepatic injury, hematologic abnormalities, cardiac dysfunction, metabolic derangements, and gastrointestinal injury, or a combination of them) [84, 88]. Although the presence of organ dysfunction increases the risk of HIE in the setting of neonatal encephalopathy, the severity of brain injury seen on neuroimaging does not always correlate with the degree of injury to other organ systems [84]. Nowadays, magnetic resonance imaging (MRI) and magnetic resonance spectroscopy (MRS), as the most sensitive neuroimaging modalities, are extensively used for the monitoring and evaluation of neonates with NE [84]. Distinct patterns of neuroimaging abnormalities, including deep nuclear gray matter or watershed cortical injury, are recognized in hypoxic-ischemic cerebral injury and have prognostic value for predicting later neurodevelopmental impairments. Early MRI obtained between 24 and 96 h of life may be more sensitive for the delineation of the timing of perinatal cerebral injury, whereas an MRI undertaken optimally at 10 days of life (with an acceptable window between 7 and 21 days of life) will best delineate the full extent of cerebral injury [84]. Use of electroencephalography (EEG) might have some limitations due to hypothermia: it may depress the amplitude-integrated EEG (aEEG) and thus limit the early predictive ability of aEEG. Improvement in aEEG tracings may be delayed until the patient undergoes rewarming and is no longer sedated [105]. Some recent investigations showed that S100B protein is a good indicator of brain damage [106]. Furthermore, the serum GFAP levels during the first week of life were increased in neonates with HIE and were predictive of brain injury on MRI. Biomarkers such as S100B and glial fibrillary acidic protein (GFAP) could help triage neonates with HIE to treatment, measure treatment efficacy, and provide prognostic information [106, 107].

According to the contemporary treatment strategy for HIE, initial resuscitation and stabilization are followed by the following steps: (1) neuroprotective strategy, (2) support of adequate ventilation and perfusion, (3) careful fluid management, (4) avoidance of hypo- and hyperglycemia, (5) avoidance of hypotension [a mean blood pressure (BP) above 35–40 mmHg is necessary to avoid decreased cerebral perfusion], and (6) treatment of seizures [108, 109].

At present, hypothermia therapy (HT) is considered as the best neuroprotective strategy for mild to moderate HIE. Mild hypothermia in the range of 33.5–35.0 °C is used. The two types of treatment are used: whole-body hypothermia and selective head cooling. Some basic studies showed far greater histological and electrophysiological protection if hypothermia was initiated within 1.5 h than if it was started 5.5 h after the cerebral insult [110]. According to recent trials, neonates undergoing earlier cooling therapy (within 180 min of birth) had better outcomes compared with those who underwent the therapy later (180–360 min after birth) [111]. The rate of death or severe disability in infants with HIE is decreased from 60% to 46% after cooling [112].

Although cooling is safe, it results in some adverse effects which include a slightly lower baseline heart rate, a marginally significant increase in the need for blood pressure support, and a platelet count below $150 \times 10^9/l$ [113]. In general, lowering the core temperature can impact hemodynamic status, respiratory physiology, fluid and electrolyte balance, and hematologic factors. In addition, pharmacokinetics and pharmacodynamics of a number of drugs commonly used in asphyxiated neonates are affected by hypothermia. Careful attention to physiologic parameters, laboratory tests, and drug dosing is essential to assure optimum outcomes for neonates undergoing hypothermia therapy [114]. There are some risks associated with return from hypothermia to normothermia as follows: (1) apnea, (2) the risk for seizures (increases due to rewarming leading to peripheral vasodilatation and the intravascular blood volume increase) [115], (3) hypotension (may occur if the vascular bed is underfilled), and (4) alteration in the cardiac function (as a result of the initial hypoxic event may play a contributing role) [110].

Importance of searching for new safe neuroprotective strategy alone or in combination with hypothermia therapy became crucial. We paid our attention to already described specific properties of E4 which were important to come up with the hypothesis that E4 might have neuroprotective effect.

4.4 Estetrol as a New Drug to Treat Neonatal HIE

4.4.1 Estetrol Attenuates Neonatal HIE

Our primary goal was to define effects of E4 in primary hippocampal cell cultures. In vitro experiments with primary hippocampal neuronal cell cultures showed impressive antioxidative and cell survival effects of different doses of E4 (notably, 650 μl, 3.25 mM, and 6.5 mM) used before or after induction of oxidative stress (Fig. 4.1a, b, c, and d, respectively) [116]. More precisely, E4 at a dose of 3.25 and 6.5 mM significantly downregulated the LDH activity in both sets of experiments (Fig. 4.2a, c), showing the dose-dependent differences at higher

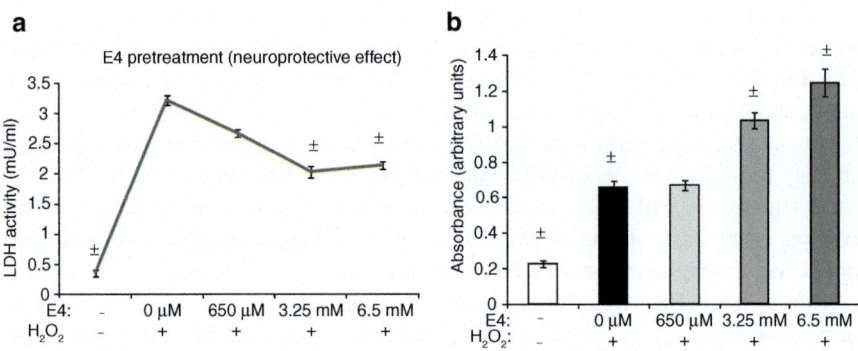

Fig. 4.1 Effect of E4 on LDH activity and the cell viability in primary hippocampal neuronal cultures subjected to the H_2O_2-induced oxidative stress. (**a, b**) E4 pretreatment. Primary hippocampal cell cultures were treated either with vehicle or with 650 μM, 3.25 mM, and 6.5 mM of E4 (1 h) before induction of oxidative stress by 100 μM of H_2O_2 (30 min). (**a**) LDH activity in untreated, H_2O_2-treated, and E4-pretreated cell cultures; (**b**) cell viability in untreated, H_2O_2-treated, and E4-pretreated groups; (**c, d**) E4 treatment. Primary hippocampal cell cultures were treated with 650 μM, 3.25 mM, and 6.5 mM of E4 (1 h) after induction of oxidative stress by 100 μM of H_2O_2 (30 min). (**c**) LDH activity in untreated, treated by H_2O_2, and E4-treated cell cultures; (**d**) cell viability in untreated cells as well as cells treated by H_2O_2 and different concentrations of E4. All measurements are expressed as mean ± SEM. *$p < 0.05$. Reproduced from *Experimental Neurology* (Tskitishvili et al., 2014, 261:298–307)

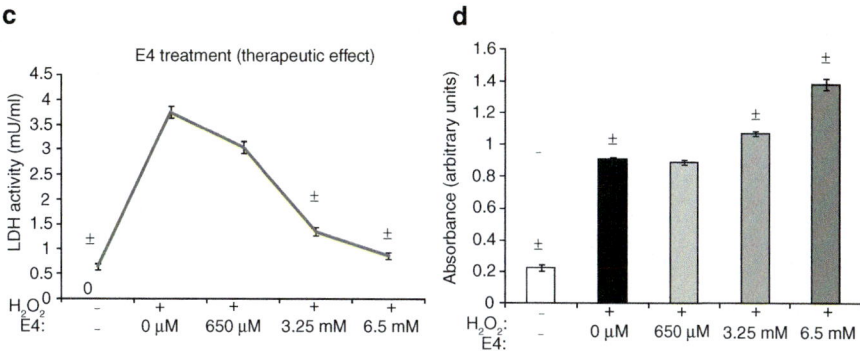

Fig. 4.1 (continued)

doses of E4 (3.25 and 6.5 mM) after induction of oxidative stress (Fig. 4.2c), whereas the same doses of E4 demonstrated significant upregulation of cell proliferation (Fig. 4.2b, d) [116].

Also our aim was to study the effect of E4 on brain damage in vivo. In vivo studies of hypoxic-ischemic brain injury were performed according to two protocols in newborn rat pups. A preventive model was tested with different doses of E4 injected to the rat pups before ischemic injury. E4 was administered intraperitoneally from postnatal day 4 (P4) to postnatal day 7 (P7). Subsequently, the left common carotid artery was ligated and cut. After recovery, the pups were exposed to low oxygen tension (8%) for 30 minutes, in a closed chamber. The therapeutic model consisted, first in the ligation at P7, of the common carotid artery and exposure to 8% oxygen for 30 minutes, to induce an hypoxic-ischemic insult (HI). The various doses of E4 were injected upon retrieval of the rat pups from the hypoxia chamber. All manipulations were performed at 37 °C. The sham group was also operated, but the carotid artery was neither ligated nor cut and the pups were not exposed to hypoxia. Rat pups recovered with their dams and reared normally until being sacrificed at P14 [116–118].

E4 did affect neither body weight nor brain weight or body temperature of the rat pups in both sets of experiments when E4 was applied before or after induction of HI events [116]. Histochemical studies of brain coronal sections revealed massive damage of the hippocampus and the cortex at the left (damaged) side of the brain (Fig. 4.2a2, b2) along with dilation of the central and the lateral ventricles in the vehicle-pretreated/treated groups [116].

Usually a good predictor of the neuroprotective activity of the compound is the counting of intact neuronal cells per visual field. Obviously, among E4-pretreated/treated groups, the hippocampus and the cortex were more preserved in sham, 5, 10, and 50 mg/kg/day E4 groups compared to the vehicle group in each region (Fig. 4.2a(1, 4–6), b(1, 4–6)). Intact cell counting was significantly different between the groups pretreated by E4 before induction of experimental hypoxic-ischemic brain injury, in the hippocampal and the cortical regions: vehicle and 5 mg/kg/day E4 groups (DG); vehicle and 5 and 10 mg/kg/day groups or sham and 1 and 50 mg/kg/day E4 groups (SGZ); sham and 1 and 10 mg/kg/day E4 groups (CA1); vehicle and sham, 50 mg/kg/day, or sham and 1 mg/kg/day E4 groups; whereas in the

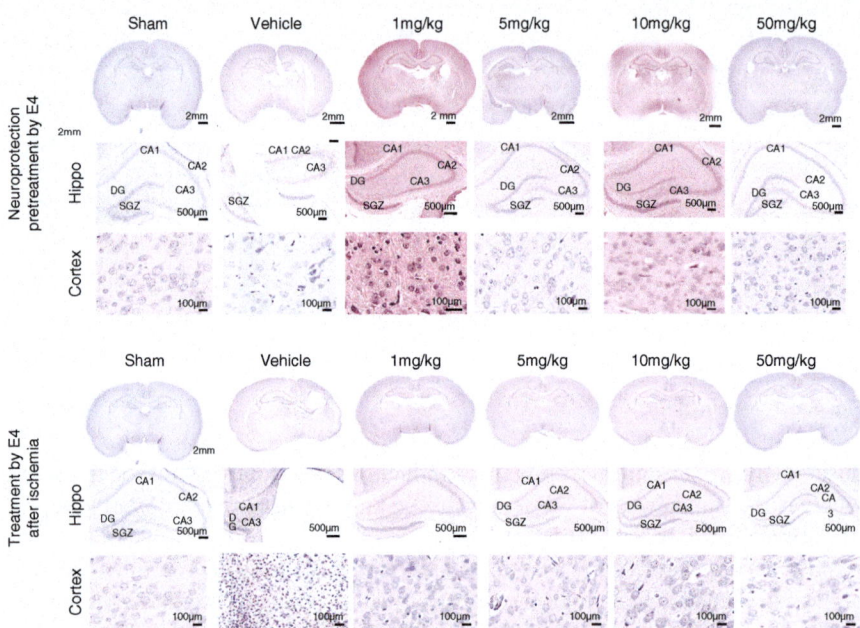

Fig. 4.2 Hematoxylin-eosin staining of coronal brain sections in the rat pups pretreated or treated with E4. Brains of the rat pups were removed upon sacrifice at P14; paraformaldehyde-fixed and paraffin-embedded samples were processed for sectioning at the hippocampus region and hematoxylin-eosin staining. Brain coronal sections of the rat pups (scale bar, 2 mm) with hippocampus region (scale bar, 500 μm) and cortex (scale bar, 100 μm) are shown. E4 pretreatment: sham, vehicle, 1 mg E4/kg/day, 5 mg E4/kg/day, 10 mg E4/kg/day, and 50 mg E4/kg/day. E4 treatment: sham, vehicle, 1 mg E4/kg/day, 5 mg E4/kg/day, 10 mg E4/kg/day, and 50 mg E4/kg/day groups. Reproduced from *Experimental Neurology* (Tskitishvili et al., 2014, 261:298–307)

cortex, the intact cell counting was significantly higher in 50 mg/kg/day E4-pretreated group (Table 4.1) like that proving impressive neuroprotective effect of E4 in the brain [116].

E4 treatment after induction of hypoxic-ischemic brain injury in newborn rat pups resulted in significant difference of intact cell counting in the hippocampal and the cortical regions between the groups as follows: vehicle and 1 mg/kg/day, sham and 5, 10, and 50 mg/kg/day E4 groups (CA1); vehicle and 10 mg/kg/day or sham and 1, 5, 10 mg/kg/day, and 50 mg/kg/day E4 groups (CA2/CA3); whereas in the cortex, the intact cell counting was significantly different between the vehicle and 1 mg/kg/day or sham and 5, 10, and 50 mg/kg/day E4 groups (Table 4.1) like that proving the importance of therapeutic effect of E4 [116].

Contemporary basic and translational research studies in the field of neurology frequently employ different technics and methodologies from proof of concept to

Table 4.1 E4 retreatment is incorrect please correct to E4 pretreatment

	E4 pretreatment						E4 treatment					
	Sham	Vehicle	1 mg/kg/day	5 mg/kg/day	10 mg/kg/day	50 mg/kg/day	Sham	Vehicle	1 mg/kg/day	5 mg/kg/day	10 mg/kg/day	50 mg/kg/day
DG	161 ± 7	85 ± 6[a]	110 ± 7	121 ± 8	114 ± 8	110 ± 9	161 ± 7	88 ± 19[b]	113 ± 9	126 ± 10	137 ± 16	137 ± 17
SGZ	61 ± 5[d]	24 ± 3[c]	35 ± 3	43 ± 4	48 ± 5	31 ± 4	61 ± 5	28 ± 7[e]	35 ± 3	46 ± 8	45 ± 7	50 ± 7
CA1	71 ± 5[f]	52 ± 4	43 ± 2	48 ± 3	57 ± 4	52 ± 4	71 ± 5[h]	28 ± 7[g]	51 ± 2	45 ± 3	46 ± 3	47 ± 5
CA2/CA3	57 ± 6[j]	29 ± 3[i]	33 ± 3	48 ± 6	39 ± 3	53 ± 5	57 ± 6[l]	14 ± 3[k]	34 ± 4	34 ± 4	35 ± 3	30 ± 3
Cortex	69 ± 5	52 ± 5[m]	52 ± 3	71 ± 5	55 ± 3	76 ± 4	69 ± 5[o]	23 ± 4[n]	42 ± 5	57 ± 7	57 ± 6	54 ± 3

Significant differences were observed:

In the DG region: [a]vehicle vs. sham, 5 mg/kg/day E4-pretreated groups; [b]vehicle vs. sham in E4-treated groups

In the SGZ: [c]vehicle vs. sham, 5, and 10 mg/kg/day E4; [d]sham vs. 1 and 50 mg/kg/day E4-pretreated groups; [e]vehicle vs. sham in E4-treated groups

In the CA1 region: [f]sham vs. 1 and 10 mg/kg/day E4-pretreated groups; [g]vehicle vs. sham, 1 mg/kg/day E4; [h]sham vs. 5, 10, and 50 mg/kg/day E4-treated groups

In the CA2/CA3 region: [i]vehicle vs. sham and 50 mg/kg/day E4; [j]sham vs. 1 mg/kg/day E4-pretreated groups; [k]vehicle vs. sham, 10 mg/kg/day; [l]sham vs. 1, 5, 10, and 50 mg/kg/day E4-treated groups

In the cortex: [m]vehicle vs. 50 mg/kg/day E4-pretreated groups; [n]vehicle vs. sham, 5, 10, and 50 mg/kg/day E4; [o]sham vs. 1 mg/kg/day E4-treated groups

Reproduced from *Experimental Neurology* (Tskitishvili et al., 2014, 261:298–307)

fully operational status. Among different issues studies of the gray and white matter and neuro- and cerebro-angiogenesis by using specific markers have paramount importance.

As it was already demonstrated earlier, microtubule-associated protein 2 (MAP-2), as a cytoskeleton protein, has its value in the growth, differentiation, and plasticity of neurons, playing key roles in neuronal responses to growth factors, neurotransmitters, synaptic activity, and neurotoxins [119]. It is frequently used as a marker of early gray matter loss in immunohistochemistry studies.

As shown in Fig. 4.3A, B in both models of in vivo hypoxic-ischemic brain injury in the vehicle groups, MAP-2 staining was negative in the hippocampus of the left hemisphere extended to the cortex (Fig. 4.3A(b), B(b)). Further calculations demonstrated that the ratio of the MAP-2-positive area was significantly higher not only in the sham-operated animals (Fig. 4.3A(a), B(a)) but in animals pretreated/treated by different concentrations of E4 (Fig. 4.3A(c)–(f), B(c)–(f)) compared to

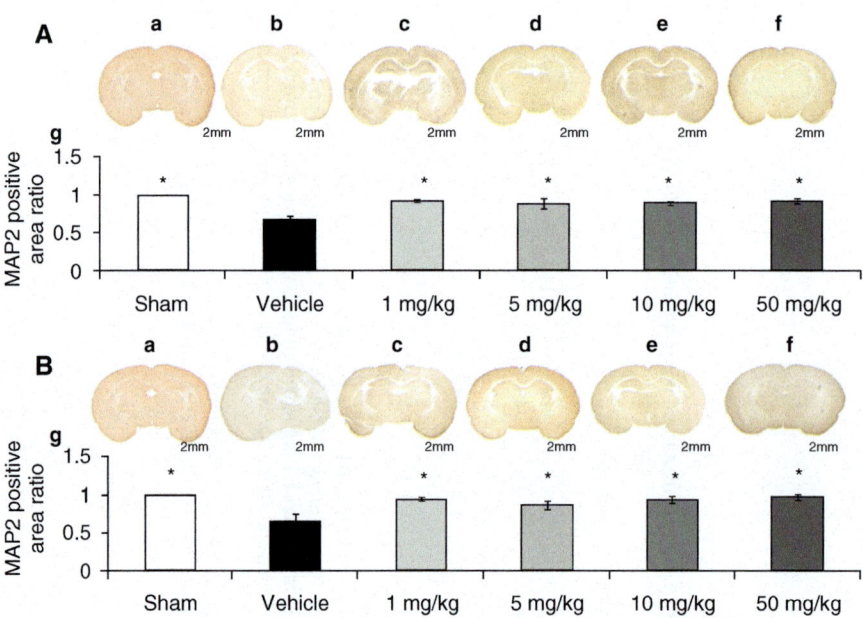

Fig. 4.3 MAP-2 staining of brain coronal sections in the rat pups pretreated or treated with E4 The sections were processed for immunohistochemical detection of neuronal cytoskeletal disruption. (**A**) E4 pretreatment: sham group (a), vehicle-treated group (b), 1 mg/kg/day E4 (c), 5 mg/kg/day E4 (d), 10 mg/kg/day E4 (e), and 50 mg/kg/day E4 (f) groups (g); (**B**) E4 treatment: sham group (a), vehicle-treated group (b), 1 mg/kg/day E4 (c), 5 mg/kg/day E4 (d), 10 mg/kg/day E4 (e), and 50 mg/kg/day E4 (f) groups. (g) The ratio of the MAP-2 positive areas was calculated as the MAP-2 positive area of the ipsilateral hemisphere divided by the MAP-2 positive area of the contralateral hemisphere. Ten samples from each group were analyzed. The ratio of the MAP-2 positive area in sham-operated animal group was considered by default as 1.0. All measurements are expressed as mean ± SEM. *$p < 0.05$. Reproduced from *Experimental Neurology* (Tskitishvili et al., 2014, 261:298–307)

the vehicle groups in both models (Fig. 4.4a(g), b(g)). Thus, E4 can preserve the early gray matter loss when administered before or after induction of experimental hypoxic-ischemic brain injury [116].

Definitely, for us, it was important to show the possible promyelinating activity of E4. Myelin basic protein (MBP), as a marker of white matter damage/demyelination, is frequently used in studies connected to brain damage [120].

There was a loss of MBP staining at the damaged left side (Figs. 4.4a and 4.5a) which was more prominent in main white matter regions [the subcortical region and the cingulum (Figs. 4.4b and 4.5b)]. Promyelinating effect of E4 was significantly upregulated in groups treated by 5 and 50 mg/kg/day E4 before induction of hypoxia-ischemia (Fig. 4.4c), whereas all the groups treated by different doses of E4 after induction of experimental brain injury had significantly higher MBP-positive area OD ratio along with the sham group (Fig. 4.5c) [118]. Significant positive correlation was observed between the myelination and the brain weights ($r = 0.707$, $p = 0.0198$) in the vehicle group of the neuroprotective in vivo model [118].

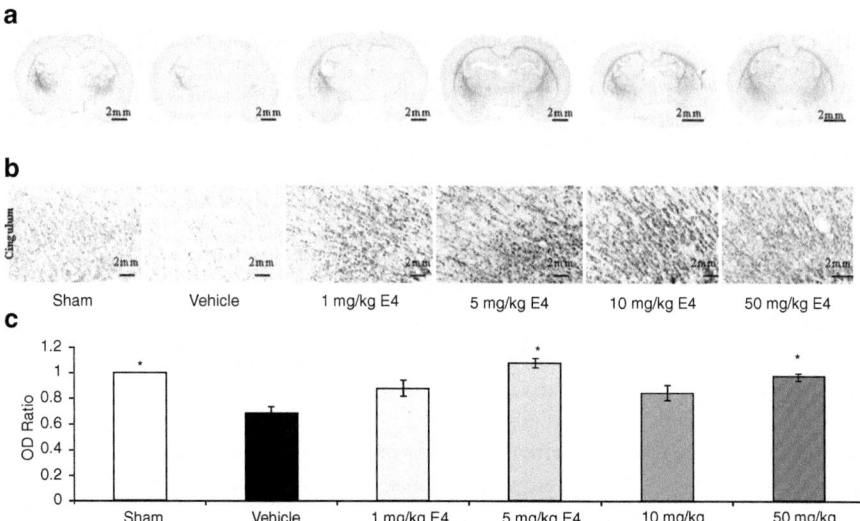

Fig. 4.4 Myelin basic protein (MBP) staining of brain coronal sections in rat pups pretreated with estetrol. (**a**) MBP staining of brain coronal sections (scale bar, 2 mm) is shown. (**b**) MBP staining of cingulum of the left hemisphere is shown (scale bar, 2 mm). (**c**) The ratio of the MBP-positive areas OD ratio was calculated as the MBP-positive area OD of the ipsilateral hemisphere divided by the MBP-positive area OD of the contralateral hemisphere. Ten samples from each study group were analyzed. The ratio of the MBP-positive area OD in the sham group was considered by default as 1.0. The MBP-positive area OD ratio was significantly higher in sham-operated animals and the 5 and 50 mg/kg/day E4-pretreated groups compared to the vehicle group. All measurements are expressed as mean ± SEM. *$p < 0.05$. Reproduced from J Endocrinol (Tskitishvili et al., 2017, 232(1):85–95)

Therapeutic effect

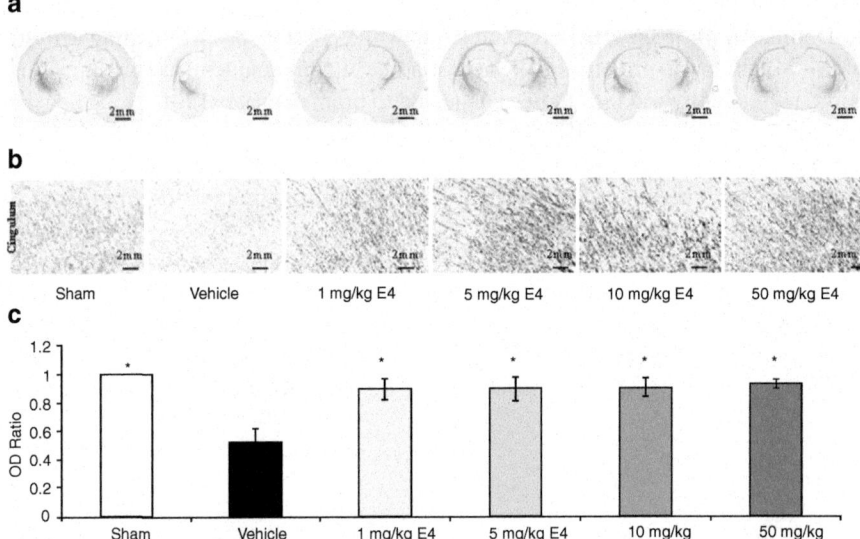

Fig. 4.5 Myelin basic protein (MBP) staining of brain coronal sections in rat pups treated with estetrol. (**a**) MBP staining of brain coronal sections (scale bar, 2 mm) is shown. (**b**) MBP staining of cingulum of the left hemisphere is shown (scale bar, 2 mm). (**c**) The ratio of the MBP-positive areas OD ratio was calculated as the MBP-positive area OD of the ipsilateral hemisphere divided by the MBP-positive area OD of the contralateral hemisphere. Ten samples from each study group were analyzed. The ratio of the MBP-positive area OD in the sham group was considered by default as 1.0. The MBP-positive area OD ratio was significantly higher in sham-operated animals and the 1, 5, 10, and 50 mg/kg/day E4-treated groups compared to the vehicle group. All measurements are expressed as mean ± SEM. *$p < 0.05$. Reproduced from J Endocrinol (Tskitishvili et al., 2017, 232(1):85–95)

Next step in studies of E4 and its neurological effects in brain was connected to the possible neurogenic- and cerebro-angiogenic effects of E4. Doublecortin (DCX), as a marker of neurogenesis, and VEGF as a marker for angiogenesis were used (Fig. 4.6). Obviously, pretreatment/treatment with different doses of E4 upregulated expression of the abovementioned markers in different regions of the brain and in different manner in all the study groups, showing co-localization of both markers in the cortical region of the 10 mg/kg/day E4-treated group (Fig. 4.4) [116]. In general, E4 pretreatment caused a significant upregulation of neurogenesis and cerebro-angiogenesis in the DG region, with 10 mg/kg for doublecortin and with all doses of E4 for VEGF (Table 4.2); in the CA1 region, in 5 mg/kg/day, 10 mg/kg/day, and 10 mg/kg/day E4 groups, respectively (Table 4.2); in the CA2/CA3 region, in 5 and 10 mg/kg/day E4 groups, respectively (Table 4.2); and in the cortex, in 10 mg/kg/day E4 (Fig. 4.4). Treatment by E4 after hypoxic-ischemic insult (Table 4.2) showed significant upregulation of neuro- and cerebro-angiogenesis in the CA1 region—in 10 and 50 mg/kg/day and in 5, 10, and 50 mg/kg/day E4 groups,

Table 4.2 Percentage of the DCX and VEGF positively stained cells in E4-pretreated/treated groups

	Sham	Vehicle	E4 pretreatment				Vehicle	E4 treatment			
			1 mg/kg/day	5 mg/kg/day	10 mg/kg/day	50 mg/kg/day		1 mg/kg/day	5 mg/kg/day	10 mg/kg/day	50 mg/kg/day
DG/DCX	43.7 ± 2.7	32.8 ± 2.6[a]	53.6 ± 5.5	50.5 ± 4.3	55.8 ± 5.7	53.8 ± 5.9	32.7 ± 3.5	37.2 ± 5.0	38.8 ± 3.2	42.6 ± 4.4	42.0 ± 2.3
CA1/DCX	18.8 ± 2.9	11.0 ± 1.5[c]	20.7 ± 3.9	35.2 ± 3.3	34.1 ± 6.7	26.7 ± 2.2	12.8 ± 4.3[e]	25.8 ± 3.2	27.7 ± 5.0	37.1 ± 3.8	37.3 ± 4.8
CA2/CA3/DCX	24.1 ± 6.1	6.42 ± 1.0[g]	17.7 ± 3.1	30.3 ± 3.7	19.7 ± 4.0	21.1 ± 4.2	10.4 ± 2.9[i]	26.3 ± 5.7	24.9 ± 5.1	42.5 ± 6.0	36.0 ± 6.1
Cortex/DCX	39.9 ± 1.6	26.0 ± 4.1[j]	32.7 ± 5.9	33.6 ± 2.6	52.1 ± 7.6	36.5 ± 6.3	23.3 ± 4.7[l]	40.8 ± 3.8	45.2 ± 3.3	49.4 ± 4.9	49.6 ± 3.1
DG/VEGF	40.1 ± 3.3	25.3 ± 2.3[b]	43.5 ± 2.1	46.0 ± 4.4	47.0 ± 5.4	46.0 ± 4.5	35.1 ± 3.6	28.9 ± 2.4	35.4 ± 2.7	42.6 ± 4.4	44.9 ± 4.3
CA1/VEGF	20.9 ± 4.1	15.2 ± 2.5[d]	27.6 ± 4.1	27.1 ± 2.8	37.4 ± 7.6	27.2 ± 3.3	15.7 ± 4.9[f]	27.2 ± 3.3	37.4 ± 4.8	37.1 ± 3.8	45.1 ± 4.7
CA2/CA3/VEGF	25.6 ± 7.9	8.8 ± 1.1[h]	34.1 ± 6.8	27.7 ± 4.8	25.5 ± 5.0	25.0 ± 2.9	15.6 ± 4.1	33.2 ± 6.2	40.5 ± 5.6	42.5 ± 6.0	44.9 ± 6.0
Cortex/VEGF	29.8 ± 4.7[m]	20.5 ± 2.4[k]	34.6 ± 5.1	28.0 ± 2.6	46.2 ± 7.6	25.9 ± 4.9	39.0 ± 4.1	30.7 ± 3.8	35.3 ± 6.2	49.4 ± 4.9	42.3 ± 2.8

Significant differences were observed:

In the DG region, E4-pretreated groups: DCX-stained cells; [a]vehicle vs. 10 mg/kg/day E4; VEGF-stained cells, [b]vehicle vs. 10 mg/kg/day E4

In the CA1 region, E4-pretreated groups: DCX-stained cells, [c]vehicle vs. 5 and 10 mg/kg/day E4; VEGF-stained cells, [d]vehicle vs. 10 mg/kg/day E4. E4-treated groups: DCX-stained cells, [e]vehicle vs. 10 and 50 mg/kg/day E4; VEGF-stained cells, [f]vehicle vs. 5, 10, and 50 mg/kg/day E4

In the CA2/CA3 region, E4-pretreated groups: DCX-stained cells, [g]vehicle vs. 5 mg/kg/day E4; VEGF-stained cells, [h]vehicle vs. 10 mg/kg/day E4. E4-treated groups: DCX-stained cells, [i]vehicle vs. 10 mg/kg/day

In the cortex, E4-pretreated groups: DCX-stained cells, [j]vehicle vs. 10 mg/kg/day E4; VEGF-stained cells, [k]vehicle vs. 10 mg/kg/day E4. E4-treated groups: DCX positively stained cells, [l]vehicle vs. 5, 10, and 50 mg/kg/day E4; VEGF-stained cells, [m]sham vs. 10 mg/kg/day E4

Reproduced from *Experimental Neurology* (Tskitishvili et al., 2014, 261:298–307)

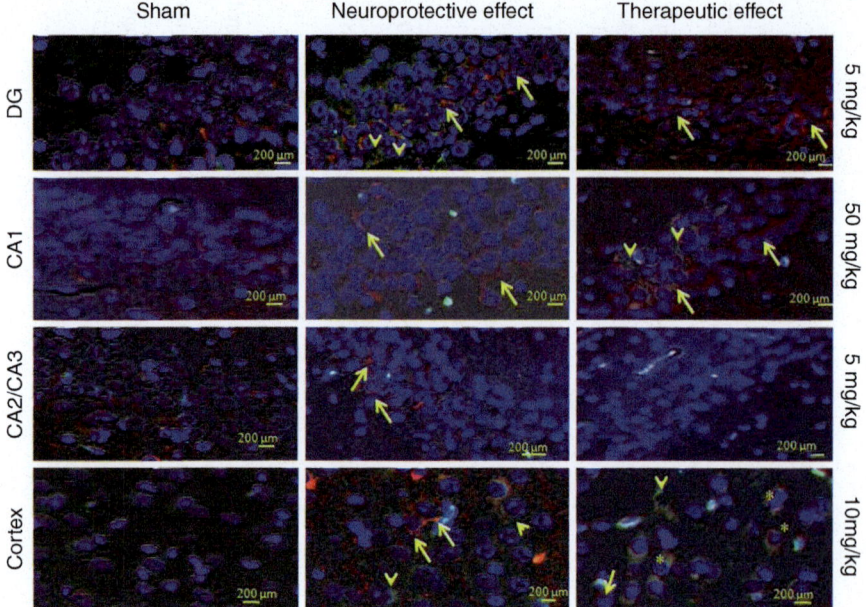

Fig. 4.6 Representative views of double-labeled immunofluorescence in the hippocampus and cortex of the rat pups pretreated or treated with E4. Double immunofluorescent staining was performed to determine the localization and expression of doublecortin (DCX) and vascular endothelial growth factor (VEGF) in different regions of hippocampus (dentate gyrus (DG), cornu ammonis 1 (CA1), cornu ammonis 2/3 (CA2/CA3), and cortex. Arrows denote DCX positively stained cells (red). Arrowheads denote VEGF positively stained cells (green). Asterisks indicate co-localization of DCX and VEGF positively stained cells. Scale bar: 200 μm. Reproduced from *Experimental Neurology* (Tskitishvili et al., 2014, 261:298–307)

respectively; in the CA2/CA3 region, neurogenesis was significantly upregulated in the 10 mg/kg/day E4 group alone, whereas in the cortex, upregulation of neuro- and cerebro-angiogenesis were more prominent in 5, 10, and 50 mg/kg/day and 10 mg/kg/day E4 groups, respectively (Table 4.2) [116] (Fig. 4.6).

Another issue was connected to the question whether pretreatment/treatment by E4 can affect the expression of brain damage markers in blood. Pretreatment by E4 in neuroprotective model resulted in significant downregulation of brain damage markers (S100B and GFAP) at a concentration of 50 mg/kg/day E4, whereas treatment by E4 after induction of experimental hypoxic-ischemic insult led to significant decrease of S100B and GFAP expression in all E4-treated groups (Table 4.3) [116].

4.4.2 Can We Use Estetrol in Combination with Other Steroids for Attenuation of HIE?

Dynamic changes in neurological field proposed new treatment strategies employing different compounds/steroids for attenuation of some neurological diseases.

Table 4.3 S100B and glial fibrillary acidic protein (GFAP) expression in blood serum of the rat pups pretreated/treated with E4

	E4 pretreatment		E4 treatment	
	S100B (pg/ml)	GFAP (pg/ml)	S100B (pg/ml)	GFAP (pg/ml)
Sham	344.6 ± 50.3[a]	407.0 ± 49.2	344.6 ± 50.3	407.6 ± 49.3
Vehicle	698.9 ± 57.3[b]	1003.9 ± 288.3[d]	1191.4 ± 211.2[e]	1762.3 ± 364.2[f]
1 mg/kg/day	560.2 ± 107.2	545.6 ± 85.4	665.7 ± 52.9	334.9 ± 23.9
5 mg/kg/day	395.0 ± 73.1	313.9 ± 36.8	628.3 ± 54.9	621.5 ± 90.7
10 mg/kg/day	715.7 ± 47.5[c]	630.4 ± 117.2	647.5 ± 41.3	479.1 ± 69.7
50 mg/kg/day	361.0 ± 32.9	300.4 ± 31.2	581.1 ± 73.5	460.0 ± 73.5

Significant differences were observed:
In E4-pretreated groups, S100B: [a]sham vs. vehicle and 10 mg/kg/day E4, [b]vehicle vs. 50 mg/kg/day E4, [c]10 mg/kg/day vs. 5 and 50 mg/kg/day E4. GFAP: [d]vehicle vs. sham and 50 mg/kg/day E4
In E4-treated groups, S100B: [e]vehicle vs. sham, 1, 5, 10, and 50 mg/kg/day E4. GFAP: [f]vehicle vs. sham, 1, 5, 10, and 50 mg/kg/day E4
Reproduced from *Experimental Neurology* (Tskitishvili et al., 2014, 261:298–307)

Like that several investigations already have demonstrated the neuroprotective efficacy of estradiol (E2) and progesterone (pregn-4-ene-3,20-dione) (P4) alone or in combination in different experimental models and clinical studies of neurological diseases: Parkinson's and Alzheimer's diseases, ischemic stroke, spinal cord injury, traumatic brain injury (TBI), and multiple sclerosis [12, 28, 29, 31, 32, 34, 37, 121–125]. P4-dependent neuroprotection is partly realized through attenuation of oxidative stress resulting from glutamate and glucose deprivation-induced toxicity [126–129]. Besides, in vitro, in primary hippocampal cell cultures, P4 might have protective effect against $FeSO_4$ and amyloid β-peptide-induced toxicity [130, 131]. Clinical studies in extremely preterm infants demonstrated reduction of the risk for cerebral palsy, spasticity, and ametropia at 5 years neurodevelopmental follow-up due to postnatal E2 and P4 combined replacement therapy [132]. Results of some studies employing combination of E2 and P4 are still controversial: though some studies have suggested that P4 does not affect the positive effects of E2 [128, 133, 134], others still argue that P4 might antagonize the positive effects of E2 [135–140].

As we know, the rat forebrain expresses high levels of progesterone receptors (PR) as early as E17–E18 in regions with important cognitive, motor, and visual functions; thus, the hippocampus has importance in establishment of early cortical circuitry. P4 neuroprotective effects are based on activation of inflammatory and oxidative mechanisms and the repair processes that usually follow the injury. As it was shown recently, the upregulation of nitric oxide synthase 2 (NOS-2), involved in production of nitric oxide free radicals, and pro-inflammatory IL-1β after ischemic events caused by MCAO is inhibited by progesterone treatment [141]. In adults after traumatic brain injury, P4 has an ability to reduce the proliferation of reactive astrocytes and inflammatory prostaglandin synthesis further leading to the reduction of edema and the blood-brain barrier leakage [122, 142]. P4 may induce a neuroprotective effect by upregulating expression of brain-derived neurotrophic factor (BDNF) or promoting increase of myelin basic protein expression (MBP)

[143], upregulating the inhibitory transmitter GABAa, and reducing the apoptosis by downregulation of NFκB [144–146]. Taken together, P4 along with E2 plays a critical role in neuronal developmental processes not only in prenatal period but in adulthood as well [147, 148].

Before starting a new stage of our studies with E4 and other steroids, it was important to define the working concentrations of P4 and E2. First, primary hippocampal neuronal cell cultures were treated after induction of the oxidative stress by P4 and E2 solely at doses starting from 1 nM until up to 1 mM. A significant downregulation of the LDH activity was observed at P4 concentration of 1 mM and E2 concentration of 100 nM (data not shown). Next we have performed treatment of primary hippocampal cell cultures after induction of oxidative stress with previously defined successful concentrations of E4 [116] which showed tremendous antioxidative and cell proliferative effects (650 μM, 3.25 mM, and 6.5 mM) alone or in combination with 1 mM PROG and/or E2 100 nM [117]. LDH activity as a marker of oxidative stress was significantly downregulated in all cultures exposed to steroids, especially in cultures exposed to different concentrations of E4 with E2 and P4 (Fig. 4.7a, b). Similar pattern of LDH activity was observed in cultures treated either by 6.5 mM E4 with E2 (Fig. 4.7a) or by different concentrations of E4 with P4 (Fig. 4.7b) compared to cultures treated by E4 alone [117]. The cell survival rate was significantly increased in cultures treated either by 6.5 mM E4 with/without E2 (Fig. 4.7c) or by 6.5 mM E4 with/without P4 (Fig. 4.7d) or by high doses of E4 with E2 and P4 (Fig. 4.7c, d). Furthermore, cells exposed to 6.5 mM E4 with/without E2 had significantly higher cell survival rate than the cultures treated by 650 μM E4 with/without E2 (Fig. 4.7c), though the dose-dependent pattern was more prominent when different concentrations of E4 were used with/without P4 (Fig. 4.7d). Cells treated by 6.5 mM E4 and P4 or treated by 6.5 mM E4 with E2 and P4 had significantly higher survival rate than the cells treated only by E4 (Fig. 4.7d) or those cells treated by 6.5 mM E4 with/without E2 (Fig. 4.7c) and by the lower doses of E4 combined with E2 and P4, respectively (Fig. 4.7c, d) [117].

Interesting observations were monitored in vivo. In neuroprotective model, when steroids were used before induction of brain injury, rectal temperature immediately after hypoxic-ischemic (HI) insult (at 0 h time point) was significantly increased only in animals from the vehicle group, whereas 2 h later the rectal temperature was significantly decreased in groups pretreated by combination of 5 mg/kg/day E4 and 1.6 mg/kg/day P4 with/without 136 ng/kg/day E2 (Fig. 4.8a) [117]. In therapeutic model, 2 h after HI insult, groups treated by combination of any dose of E4 with 16 mg/kg/day P4 plus 136 ng/kg/day E2 had significantly decreased rectal temperature than the vehicle group or the groups treated by the same doses of E4 with 1.6 mg/ kg/day P4 and E2. Combination of 10 mg/kg/day E4 with 16 mg/kg/day P4 with or without 136 ng/kg/day E2 also 10 mg/kg/day E4 alone or combined with 1.6 mg/kg/ day P4 significantly downregulated the rectal temperature (Fig. 4.8b) [117]. At 4 h

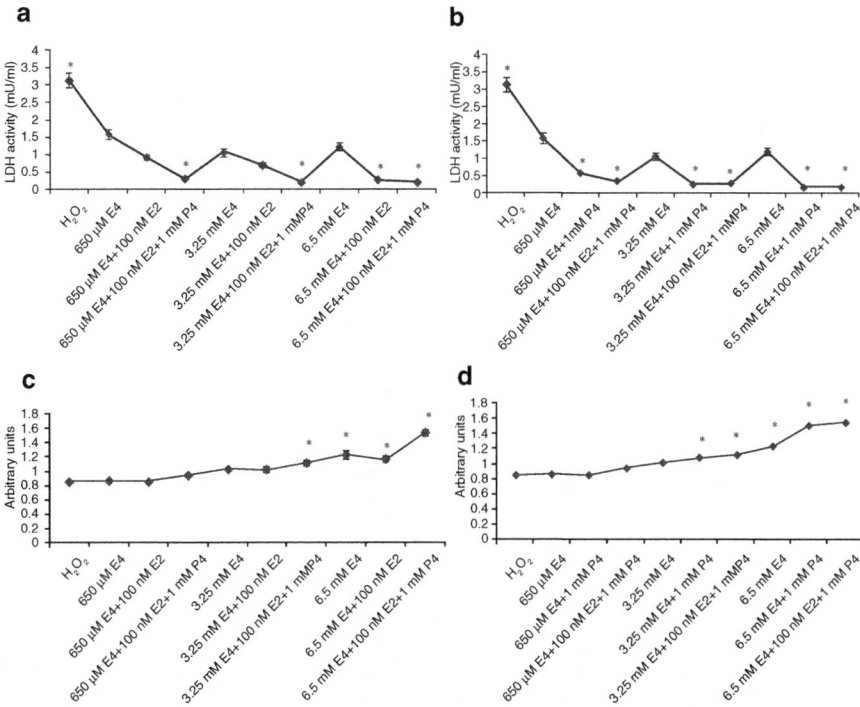

Fig. 4.7 Effect of E4 alone or in combination with P4 and/or E2 on LDH activity and cell viability in primary hippocampal cell cultures subjected to the H_2O_2-induced oxidative stress. (**a–d**) Primary hippocampal neuronal cells were treated with 650 µM, 3.25 mM, and 6.5 mM of estetrol alone or in combination with 100 nM E2 and/or 1 mM P4 for 1 h after induction of oxidative stress by 100 µM of H_2O_2 for 30 min. (**a, b**). LDH activity was significantly downregulated in all the study groups compared to the H_2O_2-treated group. The LDH activity level was significantly lower in cultures treated either with 6.5 mM E4 or 100 nM E2 (**a**) or in cultures treated by any dose of E4 along with 1 mM P4 than in cultures treated by E4 alone (**b**) as well as in cultures combinedly treated by any dose of E4 along with 1 mM P4 and 100 nM E2 than in cultures treated by E4 alone (**a, b**). (**c**) Cell survival was significantly upregulated in cultures treated by 6.5 mM E4 with/without 1 mM P4 or by 3.25 mM and 6.5 mM E4 with 100 nM E2 and 1 mM P4 in comparison with H_2O_2-treated cultures. Cells exposed to 6.5 mM E4 with/without 100 nM E2 had significantly higher cell survival rate than the cultures treated by 650 µM E4 with/without 100 nM E2. Cells combinedly treated by 6.5 mM E4 with 100 nM E2 and 1 mM P4 had significantly higher survival level than the cells treated by 6.5 mM E4 with/without 100 nM E2. (**d**) Cell survival was significantly upregulated in cultures treated by 6.5 mM E4 with/without 1 mM P4 or by 3.25 mM and 6.5 mM E4 with 100 nM E2 and 1 mM P4 than in H_2O_2-treated cultures. The dose-dependent pattern was observed when 650 µM, 3.25 mM, and 6.5 mM E4 were used with/without 1 mM P4. (**c, d**) Cell cultures combinedly treated by 6.5 mM E4 with 100 nM E2 and 1 mM P4 had significantly higher survival level than the cells treated by 650 µM and 3.25 mM E4 in combination with 100 nM E2 and 1 mM P4. All measurements are expressed as mean ± SEM. *$p \leq 0.05$. Reproduced from *Oncotarget* (Tskitishvili et al., 2016, 7(23):33722–43)

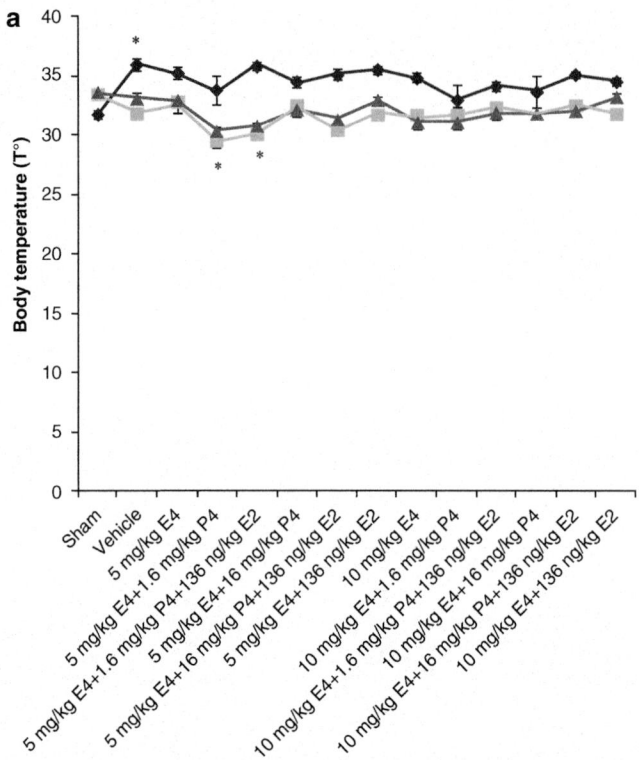

Fig. 4.8 Postoperative rectal temperature and body weight of rat pups. (**a**). In neuroprotective model, immediately after hypoxic-ischemic (HI) insult (at 0 h), the rectal temperature was significantly increased only in the vehicle group than in the sham group, whereas 2 h later the rectal temperature was significantly decreased in pretreated by 5 mg/kg/day E4 and 1.6 mg/kg/day P4 with/without 136 ng/kg/day E2 groups compared to the sham group. Four hours later no significant difference was observed among the study groups. (**b**) In therapeutic model, between the study groups immediately after HI insult, no significant differences were detected, whereas 2 h later groups treated by combination of 5 mg/kg/day or 10 mg/kg/day E4 with 16 mg/kg/day P4 plus 136 ng/kg/day E2 had significantly decreased rectal temperature than the vehicle group or the groups treated by the same doses of E4 with 1.6 mg/kg/day P4 and E2. Moreover, combination of 10 mg/kg/day E4 with 16 mg/kg/day P4 and 136 ng/kg/day E2 significantly downregulated the rectal temperature compared to the sham group or the group treated by 10 mg/kg/day E4 and 16 mg/kg/day P4 (Fig. 4.2b). Also, the groups treated by 10 mg/kg/day E4 alone or combined with 1.6 mg/kg/day P4 had significantly decreased rectal temperature compared to the group treated by 10 mg/kg/day E4 with 1.6 mg/kg/day P4 and 136 ng/kg/day E2. At 4 h after HI event, animals treated by 5 mg/kg/day or 10 mg/kg/day E4 and 136 ng/kg/day E2 with/without 16 mg/kg/day P4 had significantly decreased rectal temperature along with the sham group compared to animals treated by single doses of E4 (Fig. 4.2b). The same pattern was observed between groups treated by 10 mg/kg/day E4 with 1.6 mg/kg/day P4 and 136 ng/kg/day E2 and the group treated by E4 alone. Treatment by 5 mg/kg/day E4 with 16 mg/kg/day P4 and 136 ng/kg/day E2 significantly decreased the rectal temperature than the treatment by the same combination of compounds with 1.6 mg/kg/day P4 (Fig. 4.2b). All measurements are expressed as mean ± SEM. *$p \leq 0.05$. Reproduced from *Oncotarget* (Tskitishvili et al., 2016, 7(23):33722–43)

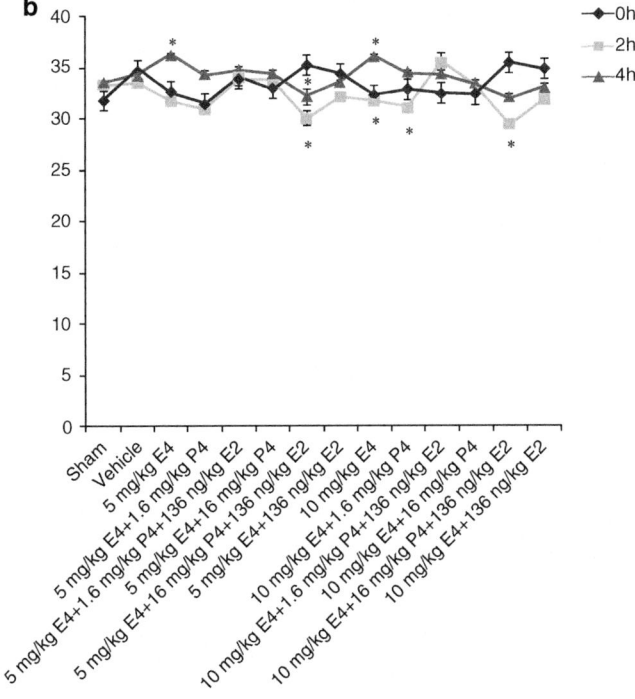

Fig. 4.8 (continued)

after HI insult, animals treated by E4 and E2 with/without 1.6 mg/kg/day/16 mg/kg/day P4 had significantly decreased rectal temperature compared to animals treated by single doses of E4 (Fig. 4.8b). Treatment by 5 mg/kg/day E4 with 16 mg/kg/day P4 and E2 significantly decreased the rectal temperature than the treatment by the same combination of compounds with 1.6 mg/kg/day P4 (Fig. 4.8b) [117].

As it is shown in Table 4.4, animals pretreated by a combination of 5 mg/kg/day E4 and 16 mg/kg/day P4 before experimental brain injury had significantly higher body weight than animals from the vehicle, sham, and combinedly pretreated by 5 mg/kg/day E4 and E2 groups, and the brain-body weight ratio was significantly higher in groups pretreated by 5 mg/kg/day E4 and 136 ng/kg/day E2 in combination either with 1.6 or 16 mg/kg/day P4. In groups treated by steroids after experimental brain damage, only animals from 10 mg/kg/day E4 group had significantly higher brain weight compared to the vehicles (Table 4.4) without affecting the brain-body weight ratio [117].

Histochemical studies of coronal sections from rat pups' brains pretreated/treated by the vehicle showed obvious injury of the hippocampus at the left carotid artery occlusion (damaged) side which was extended to the cortex at the same side (Figs. 4.9 and 4.10A(b), B(b)). It was also interesting to observe the damage of the cortex of the left hemisphere in animals that were pretreated/treated by combination of E4 and E2 (Fig. 4.9) [117].

Table 4.4 Body and brain weights of rat pups from study groups

Groups	Body weight (g)		Brain weight (g)	p
	P7	P14		
Pretreatment				
Sham	12.04 ± 0.52	26.96 ± 0.73	1.20 ± 0.01	
Vehicle	12.52 ± 0.41	27.86 ± 0.65	1.15 ± 0.01	
5 mg/kg E4	15.03 ± 0.68	24.61 ± 1.19	1.18 ± 0.03	
5 mg/kg E4 + 1.6 mg/kg P4	12.89 ± 0.46	26.63 ± 1.30	1.21 ± 0.03	
5 mg/kg E4 + 1.6 mg/kg P4 + 136 ng/kg E2	11.93 ± 0.36	22.04 ± 0.66	1.19 ± 0.03	
5 mg/kg E4 + 16 mg/kg P4	15.94 ± 0.29	25.58 ± 1.47	1.17 ± 0.02	a
5 mg/kg E4 + 16 mg/kg P4 + 136 ng/kg E2	14.27 ± 0.70	21.55 ± 0.68	1.16 ± 0.03	
5 mg/kg E4 + 136 ng/kg E2	11.94 ± 0.59	23.91 ± 1.34	1.12 ± 0.03	
10 mg/kg E4	13.35 ± 0.47	27.10 ± 0.83	1.19 ± 0.02	
10 mg/kg E4 + 1.6 mg/kg P4	12.83 ± 0.66	25.57 ± 0.99	1.25 ± 0.01	
10 mg/kg E4 + 1.6 mg/kg P4 + 136 ng/kg E2	13.59 ± 0.50	27.91 ± 1.18	1.23 ± 0.02	
10 mg/kg E4 + 16 mg/kg P4	13.55 ± 0.34	26.46 ± 1.20	1.23 ± 0.03	
10 mg/kg E4 + 16 mg/kg P4 + 136 ng/kg E2	13.15 ± 0.25	27.99 ± 1.03	1.24 ± 0.01	
10 mg/kg E4 + 136 ng/kg E2	12.47 ± 0.52	25.69 ± 0.93	1.21 ± 0.03	
Treatment				
Sham	12.04 ± 0.52	26.96 ± 0.73	1.20 ± 0.01	
Vehicle	13.43 ± 0.35	26.63 ± 0.71	1.17 ± 0.02	
5 mg/kg E4	14.14 ± 0.62	28.21 ± 1.23	1.28 ± 0.01	
5 mg/kg E4 + 1.6 mg/kg P4	14.08 ± 0.65	27.16 ± 0.66	1.23 ± 0.02	
5 mg/kg E4 + 1.6 mg/kg P4 + 136 ng/kg E2	13.66 ± 0.43	25.67 ± 0.88	1.29 ± 0.01	
5 mg/kg E4 + 16 mg/kg P4	13.51 ± 0.41	27.11 ± 1.18	1.26 ± 0.03	
5 mg/kg E4 + 16 mg/kg P4 + 136 ng/kg E2	15.03 ± 0.49	28.13 ± 1.37	1.22 ± 0.03	
5 mg/kg E4 + 136 ng/kg E2	13.93 ± 0.37	24.43 ± 2.07	1.15 ± 0.05	
10 mg/kg E4	14.25 ± 0.59	30.82 ± 0.54	1.34 ± 0.01	b
10 mg/kg E4 + 1.6 mg/kg P4	13.83 ± 0.66	24.97 ± 0.89	1.20 ± 0.02	
10 mg/kg E4 + 1.6 mg/kg P4 + 136 ng/kg E2	13.44 ± 0.47	25.48 ± 1.22	1.25 ± 0.02	
10 mg/kg E4 + 16 mg/kg P4	13.93 ± 0.39	25.98 ± 0.74	1.32 ± 0.01	
10 mg/kg E4 + 16 mg/kg P4 + 136 ng/kg E2	14.17 ± 0.51	32.41 ± 0.96	1.26 ± 0.02	
10 mg/kg E4 + 136 ng/kg E2	15.04 ± 0.42	28.64 ± 2.76	1.22 ± 0.04	

Significant differences were observed: [a]body weight at P7, 5 mg/kg/day E4 + 16 mg/kg/day P4 group vs. sham, vehicle, and 5 mg/kg/day E4 + 136 ng/kg/day E2 in pretreated groups; [b]brain weight, 10 mg/kg/day E4 vs. vehicle in treated groups

Reproduced from *Oncotarget* (Tskitishvili et al., 2016, 7(23):33722–43)

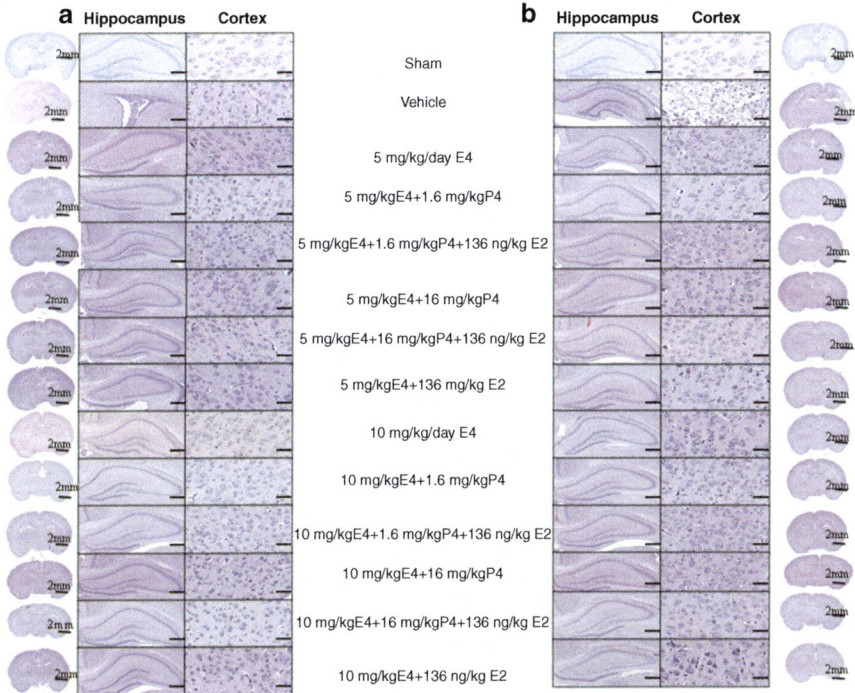

Fig. 4.9 Representative views of hematoxylin-eosin-stained brain coronal sections from rat pups pretreated/treated by E4 alone or in combination with P4 and/or E2. Paraffin-embedded brain samples were sliced into 5-µm-thick coronal sections at the hippocampus level. Sections were deparaffinized and rehydrated, and hematoxylin and eosin staining was performed. Brain coronal sections (scale bar, 2 mm) with hippocampus region (scale bar, 500 µm) and the cortex (scale bar, 100 µm) from pretreated (**a**) and treated (**b**) study groups are presented. Reproduced from *Oncotarget* (Tskitishvili et al., 2016, 7(23):33722–43)

Cell counting per visual field in pretreated groups showed (Table 4.5) that in the DG region there were significant differences between the study groups as follows: sham and the vehicle groups or groups pretreated by 5 mg/kg/day E4 and E2 with/without 16 mg/kg/day P4 (Fig. 4.9a and 4.10A(c), (d), respectively) or by 10 mg/kg/day E4 with E2 and 16 mg/kg/day P4 (Fig. 4.9a). In the same region of the hippocampus, significantly higher number of intact cells was observed in animals pretreated by 5 mg/kg/day E4 (Fig. 4.10A(c)) and 10 mg/kg/day E4 (Fig. 4.10A(f)) alone or in combination with 1.6 mg/kg/day P4 and/or E2, also in animals pretreated with 10 mg/kg/day E4 and 16 mg/kg/day P4 (Table 4.5), as well as between animals pretreated by 10 mg/kg/day E4 alone or in combination with E2 and/or any

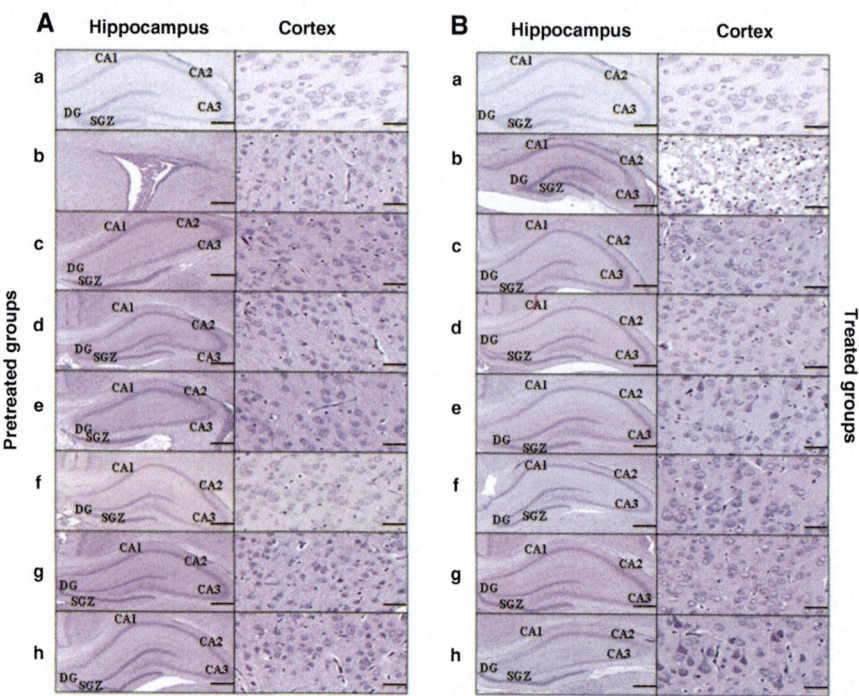

Fig. 4.10 Hematoxylin-eosin staining of the brain coronal sections from rat pups pretreated/ treated by E4 alone or in combination with P4 and/or E2. Brain coronal sections (scale bar, 2 mm) with hippocampus region (scale bar, 500 μm) and cortex (scale bar, 100 μm) from pretreated **A** and treated **B** study groups are shown: sham (a), vehicle (b), 5 mg/kg/dayE4 (c), 5 mg/kg/day E4 + 16 mg/kg/day P4 + 136 ng/kg/day E2 (d), 5 mg/kg/day E4 + 136 ng/kg/day E2 (e), 10 mg/kg/ day E4 (f), 10 mg/kg/day E4 + 16 mg/kg/day P4 (g), 10 mg/kg/day E4 + 136 ng/kg/day E2 (h). Reproduced from *Oncotarget* (Tskitishvili et al., Use of estetrol with other steroids for attenuation of neonatal hypoxic-ischemic brain injury: to combine or not to combine? *Oncotarget*. 2016, 7(23):33722–43)

concentration of P4, and the sham group (Table 4.5) [117]. In the SGZ the sham group had significantly higher intact cell counting than animals pretreated by 5 mg/ kg/day E4 with E2 (Figs. 4.9a and 4.10A(h)), whereas the number of intact cells was significantly upregulated in the groups pretreated by different doses of E4 alone or combined with 16 mg/kg/day P4. The same pattern of significant difference was observed in animals pretreated by 5 mg/kg/day E4 in combination with 16 mg/kg/ day P4 plus E2 and the vehicle group (Table 4.5) [117].

In treated groups (Figs. 4.9b and 4.10B), in the DG region, the number of intact cells was significantly different between the groups: vehicle and sham, also groups treated by combination of different doses of E4 either with any dose of P4 or E2. Intact cell number was significantly downregulated in animals combinedly treated by 10 mg/kg/day E4 and E2 (Fig. 4.10B(h)) compared to the sham group (Table 4.5). In the SGZ region, significant differences were observed between the vehicle group and the animals treated by different doses of E4 with 1.6 mg/kg/day P4 or E2, also

Table 4.5 Intact cell counting/per visual field in the hippocampus and cortex in hematoxylin-eosin-stained sections

Groups	DG	SGZ	CA1	CA2/CA3	Cortex
Pretreatment					
Sham	202.70 ± 18.28[a]	89.80 ± 8.57[f]	55.40 ± 3.34	44.70 ± 2.38	47.20 ± 3.90
Vehicle	76.30 ± 10.23[b]	33.20 ± 5.22[g]	48.30 ± 6.65	33.80 ± 3.93	33.30 ± 3.24
5 mg/kg E4	183.40 ± 11.96	72.10 ± 5.93	48.60 ± 2.57	51.80 ± 3.56	39.80 ± 2.74
5 mg/kg E4 + 1.6 mg/kg P4	168.80 ± 17.52	62.50 ± 6.97	54.00 ± 3.11	45.30 ± 2.89	36.50 ± 3.19
5 mg/kg E4 + 1.6 mg/kg P4 + 136 ng/kg E2	168.80 ± 4.71	67.7 ± 3.32	53.60 ± 3.47	40.80 ± 3.06	43.60 ± 4.02
5 mg/kg E4 + 16 mg/kg P4	148.60 ± 12.97	68.60 ± 5.15	51.70 ± 5.69	54.60 ± 7.00	41.90 ± 4.51
5 mg/kg E4 + 16 mg/kg P4 + 136 ng/kg E2	167.40 ± 13.96	73.90 ± 7.96	45.00 ± 6.07	44.40 ± 6.59	40.20 ± 3.60
5 mg/kg E4 + 136 ng/kg E2	111.40 ± 6.69	42.90 ± 3.09	56.20 ± 3.76	38.50 ± 2.85	36.50 ± 3.37
10 mg/kg E4	227.30 ± 14.18[c]	86.10 ± 5.84	64.90 ± 3.63	42.40 ± 2.49	39.60 ± 2.86
10 mg/kg E4 + 1.6 mg/kg P4	166.90 ± 11.97	64.30 ± 5.26	58.30 ± 3.53	45.30 ± 2.92	45.40 ± 5.70
10 mg/kg E4 + 1.6 mg/kg P4 + 136 ng/kg E2	123.4 ± 7.25	54.20 ± 4.84	65.90 ± 4.91	46.10 ± 7.72	41.90 ± 2.65
10 mg/kg E4 + 16 mg/kg P4	174.60 ± 12.38	73.50 ± 6.97	58.40 ± 4.74	46.30 ± 4.57	38.40 ± 5.45
10 mg/kg E4 + 16 mg/kg P4 + 136 ng/kg E2	115.70 ± 6.51	52.70 ± 2.49	45.00 ± 3.63	46.30 ± 5.02	36.90 ± 3.485
10 mg/kg E4 + 136 ng/kg E2	131.70 ± 8.94	56.30 ± 3.02	57.70 ± 2.46	43.30 ± 1.89	39.50 ± 4.37
Treatment					
Sham	202.70 ± 18.28	89.80 ± 8.57[h]	55.40 ± 3.34	44.70 ± 32.38[i]	47.20 ± 3.90
Vehicle	74.00 ± 10.61[d]	39.10 ± 6.79	41.80 ± 6.86	24.30 ± 4.15	20.30 ± 2.33[j]
5 mg/kg E4	142.90 ± 5.63	60.40 ± 3.55	56.30 ± 3.45	32.90 ± 31.62	32.70 ± 2.64
5 mg/kg E4 + 1.6 mg/kg P4	138.80 ± 14.01	45.20 ± 4.20	53.20 ± 5.67	34.60 ± 33.21	42.30 ± 3.72
5 mg/kg E4 + 1.6 mg/kg P4 + 136 ng/kg E2	160.00 ± 7.29	61.10 ± 3.94	56.50 ± 2.79	39.50 ± 31.46	41.40 ± 4.79
5 mg/kg E4 + 16 mg/kg P4	175.50 ± 7.84	61.30 ± 3.08	55.10 ± 3.85	42.5 ± 31.87	50.90 ± 4.87
5 mg/kg E4 + 16 mg/kg P4 + 136 ng/kg E2	164.00 ± 12.45	58.4 ± 4.92	57.50 ± 4.17	35.6 ± 33.45	37.00 ± 4.17
5 mg/kg E4 + 136 ng/kg E2	128.50 ± 12.15	54.10 ± 4.37	54.20 ± 4.95	38.00 ± 34.13	46.00 ± 4.51
10 mg/kg E4	150.20 ± 9.43	57.30 ± 5.19	51.20 ± 2.82	33.50 ± 0.98	46.60 ± 1.83
10 mg/kg E4 + 1.6 mg/kg P4	132.20 ± 13.68	41.90 ± 2.88	47.10 ± 6.64	37.60 ± 33.36	31.30 ± 3.83

(continued)

Table 4.5 (continued)

Groups	DG	SGZ	CA1	CA2/CA3	Cortex
10 mg/kg E4 + 1.6 mg/kg P4 + 136 ng/kg E2	156.00 ± 6.11	56.70 ± 2.45	61.50 ± 2.88	39.80 ± 31.30	38.80 ± 4.81
10 mg/kg E4 + 16 mg/kg P4	168.40 ± 4.38	65.40 ± 3.09	57.50 ± 1.73	40.40 ± 31.83	48.10 ± 4.02
10 mg/kg E4 + 16 mg/kg P4 + 136 ng/kg E2	150.00 ± 9.92	54.40 ± 4.01	50.90 ± 4.59	32.60 ± 32.82	39.10 ± 3.30
10 mg/kg E4 + 136 ng/kg E2	103.40 ± 13.47[e]	41.50 ± 5.55	48.40 ± 6.86	28.90 ± 35.34	39.10 ± 3.45

Significant differences were observed:

In the DG region

Pretreated groups: [a]sham vs. 5 mg/kg E4 + 136 ng/kg E4 + 16 mg/kg P4 + 136 ng/kg E4 + 16 mg/kg/day E2, 5 mg/kg/day E4 + 136 ng/kg/day E2, 10 mg/kg/day + 16 mg/kg/day P4 + 136 ng/kg/day E2; [b]vehicle vs. sham, 5 mg/kg/day E4, 5 mg/kg/day E4 + 1.6 mg/kg/day P4, 5 mg/kg/day E4 + 1.6 mg/kg/day P4 + 136 ng/kg/day E2, 10 mg/kg/day E4, 10 mg/kg/day E4 + 1.6 mg/kg/day P4, 10 mg/kg/day E4 + 16 mg/kg/day E4 vs. vehicle, sham, 10 mg/kg/day E4 + 1.6 mg/kg/day P4 + 136 ng/kg/day E2, 10 mg/kg/day E4 + 136 ng/kg/day E2

Treated groups: [d]vehicle vs. sham, 5 mg/kg/day E4 + 1.6 mg/kg/day P4 + 136 ng/kg/day E2, 5 mg/kg/day E4 + 16 mg/kg/day P4, 5 mg/kg/day E4 + 16 mg/kg/day P4 + 136 ng/kg/day E2, 10 mg/kg/day E4 + 1.6 mg/kg/day P4 + 136 ng/kg/day E4, 10 mg/kg/day E4 + 16 mg/kg/day P4, 10 mg/kg/day E4 + 16 mg/kg/day E4 + 16 mg/kg/day E2 vs. sham group in treated groups

In the SGZ

Pretreated groups: [f]sham vs. 5 mg/kg/day E4 + 136 ng/kg/day E2; [g]vehicle vs. sham, 5 mg/kg/day E4, 5 mg/kg/day E4 + 16 mg/kg/day P4 + 136 ng/kg/day E2, 10 mg/kg/day E4, 10 mg/kg/day E4 + 16 mg/kg/day P4

Treated groups: [h]sham vs. vehicle, 5 mg/kg/day + 136 ng/kg/day E2, 5 mg/kg/day E4 + 1.6 mg/kg/day P4, 10 mg/kg/day E4 + 1.6 mg/kg/day P4, 10 mg/kg/day E4 + 1.6 mg/kg/day P4 + 136 ng/kg/day E4 + 16 mg/kg/day E2, 10 mg/kg/day E4 + 136 ng/kg/day E2

In the CA2/CA3 region

Treated groups: [i]sham vs. vehicle in treated groups

In the cortex

Treated groups: [j]vehicle vs. sham, 5 mg/kg/day + 16 mg/kg/day + 16 mg/kg/day P4, 10 mg/kg/day, 10 mg/kg/day + 16 mg/kg/day + 16 mg/kg/day P4

Reproduced from *Oncotarget* (Tskitishvili et al., 2016, 7(23):33722–43)

the animals treated by 10 mg/kg/day E4 with E2 and different doses of P4 (Fig. 4.9b and Table 4.5). In the CA2/CA3 region, significant differences were observed only among animals from sham and the vehicle groups, whereas in the cortex, significantly higher number of intact cells was detected except for the sham group in groups treated either by different doses of E4 in combination with 16 mg/kg/day P4 or 10 mg/kg/day E4 alone (Fig. 4.10B) and the vehicle group (Table 4.5) [117].

By using the MAP staining, we have evaluated the gray matter loss in study groups. MAP-2 negatively stained areas corresponded to the damaged areas in the left hemisphere (the hippocampus and the cortex) (Fig. 4.9a, b) [117]. MAP-2 positively stained area ratio was significantly upregulated in animals pretreated by 10 mg/kg/day E4 alone along with animals from sham group (Figs. 4.11a and 4.12a), whereas after treatment with different combinations of steroids, MAP-2 positive area ratio was significantly higher in groups treated by E4 alone or in combination with 16 mg/kg/day P4 compared to the vehicle group (Figs. 4.11b and 4.12b). The similar pattern showed animals combinedly treated by 5 mg/kg/day E4 with 1.6 mg/kg/day P4 and E2. Treatment with 5 mg/kg/day E4 alone or either with 1.6 mg/kg/P4 and E2 or 16 mg/kg/day P4 restored the MAP-2 positive area ratio almost to the sham level (Figs. 4.11b and 4.12b) [117].

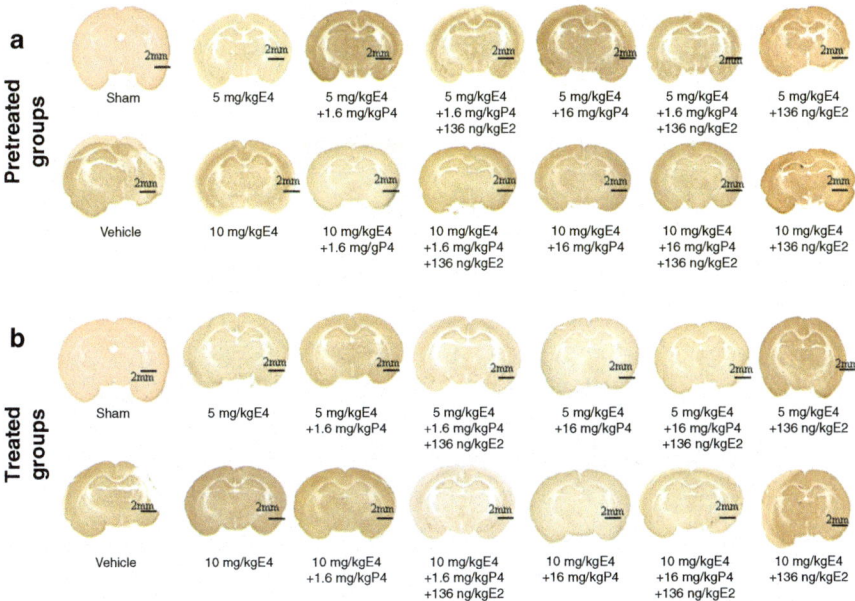

Fig. 4.11 Representative views of MAP-2-stained coronal brain sections from groups pretreated or treated with E4 alone or in combination with P4 and/or E2. From left to right are presented MAP-2-stained sections from pretreated (**a**) and treated (**b**) groups. In sections from the vehicle-pretreated/treated animals was observed an existence of MAP-2 negatively stained areas in the hippocampus and the cortex at the left, damaged side. Scale bar: 2 mm. Reproduced from *Oncotarget* (Tskitishvili et al., 2016, 7(23):33722–43)

We have also studied the possible effect of combined use of E4 with other steroids on neuro- and cerebro-angiogenesis by using specific markers DCX and VEGF, respectively, as previously (Fig. 4.13) [117]. In groups pretreated by different combinations of steroids before experimental HI insult in the DG region, neurogenesis and angiogenesis were significantly upregulated in 5 mg/kg/day E4 and 10 mg/kg/day E4 along with 1.6 mg/kg/day P4 and E2, respectively (Table 4.6); in the CA1 region, significant differences in DCX expression were observed between the sham and the vehicle groups, though VEGF expression was significantly increased in animals combinedly pretreated by 5 mg/kg/day E4 and 16 mg/kg/day P4 (Table 4.6); in the CA2/CA3 region, expressions of DCX and VEGF were significantly different only between the sham and the vehicle groups, whereas in the cortex between the sham and 5 mg/kg/day E4 plus 16 mg/kg/day P4 groups (Table 4.6) [117]. Notably, pretreatment by combination of E4 and E2 did not show any positive result for neuro- and angiogenesis (Fig. 4.13) [117].

Treatment of animals after HI insult with different combinations of steroids resulted in significant upregulation of neurogenesis in the hippocampus in animals

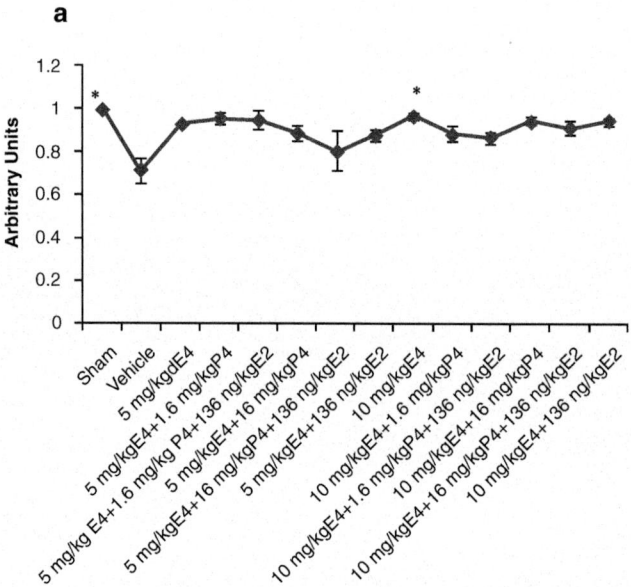

Fig. 4.12 MAP-2 staining of brain coronal sections from rat pups pretreated/treated by E4 alone or in combination with P4 and/or E2. For evaluation of gray matter loss, MAP-2 staining was performed. (**a**) Among pretreated groups the MAP-2 positively stained area ratio was significantly upregulated in animals pretreated by 10 mg/kg/day E4 alone than in the vehicles as well as in animals from sham group. (**b**) After treatment with different combinations of steroids, MAP-2-positive area ratio was significantly higher along with the sham group in groups treated by 5 or 10 mg/kg/day E4 alone or in combination with 16 mg/kg/day P4 compared to the vehicle group. The similar pattern was observed in animals combinedly treated by 5 mg/kg/day E4 with 1.6 mg/kg/day P4 and 136 ng/kg/day E2. Ten samples from each group were analyzed. The ratio of the MAP-2-positive area in sham-operated animals was considered as 1.0 by default. All measurements are expressed as mean ± SEM. *$p \leq 0.05$. Reproduced from *Oncotarget* (Tskitishvili et al., 2016, 7(23):33722–43)

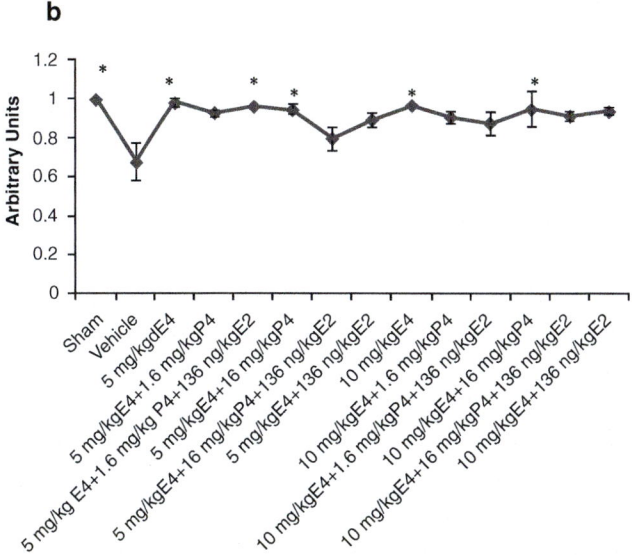

Fig. 4.12 (continued)

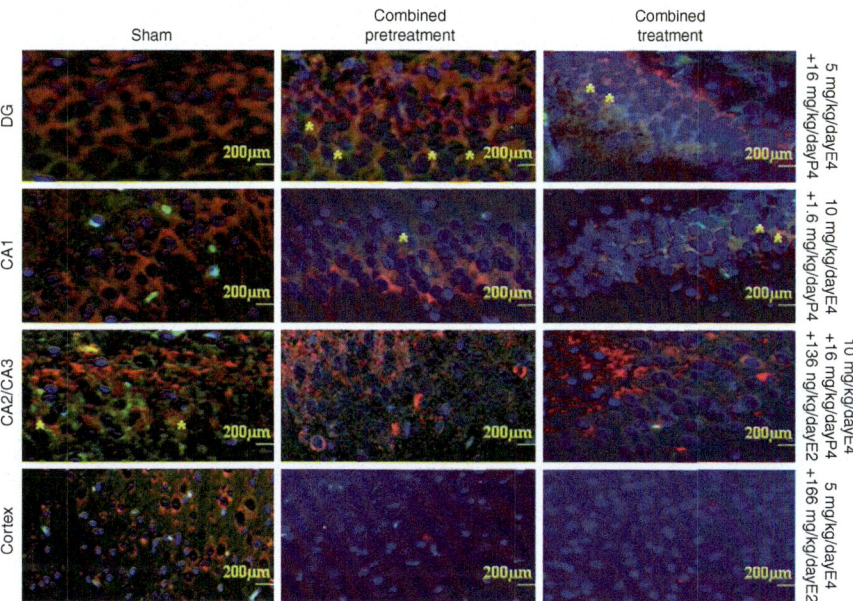

Fig. 4.13 Representative views of double-labeled immunofluorescent sections from different regions of the hippocampus and the cortex from groups pretreated/treated with E4 alone or in combination with P4 and/or E2. To determine the localization and expression of DCX and VEGF in different regions of the hippocampus and the cortex, the double immunofluorescent staining was performed. Red cells denote the DCX positively stained cells, whereas green cells denote the VEGF positively stained cells. Asterisks indicate co-localization of DCX and VEGF positively stained cells. Scale bar: 200 μm. Reproduced from *Oncotarget* (Tskitishvili et al., 2016, 7(23):33722–43)

Table 4.6 Percentage of the DCX and VEGF positively stained cells in combinedly pretreated/treated groups

Groups	DG DCX	CA1 DCX	CA2/CA3 DCX	Cortex DCX	DG VEGF	CA1 VEGF	CA2/CA3 VEGF	Cortex VEGF
Pretreatment								
Sham	59.73 ± 3.44	52.34 ± 30.99	51.25 ± 2.42	63.34 ± 2.17	52.38 ± 1.58	51.87 ± 3.68	55.79 ± 2.92	58.29 ± 2.98
Vehicle	30.90 ± 3.97[a]	16.78 ± 32.32[a]	15.97 ± 2.35[j]	29.48 ± 1.98[o]	31.25 ± 3.70[b]	20.76 ± 2.71[g]	20.05 ± 3.01[k]	28.47 ± 2.13[p]
5 mg/kg E4	60.29 ± 5.66	45.97 ± 34.40	32.38 ± 5.03[m]	51.47 ± 3.98	42.81 ± 2.68	49.99 ± 3.94	43.80 ± 3.68	46.00 ± 2.55
5 mg/kg E4 + 1.6 mg/kg P4	45.16 ± 3.26	42.67 ± 35.07	34.03 ± 5.62	51.89 ± 5.26	38.60 ± 3.32	44.96 ± 5.04	42.96 ± 3.70	40.31 ± 4.95
5 mg/kg E4 + 1.6 mg/kg P4 + 136 ng/kg E2	58.55 ± 5.37	37.08 ± 32.67	22.68 ± 2.81	53.98 ± 3.81	47.71 ± 4.36	36.17 ± 3.17	31.14 ± 2.87	39.23 ± 2.69
5 mg/kg E4 + 16 mg/kg P4	56.23 ± 4.02	51.34 ± 34.00	49.02 ± 9.09	71.46 ± 4.89	44.53 ± 2.50	59.56 ± 3.26	51.57 ± 6.77	60.22 ± 4.09
5 mg/kg E4 + 16 mg/kg P4 + 136 ng/kg E2	53.40 ± 3.56	32.41 ± 39.50	27.43 ± 9.36	53.06 ± 3.10	46.67 ± 2.59	42.49 ± 8.47	41.07 ± 7.66	49.67 ± 4.23
5 mg/kg E4 + 136 ng/kg E2	33.49 ± 4.53	42.61 ± 35.66	36.19 ± 3.25	52.05 ± 3.92	46.84 ± 2.56	50.07 ± 4.74	46.74 ± 3.87	43.20 ± 4.02
10 mg/kg E4	50.43 ± 4.56	39.96 ± 33.60	26.58 ± 2.8	56.12 ± 6.10	51.44 ± 3.29	49.21 ± 3.49	38.31 ± 4.33	52.90 ± 5.81
10 mg/kg E4 + 1.6 mg/kg P4	45.02 ± 5.92	31.59 ± 36.83	18.11 ± 3.46	44.88 ± 7.95	42.77 ± 3.97	39.57 ± 6.49	39.64 ± 6.07	46.93 ± 6.38
10 mg/kg E4 + 1.6 mg/kg P4 + 136 ng/kg E2	53.25 ± 3.17	38.75 ± 35.03	36.12 ± 4.79	56.97 ± 7.53	55.34 ± 2.35	34.83 ± 3.38	42.80 ± 5.43	52.93 ± 5.54
10 mg/kg E4 + 16 mg/kg P4	44.50 ± 2.96	32.18 ± 35.74	27.73 ± 6.12	49.22 ± 4.72	47.05 ± 3.30	32.57 ± 4.74	34.51 ± 7.05	38.10 ± 4.57
10 mg/kg E4 + 16 mg/kg P4 + 136 ng/kg E2	45.86 ± 3.28	30.73 ± 34.99	22.41 ± 4.47	53.04 ± 5.04	43.87 ± 3.22	37.30 ± 3.13	36.25 ± 6.02	38.03 ± 3.25
10 mg/kg E4 + 136 ng/kg E2	39.25 ± 1.63	41.02 ± 34.96	46.71 ± 3.76	52.02 ± 3.34	48.40 ± 2.66	49.99 ± 3.20	51.74 ± 5.20	45.40 ± 3.63
Treatment								
Sham	59.73 ± 3.44[d]	52.43 ± 0.99	51.25 ± 2.42	63.34 ± 2.17	52.38 ± 1.58	51.87 ± 3.68	55.79 ± 2.92	58.29 ± 2.98
Vehicle	30.25 ± 4.90[c]	23.17 ± 4.43[h]	16.96 ± 3.67[l]	31.01 ± 3.90[q]	29.87 ± 2.88[c]	21.95 ± 2.48[j]	22.93 ± 2.37[m]	27.85 ± 2.80[r]
5 mg/kg E4	55.72 ± 2.91	36.63 ± 4.00	15.09 ± 2.12	61.28 ± 6.10	54.05 ± 3.51	36.54 ± 3.15	34.12 ± 3.54	40.72 ± 4.85
5 mg/kg E4 + 1.6 mg/kg P4	37.27 ± 3.44	34.00 ± 5.20	24.45 ± 5.83	52.05 ± 6.93	43.07 ± 3.66	36.96 ± 7.55	40.78 ± 9.06	44.91 ± 5.89
5 mg/kg E4 + 1.6 mg/kg P4 + 136 ng/kg E2	34.85 ± 2.10	36.95 ± 3.00	30.95 ± 3.64	53.75 ± 4.25	41.34 ± 2.37	35.08 ± 3.94	33.83 ± 5.17	45.44 ± 3.91

5 mg/kg E4 + 16 mg/kg P4	53.06 ± 2.55	43.67 ± 3.16	46.37 ± 3.61	47.08 ± 5.96	54.97 ± 3.07	49.78 ± 2.58	52.41 ± 4.25	45.84 ± 5.02
5 mg/kg E4 + 16 mg/kg P4 + 136 ng/kg E2	41.97 ± 2.02	43.27 ± 2.84	38.16 ± 3.91	39.14 ± 3.92	42.71 ± 3.02	44.08 ± 4.12	35.17 ± 3.88	34.58 ± 3.06
5 mg/kg E4 + 136 ng/kg E2	41.69 ± 2.75	54.47 ± 4.17	43.03 ± 5.13	53.37 ± 3.72	40.10 ± 4.40	50.32 ± 3.00	43.75 ± 3.83	36.50 ± 3.17
10 mg/kg E4	43.67 ± 2.26	41.08 ± 2.47	36.18 ± 3.70	53.88 ± 3.90	44.65 ± 3.38	46.16 ± 2.96	49.14 ± 3.84	46.66 ± 3.90
10 mg/kg E4 + 1.6 mg/kg P4	49.64 ± 4.35	45.286 ± 4.01	52.53 ± 5.02	44.61 ± 5.31	43.31 ± 3.97	51.91 ± 1.57	49.58 ± 4.25	41.96 ± 6.01
10 mg/kg E4 + 1.6 mg/kg P4 + 136 ng/kg E2	37.73 ± 3.38	44.74 ± 7.93	31.47 ± 6.98	47.19 ± 6.10	46.97 ± 3.91	39.40 ± 3.79	40.78 ± 4.16	34.81 ± 3.12
10 mg/kg E4 + 16 mg/kg P4	41.10 ± 4.00	48.83 ± 2.69	46.83 ± 3.53	62.66 ± 3.74	46.85 ± 3.19	50.72 ± 3.83	52.68 ± 3.94	48.70 ± 3.76
10 mg/kg E4 + 16 mg/kg P4 + 136 ng/kg E2	33.53 ± 1.70	30.11 ± 2.24	27.84 ± 4.31	42.81 ± 2.93	45.08 ± 1.75	40.39 ± 3.51	39.24 ± 4.96	37.98 ± 3.76
10 mg/kg E4 + 136 ng/kg E2	39.89 ± 3.20	38.39 ± 6.74	42.00 ± 5.22	46.20 ± 3.74	47.03 ± 3.82	44.97 ± 8.41	40.61 ± 6.51	39.07 ± 3.32

Significant differences were observed:

In the DG region

Pretreated groups: DCX-stained cells—[a]*vehicle vs. sham, 5 mg/kg E4; VEGF-stained cells*—[b]*vehicle vs. sham, 5 mg/kg E4 + 16 mg/kg P4*

Treated groups: DCX-stained cells—[c]*vehicle vs. sham, 5 mg/kg/day E4, 5 mg/kg/day E4 + 16 mg/kg/day P4, 5 mg/kg/day E4 + 1.6 mg/kg/day P4, 5 mg/kg/day E4 + 1.6 mg/kg/day P4 + 136 ng/kg/day E2, 10 mg/kg/day E4 + 1.6 mg/kg/day P4 + 136 ng/kg/day E2, 10 mg/kg/day E4 + 16 mg/kg/day P4; VEGF-stained cells*—[c]*vehicle vs. sham, 5 mg/kg/day E4, 5 mg/kg/day E4 + 16 mg/kg/day P4*

In the CA1 region

Pretreated groups: DCX-stained cells—[f]*vehicle vs. sham; VEGF-stained cells*—[g]*vehicle vs. sham, 5 mg/kg/day + 16 mg/kg/day P4*

Treated groups: DCX-stained cells—[h]*vehicle vs. sham, 5 mg/kg/day E4 + 136 ng/kg/day E2; VEGF-stained cells*—[i]*vehicle vs. sham, 10 mg/kg/day E4 + 1.6 mg/kg/day E4 + 16 mg/kg/day P4*

In the CA2/CA3 region

Pretreated groups: DCX-stained cells—[j]*vehicle vs. sham; VEGF-stained cells*—[k]*vehicle vs. sham; VEGF-stained cells*—[m]*5 mg/kg/day E4 vs. sham, 5 mg/kg/day E4 + 16 mg/kg/day P4*

Treated groups: DCX-stained cells—[l]*vehicle vs. sham, 10 mg/kg/day E4 + 1.6 mg/kg/day E4 vs. sham, 5 mg/kg/day E4 + 16 mg/kg/day P4; VEGF-stained cells*—[m]*5 mg/kg/day E4 vs. sham, 5 mg/kg/day E4 + 16 mg/kg/day P4; VEGF-stained cells*—[n]*vehicle vs. sham*

In the cortex

Pretreated groups: DCX-stained cells—[o]*vehicle vs. sham, 5 mg/kg/day E4 + 16 mg/kg/day P4*

Treated groups: DCX-stained cells—[q]*vehicle vs. sham; VEGF-stained cells*—[r]*vehicle vs. sham*

Reproduced from Oncotarget (Tskitishvili et al., 2016, 7(23):33722–43) treated by 5 mg/kg/day E4 alone or with 16 mg/kg/day P4 (Fig. 4.13). Also, sham group showed significantly higher number of DCX positively stained cells than the groups combinedly treated either by 5 mg/kg/day with 1.6 mg/kg/day P4 or 10 mg/kg/day E4 with 16 mg/kg/day P4 and E2 as well as groups treated by E4 in combination with 1.6 mg/kg/day P4 and E2 (Table 4.6) [117]. In the same region, angiogenesis was significantly upregulated in the sham-operated animals and in groups treated by 5 mg/kg/day E4 alone or in combination with 16 mg/kg/day P4; in the CA1 region, neurogenesis was significantly upregulated along with the sham group in animals treated by 5 mg/kg/day E4 along with E2 than in the vehicles, whereas angiogenesis was significantly upregulated in sham group and in animals treated by 10 mg/kg/day E4 with 1.6 mg/kg/day P4 (Table 4.6) [117]; In the CA2/CA3 region expressions of DCX and VEGF were significantly different between sham and the vehicle groups. In the CA2/CA3 region significant differences in DCX expression was detected between sham group, the animals treated by 10mg/kg/d E4 with 1.6mg/kg/d P4 and the vehicles as well as between sham group, the animals treated by 5mg/kg/d E4 with 16mg/kg/d P4 and the group treated by 5mg/kg/d E4 alone (Table 4.6); in the same region, VEGF was significantly more expressed in sham group than in the vehicles; in the cortex neuro- and angiogenesis were significantly more upregulated only in sham group compared to the vehicle group (Table 4.6); in general, combination of E4 with E2 resulted in low DCX and VEGF expression levels in the cortex (Fig. 4.13) [117].

The next step was evaluation of brain damage marker (GFAP) as it was discussed previously [117]. Combined pretreatment by 5 mg/kg/day E4 with P4 and E2 resulted in significant downregulation of GFAP expression compared to the vehicle group (Table 4.7). Different patterns of GFAP expression were observed in different groups. Significant downregulation of GFAP concentration was also observed in animals pretreated either by 5 mg/kg/day E4 alone or in combination with different doses of P4 and E2 or combined with 16 mg/kg/day P4 and in sham group than in animals pretreated by 5 mg/kg/day E4 and E2 (Table 4.7), also between groups pretreated by 10 mg/kg/day E4 alone or in combination with different doses of P4 and E2 or with 16 mg/kg/day P4 than in animals pretreated by 10 mg/kg/day E4 and E2 (Table 4.7) [117]. Treatment by E4 with P4 and/or E2 resulted in significant decrease of GFAP protein concentration in 10 mg/kg/day E4 along with the sham groups compared to animals treated by combination of 10 mg/kg/day E4 and E2 (Table 4.7). In vivo, in pretreated/treated groups, the combination of E4 and E2 showed significantly higher levels of GFAP, suggesting a negative cooperativity of these steroids upon cell survival (Table 4.7) [118].

After taking into account all the observations and experimental results, we have defined that combined use of E4 with other steroids has no benefit over the single use of E4 [117].

Table 4.7 Glial fibrillary acidic protein (GFAP) expression in blood serum (pg/ml) of the combinedly pretreated/treated rat pups

Group	Combined pretreatment		Combined treatment	
	pg/ml	N of samples	pg/ml	N of samples
Sham	2393.40 ± 1454.429[a]	8	2393.40 ± 1454.43[e]	8
Vehicle	23,915.91 ± 3158.84[b]	10	28,901.155 ± 4480.30	11
5 mg/kg E4	6220.49 ± 1763.17	11	6380.10 ± 4062.591	10
5 mg/kg E4 + 1.6 mg/kg P4	12,548.31 ± 2280.50	10	8146.34 ± 3596.07	10
5 mg/kg E4 + 1.6 mg/kg P4 + 136 ng/kg E2	1011.42 ± 55.32	13	19,226.69 ± 2559.70	10
5 mg/kg E4 + 16 mg/kg P4	5113.67 ± 1733.57	10	25,919.72 ± 4487.50	10
5 mg/kg E4 + 16 mg/kg P4 + 136 ng/kg E2	737.01 ± 69.82	11	17,476.73 ± 2643.53	10
5 mg/kg E4 + 136 ng/kg E2	28,442.46 ± 3457.11[c]	11	32,354.42 ± 5946.66	10
10 mg/kg E4	12,413.45 ± 2243.05	12	10,806.52 ± 1915.19[f]	10
10 mg/kg E4 + 1.6 mg/kg P4	27,225.88 ± 8442.88	7	18,796.20 ± 4279.45	10
10 mg/kg E4 + 1.6 mg/kg P4 + 136 ng/kg E2	9672.46 ± 2461.11	12	20,470.58 ± 1468.47	14
10 mg/kg E4 + 16 mg/kg P4	12,037.18 ± 3726.66	12	15,974.26 ± 2111.42	11
10 mg/kg E4 + 16 mg/kg P4 + 136 ng/kg E2	11,202.39 ± 2765.16	11	22,202.18 ± 2624.61	11
10 mg/kg E4 + 136 ng/kg E2	32,898.22 ± 3437.25[d]	11	26,660.81 ± 4870.81	10

Significant differences were observed:

In pretreated groups: [a]sham vs. vehicle, 10 mg/kg/day E4 + 136 ng/kg/day E2, 10 mg/kg/day E4 + 1.6 mg/kg/day P4; [b]vehicle vs. 5 mg/kg/day E4 + 1.6 mg/kg/day P4 + 136 ng/kg/day E2, 5 mg/kg/day E4 + 16 mg/kg/day P4 + 136 ng/kg/day E2; [c]5 mg/kg/day E4 + 136 ng/kg/day E2 vs. sham, 5 mg/kg/day E4, 5 mg/kg/day E4 + 1.6 mg/kg/day P4 + 136 ng/kg/day E2, 5 mg/kg/day E4 + 16 mg/kg/day P4, 5 mg/kg/day E4 + 16 mg/kg/day P4 + 136 ng/kg/day E2; [d]10 mg/kg/day E4 + 136 ng/kg/day vs. sham, 10 mg/kg/day E4, 10 mg/kg/day E4 + 1.6 mg/kg/day P4 + 136 ng/kg/day E2, 10 mg/kg/day E4 + 16 mg/kg/day P4, 10 mg/kg/day E4 + 16 mg/kg/day P4 + 136 ng/kg/day E2

In treated groups: [e]sham vs. vehicle, 5 mg/kg/day E4 + 136 ng/kg/day E2, 10 mg/kg/day E4 + 136 ng/kg/day E2; [f]10 mg/kg/day E4 vs. 10 mg/kg/day E4 + 136 ng/kg/day E2

Reproduced from *Oncotarget* (Tskitishvili et al., 2016, 7(23):33722–43)

4.4.3 How E4 Is Realizing Its Neuroprotective Effects?

Recent studies in different cells and tissues showed that E4 acts as a selective estrogen receptor modulator (SERM) by activating the nuclear ERα, inhibiting its membrane form and blocking the membrane initiated steroid signaling by E2 [149]. E4 may have a synergistic role with E2 (through activation of nuclear ERα) or an antiestrogenic effect by blocking membrane ERα and its activation by E2 depending on the respective role of nuclear and membrane forms of ERα in target organs. Thus, E4 has biological activities distinct from E2, depending on the tissues and cells and the selective binding to the nuclear/membrane form of ERα [149]. In general, palmitoylation regulates 17β-estradiol-induced ERα degradation and transcriptional activity [150] and may explain the ability of ERα to associate to plasma membrane making possible E2-dependent rapid functions [151], and the same might be plausible for E4-dependent rapid functions. Recent studies also have shown that ERβ expression in oligodendrocytes is important for the attenuation of clinical disease by an ERβ ligand, like that pointing an importance of this receptor in myelination [152].

As far we were going in our research as meticulously, we were trying to identify the exact mechanism of E4-dependent neuroprotective actions. Recent studies showed that, in general, the neuroprotective actions of estrogens among other factors also depend on their strong antioxidant properties. All estrogens have a phenolic moiety in their structure, the free phenolic OH group, which has been considered the quintessential feature in conferring protection against oxidative stress [153]. E4 has the highest number (four) of free phenolic hydroxyl groups in its structure, thus pointing out the possibility to have stronger antioxidant properties than other estrogens. Thus, one more explanation for E4 neuroprotective effect might be attributed to its strong antioxidant effect as well, which is demonstrated by our previous studies [116, 117], but it is not enough to explain the full spectrum of impressive results of action of E4 in the CNS.

For in vitro studies, we have used one of the most successful concentrations of E4 (3.25 mM) already defined from our previous research [116] alone or in combination with different estrogen receptor inhibitors and/or palmitoylation inhibitor after induction of oxidative stress in primary hippocampal neuronal cell cultures. The antioxidative activity of E4 and the expression of LDH were completely blocked only by concomitant treatment of cells with E4, MPP (inhibitor of ERα), and PHTTP (inhibitor of ERβ) (Fig. 4.14a, b) [118]. Inhibition of palmitoylation alone with 2-BR or in combination with MPP significantly decreased LDH activity, suggesting that the combined blockage of ERα and palmitoylation is not sufficient to inhibit the E4-dependent effects (Fig. 4.14c), whereas combination of E4 with 2-BR, MPP, and PHTTP completely blocked the antioxidative effects of E4 once again suggesting the role of both receptors, ERα and ERβ (Fig. 4.14c). Inhibition of GPR30 receptor did not block the E4 actions (Fig. 4.14d) [118].

Cell survival rate was significantly downregulated only by inhibition of ERβ alone (Fig. 4.15b). All cells treated either by E4 alone or in combination with different combinations of 2-BR, MPP, and PHTTP had significantly higher cell survival rate, and inhibition of palmitoylation along with inhibition of ERα activity resulted in a significantly higher cell survival rate suggesting that ERα (probably membrane form of the receptor) does not affect the E4-dependent cell survival/proliferation actions (Fig. 4.15c). Inhibition of GPER did not affect the cell survival rate (Fig. 4.15d) [118].

As we have already discussed earlier, the expression of ERα and ERβ displays different spatial-temporal patterns during human cortical and hippocampal

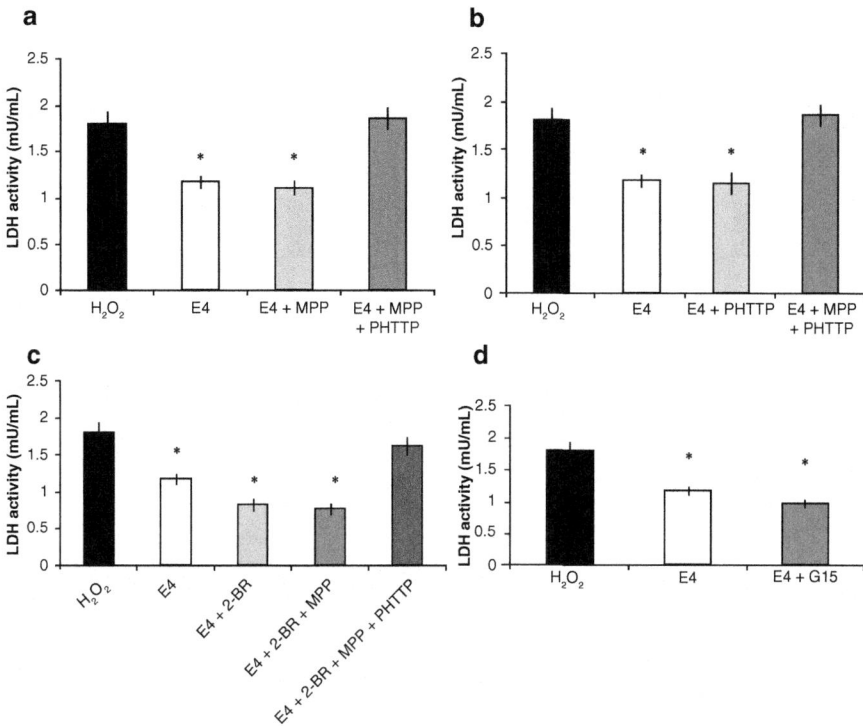

Fig. 4.14 Effect of E4 in combination with different receptor inhibitors on LDH activity in primary hippocampal neuronal cultures subjected to the H_2O_2-induced oxidative stress. Primary hippocampal cell cultures were exposed to 3.25 mM E4 alone or in combination with MPP, PHTTP, G15, and/ or 2-BR after induction of oxidative stress. (**a**) LDH activity was significantly decreased by treatment with E4 alone or in combination with ERα inhibitor MPP compared to the H_2O_2-treated cell cultures or cultures combinedly treated by E4 + MPP + PHTTP. Combined use of MPP and PHTTP significantly increased the LDH activity compared to the cells treated by E4 alone or in combination with MPP. (**b**) LDH activity was significantly decreased by treatment with E4 alone or in combination with ERβ inhibitor PHTTP compared to the H_2O_2-treated cell cultures or cultures combinedly treated by E4 + MPP + PHTTP. Combined use of MPP and PHTTP significantly increased the LDH compared to the cell cultures treated by E4 alone or in combination with PHTTP. (**c**) Inhibition of palmitoylation alone or in combination with MPP significantly downregulated LDH activity compared to the H_2O_2-treated cells or to those treated by E4 alone. Combination of E4 with 2-BR, MPP, and PHTTP significantly upregulated LDH activity compared to the cell cultures treated by E4 or 2-BR alone or in combination with MPP. (**d**) Cell cultures treated by E4 alone or in combination with GPR30 inhibitor G15 had significantly lower LDH activity compared to the cultures treated by H_2O_2 alone. No significant difference was observed between the cells treated by E4 alone or in combination with G15. Reproduced from J Endocrinol (Tskitishvili et al., 2017, 232(1):85–95)

development, and knowledge of the region-specific expression of each ER subtype is critical to better understand the actions of estrogens on the human brain [3]. Even though, the genomic effects of ERs are mostly studied, we have to pay attention to the rapid cellular signaling (non-genomic) effects that are thought to be mediated primarily by membrane-associated forms of these receptors [154]. These

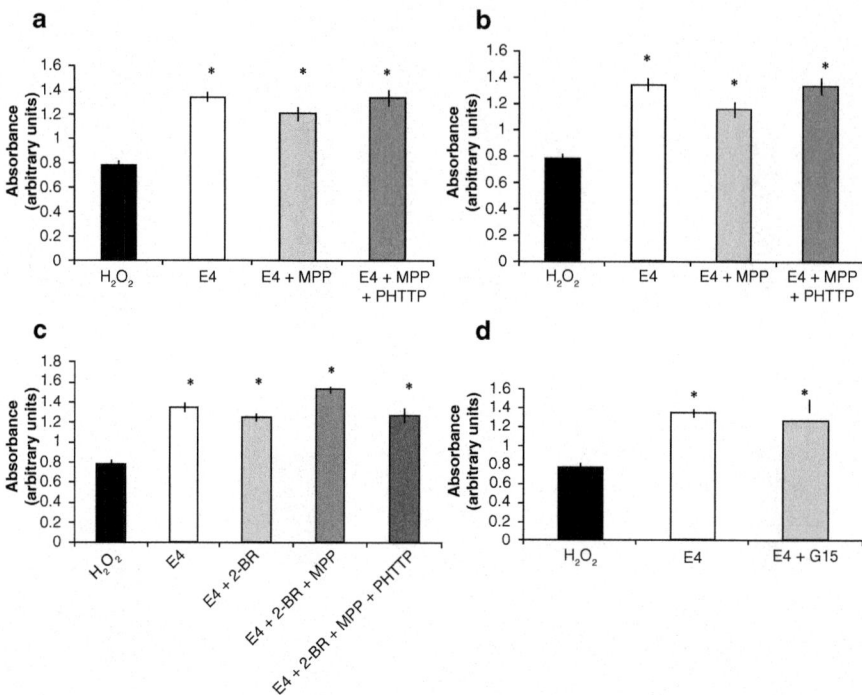

Fig. 4.15 Effect of E4 in combination with different receptor inhibitors on cell survival in primary hippocampal neuronal cultures subjected to the H_2O_2-induced oxidative stress. Primary hippocampal cell cultures were exposed to 3.25 mM E4 alone or in combination with MPP, PHTTP, G15, and/or 2-BR after induction of oxidative stress. (**a**) Cell survival rate was significantly upregulated in cells treated by E4 alone or in combination either with MPP or MPP + PHTTP compared to cells solely treated by H_2O_2. (**b**) Cultures treated either by E4 alone or with PHTTP with/without MPP had significantly upregulated cell survival rate compared to cells treated by H_2O_2 alone. Cells combinedly treated by E4 with PHTTP had significantly lower cell survival rate than the cell cultures treated by E4 alone. (**c**) Cells treated either by E4 alone or in combination with 2-BR, MPP, and/or PHTTP had significantly higher cell survival rate compared to the cells solely treated by H_2O_2. Treatment of cultures by E4 and 2-BR along with MPP resulted in significant upregulation of cell survival compared to the cultures treated by 2-BR alone or in combination with MPP and PHTTP. No significant difference was observed between the cells treated by E4 alone or those treated by different combinations of E4, 2-BR, MPP, and/or PHTTP. (**d**) Treatment of cell cultures by E4 alone or in combination with G15 significantly upregulated the cell survival rate compared to cell cultures treated by H_2O_2. No significant difference was observed between cells treated by E4 alone or in combination with G15. Reproduced from J Endocrinol (Tskitishvili et al., 2017, 232(1):85–95)

non-genomic signaling events are dependent to the estrogen-binding sites on intracellular membranes, whereas some reports suggest that palmitoylation or phosphorylation [150] may target classical ERs to the cytoplasmic side of the plasma membrane. In general, palmitoylation is necessary for ERα transcriptional activity, and inhibition of ERα palmitoylation constitutively addresses ERα to the nuclear matrix resulting in the basal degradation of the neo-synthesized ERα [155], though we did not observe any significant effect of palmitoylation inhibition on cell survival/proliferation [118].

It was already defined that the potential role of ERβ expression in cells of oligodendrocyte (OL) lineage in ERβ ligand-mediated neuroprotection is important, and it results in the upregulation of myelination [152]. Also, neuroprotection might be mediated through ERα in astrocytes exclusively [156]. Our studies prove that the E4-mediated activities in the CNS are realized through ERα and ERβ, like that enlightening the important role of E4 as a selective estrogen receptor modulator (SERM) with neurosteroid actions.

4.5 Conclusion

Summarizing our findings we can admit that for the first time we proved impressive antioxidative, neuroprotective, promyelinating, and neuro-, and angiogenesis effects of estetrol in the CNS by employing in vitro and in vivo studies. We believe that our investigation will open new horizons for the development of new perinatal treatment strategies not only for HIE but for periventricular leukomalacia (PVL) as well. Our research could also contribute to a better understanding of the pathophysiology and treatment of other neurological diseases such as Alzheimer's and Parkinson's diseases, traumatic brain injury, and multiple sclerosis.

References

1. Charles H. Rodeck, Martin J. Whittle, Fetal medicine: basic science and clinical practice. 2nd edition, 2009, Elsevier Health Sciences, London.
2. Shiota K. Prenatal development of the human central nervous system, normal and abnormal. Donald School J Ultrasound Obstet Gynecol. 2015;9(1):61–6.
3. Gonzalez M, Cabrera-Socorro A, Perez-Garcia CG, Fraser JD, Lopez FJ, Alonso R, et al. Distribution patterns of estrogen receptor alpha and beta in the human cortex and hippocampus during development and adulthood. J Comp Neurol. 2007;503(6):790–802. https://doi.org/10.1002/cne.21419.
4. Hart SA, Patton JD, Woolley CS. Quantitative analysis of ER alpha and GAD colocalization in the hippocampus of the adult female rat. J Comp Neurol. 2001;440:144–55. https://doi.org/10.1002/cne.1376.
5. Shughrue PJ, Merchenthaler I. Evidence for novel estrogen binding sites in the rat hippocampus. Neuroscience. 2000;99:605–12. https://doi.org/10.1210/endo.139.12.6525.
6. O'Keefe JA, Li Y, Burgess LH, Handa RJ. Estrogen receptor mRNA alterations in the developing rat hippocampus. Brain Res Mol Brain Res. 1995;30:115–24. https://doi.org/10.1016/0169-328X(94)00284-L.
7. Solum DT, Handa RJ. Localization of estrogen receptor alpha (ER-alpha) in pyramidal neurons of the developing rat hippocampus. Brain Res Dev Brain Res. 2001;28:165–75. https://doi.org/10.1016/S0165-3806(01)00171-7.
8. Nomura M, Korach KS, Pfaff DW, Ogawa S. Estrogen receptor b (ERb) protein levels in neurons depend on estrogen receptor a (ERa) gene expression and on its ligand in a brain region-specific manner. Mol Brain Res. 2003;110(2003):7–14. https://doi.org/10.1016/S0169-328X(02)00544-2.
9. Van der Knaap MS, Valk J. Magnetic resonance of myelin, myelination and myelin disorders. 2nd ed. Berlin: Springer; 1995.

10. Oakey RE. The progressive increase in oestrogen production in human pregnancy: an appraisal of the factors responsible. Vitam Horm. 1970;28:1.
11. Levitz M, Young BK. Estrogens in pregnancy. Vitam Horm. 1977;35:109.
12. Brann DW, Dhandapani K, Wakade C, Mahesh VB, Khan MM. Neurotrophic and neuroprotective actions of estrogen: basic mechanisms and clinical implications. Steroids. 2007;72:381–405. https://doi.org/10.1016/j.steroids.2007.02.003.
13. McCarty MM. Estradiol and the developing brain. Physiol Rev. 2008;88(1):91–124.
14. Lee HS, Han J, Baim HJ, Kim KW. Brain angiogenesis in developmental and pathological processes: regulation, molecular and cellular communication at the neurovascular interface. FEBS J. 2009;276(17):4622–35. https://doi.org/10.1111/j.1742-4658.2009.07174.x.
15. Park JA, Choi KS, Kim SY, Kim KW. Coordinated interaction of the vascular and nervous systems: from molecule- to cell-based approaches. Biochem Biophys Res Commun. 2003;311:247–53. https://doi.org/10.1016/j.bbrc.2003.09.129.
16. Gordon GR, Mulligan SJ, MacVicar BA. Astrocyte control of the cerebrovasculature. Glia. 2007;55:1214–21. https://doi.org/10.1002/glia.20543.
17. Mulligan SJ, MacVicar BA. Calcium transients in astrocyte endfeet cause cerebrovascular constrictions. Nature. 2004;431:195–9. https://doi.org/10.1038/nature02827.
18. Zonta M, Angulo MC, Gobbo S, Rosengarten B, Hossmann KA, Pozzan T, et al. Neuron-to-astrocyte signaling is central to the dynamic control of brain microcirculation. Nat Neurosci. 2003;6:43–50. https://doi.org/10.1038/nn980.
19. Krause DN, Duckles SP, Pelligrino DA. Influence of sex steroid hormones on cerebrovascular function. J Appl Physiol. 2006;101(4):1252–61. https://doi.org/10.1152/japplphysiol.01095.2005.
20. Barouk S, Hintz T, Li P, Duffy AM, MacLusky NJ, Scharfman HE. 17β-estradiol increases astrocytic vascular endothelial growth factor (VEGF) in adult female rat hippocampus. Endocrinology. 2011;152(5):1745–51. https://doi.org/10.1210/en.2010-1290.
21. Jin K, Zhu Y, Sun Y, Mao XO, Xie L, Greenberg DA. Vascular endothelial growth factor (VEGF) stimulates neurogenesis in vitro and in vivo. Proc Natl Acad Sci U S A. 2002;99(18):11946–50. https://doi.org/10.1073/pnas.182296499.
22. Zhu Y, Jin K, Mao XO, Greenberg DA. Vascular endothelial growth factor promotes proliferation of cortical neuron precursors by regulating E2F expression. FASEB J. 2003;17(2):186–93. https://doi.org/10.1096/fj.02-0515com.
23. Ogunshola OO, Stewart WB, Mihalcik V, Solli T, Madri JA, Ment LR. Neuronal VEGF expression correlates with angiogenesis in postnatal developing rat brain. Brain Res Dev Brain Res. 2000;119(1):139–53. https://doi.org/10.1016/S0165-3806(99)00125-X.
24. Haigh JJ, Morelli PI, Gerhardt H, Haigh K, Tsien J, Damert A, et al. Cortical and retinal defects caused by dosage-dependent reductions in VEGFA paracrine signaling. Dev Biol. 2003;262:225–41. https://doi.org/10.1016/S0012-1606(03)00356-7.
25. Raab S, Beck H, Gaumann A, Yüce A, Gerber HP, Plate K, et al. Impaired brain angiogenesis and neuronal apoptosis induced by conditional homozygous inactivation of vascular endothelial growth factor. Thromb Haemost. 2004;91:595–605. https://doi.org/10.1160/TH03-09-0582.
26. Wise PM. Estrogens and neuroprotection. Trends Endocrinol Metab. 2002;6:229–30.
27. Dubal DB, Wisel PM. Estrogen and neuroprotection: from clinical observations to molecular mechanisms. Dialogues Clin Neurosci. 2002;4(2):149–61.
28. Cho JJ, Iannucci FA, Fraile M, Franco J, Alesius TN, Stefano GB. The role of the estrogen in neuroprotection: implications for neurodegenerative diseases. Neuro Endocrinol Lett. 2003;24:141–7.
29. Garcia-Segura LM, Azcoitia I, DonCarlos LL. Neuroprotection by estradiol. Prog Neurobiol. 2001;63:29–60. https://doi.org/10.1016/S0301-0082(00)00025-3.
30. Gold SM, Voskuhl RR. Estrogen treatment in multiple sclerosis. J Neurol Sci. 2009;286(1–2):99–103. https://doi.org/10.1016/j.jns.2009.05.028.
31. Samantaray S, Matzelle DD, Ray SK, Banik NL. Physiological low dose of estrogen-protected neurons in experimental spinal cord injury. Ann N Y Acad Sci. 2010;1199:86–9. https://doi.org/10.1111/j.1749-6632.2009.05360.x.

32. Suzuki S, Brown CM, Wise PM. Neuroprotective effects of estrogens following ischemic stroke. Front Neuroendocrinol. 2009;30:201–11. https://doi.org/10.1016/j.yfrne.2009.04.007.
33. Henderson VW, Benke KS, Green RC, Cupples LA, Farrer LA, MIRAGE study Group. Postmenopausal hormone therapy and Alzheimer's disease risk: interaction with age. J Neurol Neurosurg Psychiatry. 2005;76:103–5. https://doi.org/10.1136/jnnp.2003.024927.
34. Currie LJ, Harrison MB, Trugman JM, Bennett JP, Wooten JF. Postmenopausal estrogen use affects risk for Parkinson disease. Arch Neurol. 2004;61:886–8. https://doi.org/10.1001/archneur.61.6.886.
35. Gardiner SA, Morrison MF, Mozley PD, Mozley LH, Brensinger C, Bilker W. Pilot study on the effect of estrogen replacement therapy on brain dopamine transporter availability in healthy, postmenopausal women. Am J Geriatr Psychiatry. 2004;12:621–30. https://doi.org/10.1176/appi.ajgp.12.6.621.
36. Li R, Shen Y, Yang LB, Lue LF, Finch C, Rogers J. Estrogen enhances uptake of amyloid beta-protein by microglia derived from the human cortex. J Neurochem. 2000;75:1447–54. https://doi.org/10.1046/j.1471-4159.2000.0751447.x.
37. Xu H, Gouras GK, Greenfield JP, Vincent B, Naslund J, Mazzarelli L, et al. Estrogen reduces neuronal generation of Alzheimer beta-amyloid peptides. Nat Med. 1998;4:447–51.
38. Kenchappa RS, Diwakar L, Annepu J, Ravindranath V. Estrogen and neuroprotection: higher constitutive expression of glutaredoxin in female mice offers protection against MPTP-mediated neurodegeneration. FASEB J. 2004;18:1102–4. https://doi.org/10.1096/fj.03-1075fje.
39. Ramirez AD, Liu X, Menniti FS. Repeated estradiol treatment prevents MPTP-induced dopamine depletion in male mice. Neuroendocrinology. 2003;77:223–31. https://doi.org/10.1159/000070277.
40. Nilsen J. Estradiol and neurodegenerative oxidative stress. Front Neuroendocrinol. 2008;9(4):463–75. https://doi.org/10.1016/j.yfrne.2007.12.005.
41. Zhang QG, Wang RM, Scott E, Han D, Dong Y, Tu JY, et al. C terminus of Hsc70-interacting protein (CHIP)-mediated degradation of hippocampal estrogen receptor-alpha and the critical period hypothesis of estrogen neuroprotection. Proc Natl Acad Sci U S A. 2011;108:E617–E24. https://doi.org/10.1093/brain/awt046.
42. Arevalo MA, Santos-Galindo M, Bellini M, Azcoitia I, Garcia-Segura LM. Actions of estrogens on glial cells: implications for neuroprotection. Biochim Biophys Acta. 2010;1800:1106–12. https://doi.org/10.1016/j.bbagen.2009.10.002.
43. Dhandapani KM, Brann DW. Role of astrocytes in estrogen-mediated neuroprotection. Exp Gerontol. 2007;42(1–2):70–5. https://doi.org/10.1016/j.exger.2006.06.032.
44. Brinton RD. The healthy cell bias of estrogen action: mitochondrial bioenergetics and neurological implications. Trends Neurosci. 2008;31(10):529–37. https://doi.org/10.1016/j.tins.2008.07.003.
45. Irwin RW, Yao J, Hamilton RT, Cadenas E, Brinton RD, Nilsen J. Progesterone and estrogen regulate oxidative metabolism in brain mitochondria. Endocrinology. 2008;149(6):3167–75. https://doi.org/10.1210/en.2007-1227.
46. Nilsen J, Brinton RD. Mitochondria as therapeutic targets of estrogen action in the central nervous system. Curr Drug Targets CNS Neurol Disord. 2004;3(4):297–13.
47. Nilsen J, Chen S, Irwin RW, Iwamoto S, Brinton RD. Estrogen protects neuronal cells from amyloid beta-induced apoptosis via regulation of mitochondrial proteins and function. BMC Neurosci. 2006;7:74. https://doi.org/10.1186/1471-2202-7-74.
48. Nilsen J, Irwin RW, Gallaher TK, Brinton RD. Estradiol in vivo regulation of brain mitochondrial proteome. J Neurosci. 2007;27:14069–77. https://doi.org/10.1523/JNEUROSCI.4391-07.2007.
49. Brinton RD. Estrogen regulation of glucose metabolism and mitochondrial function: therapeutic implications for prevention of Alzheimer's disease. Adv Drug Deliv Rev. 2008;60(13–14):1504–11. https://doi.org/10.1016/j.addr.2008.06.003.
50. Sakamoto H, Matsuda K, Hosokawa K, Nishi M, Morris JF, Prossnitz ER, et al. Expression of G protein-coupled receptor-30, a G protein-coupled membrane estrogen receptor, in oxytocin neurons of the rat paraventricular and supraoptic nuclei. Endocrinology. 2007;148(12):5842–50. https://doi.org/10.1210/en.2007-0436.

51. Revankar CM, Cimino DF, Sklar LA, Arterburn JB, Prossnitz ER. A transmembrane intracellular estrogen receptor mediates rapid cell signaling. Science. 2005;307(5715):1625–30. https://doi.org/10.1126/science.1106943.

52. Funakoshi T, Yanai A, Shinoda K, Kawano MM, Mizukami Y. G protein-coupled receptor 30 is an estrogen receptor in the plasma membrane. Biochem Biophys Res Commun. 2006;46(3):904–10. https://doi.org/10.1016/j.bbrc.2006.05.191.

53. Xu H, Qin S, Carrasco GA, Dai Y, Filardo EJ, Prossnitz ER, et al. Extra-nuclear estrogen receptor GPR30 regulates serotonin function in rat hypothalamus. Neuroscience. 2009;158(4):1599–607. https://doi.org/10.1016/j.neuroscience.2008.11.028.

54. Alyea RA, Laurence SE, Kim SH, Katzenellenbogen BS, Katzenellenbogen JA, Watson CS. The roles of membrane estrogen receptor subtypes in modulating dopamine transporters in PC-12 cells. J Neurochem. 2008;106(4):1525–33. https://doi.org/10.1111/j.1471-4159.2008.05491.x.

55. Kuhn J, Dina OA, Goswami C, Suckow V, Levine JD, Hucho T. GPR30 estrogen receptor agonists induce mechanical hyperalgesia in the rat. Eur J Neurosci. 2008;27(7):1700–9. https://doi.org/10.1111/j.1460-9568.2008.06131.x.

56. Qiu J, Bosch MA, Tobias SC, Krust A, Graham SM, Murphy SJ, et al. A G-protein-coupled estrogen receptor is involved in hypothalamic control of energy homeostasis. J Neurosci. 2006;26(21):5649–55. https://doi.org/10.1523/JNEUROSCI.0327-06.2006.

57. Delaunay F, Pettersson K, Tujague M, Gustafsson JA. Functional differences between the amino-terminal domains of estrogen receptors alpha and beta. Mol Pharmacol. 2000;58(3):584–90. https://doi.org/10.1124/mol.58.3.584.

58. He S, Nelson ER. 27-Hydroxycholesterol, an endogenous selective estrogen receptor modulator. Maturitas. 2017;104:29–35. https://doi.org/10.1016/j.maturitas.2017.07.014.

59. Li X, Schwartz PE, Rissman EF. Distribution of estrogen receptor β-like immunoreactivity in rat forebrain. Neuroendocrinology. 1997;66:63–7.

60. Shughrue PJ, Lane MV, Merchenthaler I. Comparative distribution of estrogen receptor-α and -β mRNA in the rat central nervous system. J Comp Neurol. 1997;388:507–25. https://doi.org/10.1002/(SICI)1096-9861(19971201)388:4<507::AID-CNE1>3.0.CO;2-6.

61. Zhang JQ, Cai WQ, Zhou de S, Su BY. Distribution and differences of estrogen receptor beta immunoreactivity in the brain of adult male and female rats. Brain Res. 2002;935(1–2):73–80. https://doi.org/10.1016/S0006-8993(02)02460-5.

62. Mitra SW, Hoskin E, Yudkovitz J, Pear L, Wilkinson HA, Hayashi S, et al. Immunolocalization of estrogen receptor-α in the mouse brain: comparison with estrogen receptor β. Endocrinology. 2003;144(5):2055–67. https://doi.org/10.1210/en.2002-221069.

63. Brinton RD. Estrogen-induced plasticity from cells to circuits: predictions for cognitive function. Trends Pharmacol Sci. 2009;30(4):212–22. https://doi.org/10.1016/j.tips.2008.12.006.

64. Hajszan T, Milner TA, Leranth C. Sex steroids and the dentate gyrus. Prog Brain Res. 2007;163:399–416. https://doi.org/10.1016/S0079-6123(07)63023-4.

65. Dan P, Cheung JC, Scriven DR, Moore ED. Epitope-dependent localization of estrogen receptor-alpha, but not -beta, in en face arterial endothelium. Am J Physiol Heart Circ Physiol. 2003;284:H1295–306. https://doi.org/10.1152/ajpheart.00781.2002.

66. Mazzucco CA, Lieblich SE, Bingham BI, Williamson MA, Viau V, Galea LAM. Both estrogen receptor alpha and estrogen receptor beta agonists enhance cell proliferation in the dentate gyrus of adult female rats. Neuroscience. 2006;141(4):1793–800. https://doi.org/10.1016/j.neuroscience.2006.05.032.

67. Alkayed NJ, Murphy SJ, Traystman RJ, Hurn PD, Miller VM. Neuroprotective effects of female gonadal steroids in reproductively senescent female rats. Stroke. 2000;31(1):161–8. https://doi.org/10.1161/01.STR.31.1.161.

68. Kuan CY, Roth KA, Flavell RA, Rakic P. Mechanisms of programmed cell death in the developing brain. Trends Neurosci. 2000;23(7):291–7. https://doi.org/10.1016/S0166-2236(00)01581-2.

69. Singh M. Ovarian hormones elicit phosphorylation of Akt and extracellular-signal regulated kinase in explants of the cerebral cortex. Endocrine. 2001;14(3):407–15. https://doi.org/10.1385/ENDO:14:3:407.

70. Zaidi AU, D'Sa-Eipper C, Brenner J, Kuida K, Zheng TS, Flavell RA, et al. Bcl-X(L)-caspase-9 interactions in the developing nervous system: evidence for multiple death pathways. J Neurosci. 2001;21(1):169–75.
71. Wade CB, Dorsa DM. Estrogen activation of cyclic adenosine 5′-monophosphate response element-mediated transcription requires the extracellularly regulated kinase/mitogen-activated protein kinase pathway. Endocrinology. 2003;144:832–8. https://doi.org/10.1210/en.2002-220899.
72. Quesada A, Micevych PE. Estrogen interacts with the IGF-1 system to protect nigrostriatal dopamine and maintain motoric behavior after 6-hydroxydopamine lesions. J Neurosci Res. 2004;75(1):107–16. https://doi.org/10.1002/jnr.10833.
73. Hagen AA, Barr M, Diczfalusy E. Metabolism of 17β-oestradiol-4-14C in early infancy. Acta Endocrinol. 1965;49:207–20. https://doi.org/10.1530/acta.0.0490207.
74. Warmerdam EG, Visser M, Coeling Bennink HJ, Groen M. A new route of synthesis of estetrol. Climacteric. 2008;11(Suppl 1):59–63. https://doi.org/10.1080/13697130802054078.
75. Holinka CF, Diczfalusy E, Coeling Bennink HJTC. Estetrol: a unique steroid in human pregnancy. J Steroid Biochem Mol Biol. 2008;110(1–2):138–43. https://doi.org/10.1016/j.jsbmb.2008.03.027.
76. Visser M, Foidart J-M, Coelingh Bennink HJT. In vitro effects of estetrol on receptor binding, drug targets and human liver cell metabolism. Climacteric. 2008;11(Suppl 1):64–8. https://doi.org/10.1080/13697130802050340.
77. Coeling Bennink HJTC, Skouby S, Bouchard P, Holinka CF. Ovulation inhibition by estetrol in an in vivo model. Contraception. 2008;77(3):186–90. https://doi.org/10.1016/j.contraception.2007.11.014.
78. Coelingh Bennink HJTC, Holinka CF, Diczfalusy E. Estetrol review: profile and potential clinical applications. Climacteric. 2008;11(Suppl 1):47–58. https://doi.org/10.1080/13697130802040077.
79. Hirano S, Furutama D, Hanafusa T. Physiologically high concentrations of 17beta-estradiol enhance NF-kappaB activity in human T cells. Am J Physiol Regul Integr Comp Physiol. 2007;292(4):R1465–71. https://doi.org/10.1152/ajpregu.00778.2006.
80. Koh KK, Yoon BK. Controversies regarding hormone therapy: insights from inflammation and hemostasis. Cardiovasc Res. 2006;70(1):22–30. https://doi.org/10.1016/j.cardiores.2005.12.004.
81. Herrington DM, Klein KP. Invited review: Pharmacogenetics of estrogen replacement therapy. J Appl Physiol (1985). 2001;91(6):2776–84. https://doi.org/10.1152/jappl.2001.91.6.2776.
82. Arnal JF, Valéra MC, Payrastre B, Lenfant F, Gourdy P. Structure-function relationship of estrogen receptors in cardiovascular pathophysiological models. Thromb Res. 2012;130(Suppl 1):S7–11. https://doi.org/10.1016/j.thromres.2012.08.261.
83. Deroo BJ, Korach KS. Estrogen receptors and human disease: an update. Arch Toxicol. 2012;86(10):1491–504. https://doi.org/10.1007/s00204-012-0868-5.
84. ACOG. Executive summary: Neonatal encephalopathy and neurologic outcome, second edition. Report of the American College of Obstetricians and Gynecologists' Task Force on Neonatal Encephalopathy. Obstet Gynecol. 2014;123(4):896–901.
85. Gluckman PD, Wyatt JS, Azzopardi D, Ballard R, Edwards AD, Ferriero DM, et al. Selective head cooling with mild systemic hypothermia after neonatal encephalopathy: multicenter randomised trial. Lancet. 2005;65(9460):663–70. https://doi.org/10.1016/S0140-6736(05)17946-X.
86. Shankaran S, Laptook AR, Ehrenkranz RA, Tyson JE, McDonald SA, Donovan EF, et al. Whole-body hypothermia for neonates with hypoxic-ischemic encephalopathy. N Engl J Med. 2005;353(15):1574–84. https://doi.org/10.1056/NEJMcps050929.
87. Robertson CM, Perlman M. Follow-up of the term infant after hypoxic-ischemic encephalopathy. Paediatr Child Health. 2006;11(5):278–82.
88. Zanelli SA. http://emedicine.medscape.com/article/973501-overview?src=refgatesrc1#a5. Accessed 16 Jan 2015.

89. Bryce J, Boschi-Pinto C, Shibuya K, Black RE, WHO Child Health Epidemiology Reference Group. WHO estimates of the causes of death in children. Lancet. 2005;365(9465): 1147–52.
90. Badawi N, Kurinczuk JJ, Keogh JM, Alessandri LM, O'Sullivan F, Burton PR, et al. Antepartum risk factors for newborn encephalopathy: the Western Australian case-control study. BMJ. 1998;317(7172):1549–53. https://doi.org/10.1136/bmj.317.7172.1549.
91. Badawi N, Kurinczuk JJ, Keogh JM, Alessandri LM, O'Sullivan F, Burton PR, et al. Intrapartum risk factors for newborn encephalopathy: the Western Australian case-control study. BMJ. 1998;317(7172):1554–8. https://doi.org/10.1136/bmj.317.7172.1554.
92. Graham EM, Ruis KA, Hartman AL, Northington FJ, Fox HE. A systematic review of the role of intrapartum hypoxia-ischemia in the causation of neonatal encephalopathy. Am J Obstet Gynecol. 2008;199(6):587–95. https://doi.org/10.1016/j.ajog.2008.06.094.
93. Ankarcrona M, Dypbukt JM, Bonfoco E, Zhivotovsky B, Orrenius S, Lipton SA, et al. Glutamate-induced neuronal death: a succession of necrosis or apoptosis depending on mitochondrial function. Neuron. 1995;15(4):961–73. https://doi.org/10.1016/0896-6273(95)90186-8.
94. Pacher P, Beckman JS, Liaudet L. Nitric oxide and peroxynitrite in health and disease. Physiol Rev. 2007;87(1):315–424. https://doi.org/10.1152/physrev.00029.2006.
95. Chang YC, Huang CC. Perinatal brain injury and regulation of transcription. Curr Opin Neurol. 2006;19(2):141–7. https://doi.org/10.1097/01.wco.0000218229.73678.a8.
96. Domoki F, Kis B, Nagy K, Farkas E, Busija DW, Bari F. Diazoxide preserves hypercapnia-induced arteriolar vasodilation after global cerebral ischemia in piglets. Am J Physiol Heart Circ Physiol. 2005;289:H368–73. https://doi.org/10.1152/ajpheart.00887.2004.
97. Gerosa C, Fanni D, Puddu M, Locci G, Obinu E, Fanos V, et al. Histological markers of neonatal asphyxia: the relevant role of vascular changes. J Pediatr Neonat Individual Med. 2014;3(2):e030275.
98. Olah O, Toth-Szuki V, Temesvari P, Bari F, Domoki F. Delayed neurovascular dysfunction is alleviated by hydrogen in asphyxiated newborn pigs. Neonatology. 2013;104:79–86. https://doi.org/10.1159/000348445.
99. Ireland Z, Castillo-Melendez M, Dickinson H, Snow R, Walker DW. A maternal diet supplemented with creatine from mid-pregnancy protects the newborn spiny mouse brain from birth hypoxia. Neuroscience. 2011;194:372–9. https://doi.org/10.1016/j.neuroscience.2011.05.012.
100. Fleiss B, Coleman HA, Castillo-Melendez M, Ireland Z, Walker DW, Parkington HC. Effects of birth asphyxia on neonatal hippocampal structure and function in the spiny mouse. Int J Dev Neurosci. 2011;29:757–66. https://doi.org/10.1016/j.ijdevneu.2011.05.006.
101. Schiering IA, de Haan TR, Niermeijer JM, Koelman JH, Majoie CB, Reneman L, et al. Correlation between clinical and histologic findings in the human neonatal hippocampus after perinatal asphyxia. J Neuropathol Exp Neurol. 2014;73:324–34. https://doi.org/10.1097/NEN.0000000000000056.
102. Okereafor A, Allsop J, Counsell SJ, Fitzpatrick J, Azzopardi D, Rutherford MA, et al. Patterns of brain injury in neonates exposed to perinatal sentinel events. Pediatrics. 2008;121(5):906–14. https://doi.org/10.1542/peds.2007-0770.
103. Sarnat HB, Sarnat MS. Neonatal encephalopathy following fetal distress: a clinical and electroencephalographic study. Arch Neurol. 1976;33(10):696–705. https://doi.org/10.1001/archneur.1976.00500100030012.
104. Douglas-Escobar M, Weiss MD. Hypoxic-ischemic encephalopathy: a review for the clinician. JAMA Pediatr. 2015;169(4):397–403. https://doi.org/10.1001/jamapediatrics.2014.3269.
105. Thoresen M, Hellstrom-Westas L, Liu X, de Vries LS. Effect of hypothermia on amplitude-integrated electroencephalogram in infants with asphyxia. Pediatrics. 2010;126(1):e131–9. https://doi.org/10.1542/peds.2009-2938.
106. Rothermundt M, Peters M, Prehn JH, Arolt V. S100B in brain damage and neurodegeneration. Microsc Res Tech. 2003;60(6):614–32. https://doi.org/10.1002/jemt.10303.

107. Ennen CS, Huisman TA, Savage WJ, Northington FJ, Jennings JM, Everett AD, et al. Glial fibrillary acidic protein as a biomarker for neonatal hypoxic-ischemic encephalopathy treated with whole-body cooling. Am J Obstet Gynecol. 2005;205(3):251.e1–7. https://doi.org/10.1016/j.ajog.2011.06.025.
108. Shankaran S. The postnatal management of the asphyxiated term infant. Clin Perinatol. 2002;29(4):675–92.
109. Stola A, Perlman J. Post-resuscitation strategies to avoid ongoing injury following intrapartum hypoxia-ischemia. Semin Fetal Neonatal Med. 2008;13(6):424–31. https://doi.org/10.1016/j.siny.2008.04.011.
110. Hoehn T, Hansmann G, Bührer C, Simbruner G, Gunn AJ, Yager J, et al. Therapeutic hypothermia in neonates. Review of current clinical data, ILCOR recommendations and suggestions for implementation in neonatal intensive care units. Resuscitation. 2008;78:7–12. https://doi.org/10.1016/j.resuscitation.2008.04.027.
111. Thoresen M, Tooley J, Liu X, Jary S, Fleming P, Luyt K, et al. Time is brain: starting therapeutic hypothermia within three hours after birth improves motor outcome in asphyxiated newborns. Neonatology. 2013;104(3):228–33. https://doi.org/10.1159/000353948.
112. Edwards DA, Azzopardi DV, Gunn AJ. Neonatal neural rescue: a clinical guide. Cambridge, UK: Cambridge University Press; 2013.
113. Ballot DE. Cooling for newborns with hypoxic ischaemic encephalopathy: RHL commentary (last revised: 1 October 2010). The WHO Reproductive Health Library. Geneva: World Health Organization (WHO).
114. Zanelli S, Buck M, Fairchild K. Physiologic and pharmacologic considerations for hypothermia therapy in neonates. J Perinatol. 2011;31(6):377–86. https://doi.org/10.1038/jp.2010.146.
115. Thoresen M, Whitelaw A. Therapeutic hypothermia for hypoxic-ischaemic encephalopathy in the newborn infant. Curr Opin Neurol. 2005;18(2):111–6. https://doi.org/10.1097/01.wco.0000162850.44897.c6.
116. Tskitishvili E, Nisolle M, Munaut C, Pequeux C, Gerard C, Noel A, et al. Neonatal estetrol attenuates neonatal hypoxic-ischemic brain injury. Exp Neurol. 2014;261:298–307. https://doi.org/10.1016/j.expneurol.2014.07.015.
117. Tskitishvili E, Pequeux C, Munaut C, Viellevoye R, Nisolle M, Noël A, et al. Use of estetrol with other steroids for attenuation of neonatal hypoxic-ischemic brain injury: to combine or not to combine? Oncotarget. 2016;7(23):33722–43. https://doi.org/10.18632/oncotarget.9591.
118. Tskitishvili E, Pequeux C, Munaut C, Viellevoye R, Nisolle M, Noël A, et al. Estrogen receptors and estetrol-dependent neuroprotective actions: a pilot study. J Endocrinol. 2017;232(1):85–95. https://doi.org/10.1530/JOE-16-0434.
119. Johnson GV, Jope RS. The role of microtubule-associated protein 2 (MAP-2) in neuronal growth, plasticity, and degeneration. J Neurosci Res. 1992;33(4):505–12. https://doi.org/10.1002/jnr.490330402.
120. Bartosik-Psujek H, Stelmasiak Z. Biochemical markers of damage of the central nervous system in multiple sclerosis. Ann Univ Mariae Curie Sklodowska Med. 2001;56:389–92.
121. Roof RL, Duvdevani R, Braswell L, Stein DG. Progesterone facilitates cognitive recovery and reduces secondary neuronal loss caused by cortical contusion injury in male rats. Exp Neurol. 1994;129:64–9. https://doi.org/10.1006/exnr.1994.1147.
122. Roof RL, Hoffman SW, Stein DG. Progesterone protects against lipid peroxidation following traumatic brain injury in rats. Mol Chem Neuropathol. 1997;31(1):1–11.
123. Roof RL, Hall E. Gender differences in acute CNS trauma and stroke: neuroprotective effects of estrogen and progesterone. J Neurotrauma. 2000;17(5):367–88. https://doi.org/10.1089/neu.2000.17.367.
124. Stein D. Brain damage, sex hormones and recovery: a new role for progesterone and estrogen? Trends Neurosci. 2001;24(7):386–91. https://doi.org/10.1016/S0166-2236(00)01821-X.

125. Gold SM, Voskuhl RR. Estrogen and testosterone therapies in multiple sclerosis. Prog Brain Res. 2009;175:239–51. https://doi.org/10.1016/S0079-6123(09)17516-7.

126. Kaur P, Jodhka PK, Underwood WA, Bowles CA, de Fiebre NC, de Fiebre CM, et al. Progesterone increases brain-derived neurotrophic factor expression and protects against glutamate toxicity in a mitogen-activated protein kinase- and phosphoinositide-3 kinase-dependent manner in cerebral cortical explants. J Neurosci Res. 2007;85(11):2441–9. https://doi.org/10.1002/jnr.21370.

127. Nilsen J, Brinton RD. Impact of progestins on estradiol potentiation of the glutamate calcium response. Neuroreport. 2002;13(6):825–30.

128. Nilsen J, Brinton RD. Impact of progestins on estrogen induced neuroprotection: synergy by progesterone and 19-norprogesterone and antagonism by medroxyprogesterone acetate. Endocrinology. 2002;143(1):205–12. https://doi.org/10.1210/endo.143.1.8582.

129. Nilsen J, Brinton RD. Divergent impact of progesterone and medroxyprogesterone acetate (Provera) on nuclear mitogen activated protein kinase signaling. Proc Natl Acad Sci U S A. 2003;100(18):10506–11. https://doi.org/10.1073/pnas.1334098100.

130. Goodman Y, Bruce AJ, Cheng B, Mattson MP. Estrogens attenuate and corticosterone exacerbates excitotoxicity, oxidative injury, and amyloid beta-peptide toxicity in hippocampal neurons. J Neurochem. 1996;66:1836–44. https://doi.org/10.1046/j.1471-4159.1996.66051836.x.

131. Singh M, Su C. Progesterone and neuroprotection. Horm Behav. 2013;63(2):284–90. https://doi.org/10.1016/j.yhbeh.2012.06.003.

132. Trotter A, Steinmacher J, Kron M, Pohlandt F. Neurodevelopmental follow-up at five years corrected age of extremely low birth weight infants after postnatal replacement of 17-estradiol and progesterone. J Clin Endocrinol Metab. 2012;97(3):1041–7. https://doi.org/10.1210/jc.2011-2612.

133. Lorenz L, Dang J, Misiak M, Tameh Abolfazl A, Beyer C, Kipp M. Combined 17beta-oestradiol and progesterone treatment prevents neuronal cell injury in cortical but not midbrain neurones or neuroblastoma cells. J Neuroendocrinol. 2009;21(10):841–9. https://doi.org/10.1111/j.1365-2826.2009.01903.x.

134. Mannella P, Sanchez AM, Giretti MS, Genazzani AR, Simoncini T. Oestrogen and progestins differently prevent glutamate toxicity in cortical neurons depending on prior hormonal exposure via the induction of neural nitric oxide synthase. Steroids. 2009;74(8):650–6. https://doi.org/10.1210/me.2008-0408.

135. Aguirre CC, Baudry M. Progesterone reverses 17betaestradiol-mediated neuroprotection and BDNF induction in cultured hippocampal slices. Eur J Neurosci. 2009;29(3):447–54. https://doi.org/10.1111/j.1460-9568.2008.06591.x.

136. Aguirre C, Jayaraman A, Pike C, Baudry M. Progesterone inhibits estrogen-mediated neuroprotection against excitotoxicity by down-regulating estrogen receptor-beta. J Neurochem. 2010;115(5):1277–87. https://doi.org/10.1111/j.1471-4159.2010.07038.x.

137. Carroll JC, Rosario ER, Pike CJ. Progesterone blocks estrogen neuroprotection from kainate in middle-aged female rats. Neurosci Lett. 2008;445(3):229–32. https://doi.org/10.1016/j.neulet.2008.09.010.

138. Jayaraman A, Pike CJ. Progesterone attenuates oestrogen neuroprotection via downregulation of oestrogen receptor expression in cultured neurones. J Neuroendocrinol. 2009;21(1):77–81. https://doi.org/10.1111/j.1365-2826.2008.01801.x.

139. Rosario ER, Ramsden M, Pike CJ. Progestins inhibit the neuroprotective effects of estrogen in rat hippocampus. Brain Res. 2006;1099(1):206–10. https://doi.org/10.1016/j.brainres.2006.03.127.

140. Yao J, Chen S, Cadenas E, Brinton RD. Estrogen protection against mitochondrial toxin-induced cell death in hippocampal neurons: antagonism by progesterone. Brain Res. 2011;1379:2–10. https://doi.org/10.1016/j.brainres.2010.11.090.

141. Gibson C, Constantin D, Prior M, Bath P, Murphy S. Progesterone suppresses the inflammatory response and nitric oxide synthase-2 expression following cerebral ischemia. Exp Neurol. 2005;193(2):522–30. https://doi.org/10.1016/j.expneurol.2005.01.009.

142. Grossman K, Goss C, Stein D. Effects of progesterone on the inflammatory response to brain injury in the rat. Brain Res. 2004;1008(1):29–39. https://doi.org/10.1016/j. brainres.2004.02.022.
143. Labombarda F, Gonzalez S, Gonzalez Deniselle MC, Garay L, Guennoun R, Schumacher M, et al. Progesterone increases the expression of myelin basic protein and the number of cells showing NG2 immunostaining in the lesioned spinal cord. J Neurotrauma. 2006;23(2): 181–92. https://doi.org/10.1089/neu.2006.23.181.
144. Pierson RC, Lyons AM, Greenfield LJ Jr. Gonadal steroids regulate GABAA receptor subunit mRNA expression in NT2-Nneurons. Brain Res Mol Brain Res. 2005;138(2):105–15. https:// doi.org/10.1016/j.molbrainres.2004.10.047.
145. Mani SK. Signaling mechanisms in progesterone neurotransmitter interactions. Neuroscience. 2006;138(3):773–81. https://doi.org/10.1016/j.neuroscience.2005.07.034.
146. Pettus EH, Wright DW, Stein DG, Hoffman SW. Progesterone treatment inhibits the inflammatory agents that accompany traumatic brain injury. Brain Res. 2005;1049(1):112–9. https://doi.org/10.1016/j.brainres.2005.05.004.
147. Quadros PS, Pfau JL, Wagner CK. Distribution of progesterone receptor immunoreactivity in the fetal and neonatal rat forebrain. J Comp Neurol. 2007;504(1):42–56.
148. Jahagirdar V, Wagner CK. Ontogeny of progesterone receptor expression in the subplate of fetal and neonatal rat cortex. Cereb Cortex. 2010;20(5):1046–52. https://doi.org/10.1002/cne.21427.
149. Abot A, Fontaine C, Buscato M, Solinhac R, Flouriot G, Fabre A, et al. The uterine and vascular actions of estetrol delineate a distinctive profile of estrogen receptor modulation, uncoupling nuclear and membrane activation. EMBO Mol Med. 2014;6(10):1328–46. https://doi.org/10.15252/emmm.201404112.
150. La Rosa P, Pesiri V, Leclerq G, Marino M, Acconcia F. Palmitoylation regulates 17β-estradiol-induced estrogen receptor-α degradation and transcriptional activity. Mol Endocrinol. 2012;26(5):762–74. https://doi.org/10.1210/me.2011-1208.
151. Acconcia F, Ascenzi P, Fabozzi G, Visca P, Marino M. S-palmitoylation modulates human estrogen receptor-alpha functions. Biochem Biophys Res Commun. 2004;316:878–83. https://doi.org/10.1016/j.bbrc.2004.02.129.
152. Khalaj AJ, Yoon J, Nakai J, Winchester Z, Moore SM, Yoo T, et al. Estrogen receptor (ER) β expression in oligodendrocytes is required for attenuation of clinical disease by an ERβ ligand. Proc Natl Acad Sci U S A. 2013;110(47):19125–30. https://doi.org/10.1073/pnas.1311763110.
153. Prokai L, Prokai-Tatrai K, Perjesi P, Simpkins JW. Mechanistic insights into the direct antioxidant effects of estrogens. Drug Dev Res. 2005;66(2):118–25. https://doi.org/10.1002/ddr.20050.
154. Hammes SR, Levin ER. Extranuclear steroid receptors: nature and actions. Endocr Rev. 2007;28:726–41. https://doi.org/10.1210/er.2007-0022.
155. Suzuki S, Gerhold LM, Bottner M, Rau SW, Dela Cruz C, Yang E, et al. Estradiol enhances neurogenesis following ischemic stroke through estrogen receptors a and b. J Comp Neurol. 2007;500:1064–75. https://doi.org/10.1002/cne.21240.
156. Spence RD, Hamby ME, Umeda E, Itoh N, Du S, Wisdom AJ, et al. Neuroprotection mediated through estrogen receptor-α in astrocytes. Proc Natl Acad Sci U S A. 2011;108:8867–72. https://doi.org/10.1073/pnas.1103833108.

Adrenal Androgens Impact on Neurosteroids

5

Marta Caretto, Andrea Giannini, Tommaso Simoncini, and Andrea R. Genazzani

5.1 Androgens and Aging

The human adrenal produces a variety of 19 carbon (C_{19}) steroids, such as dehydro-epiandrosterone (DHEA), DHEA sulfate (DHEAS), androstenedione (A4), androstenediol, and 11β-hydroxyandrostenedione (11OHA). These steroids have an androgenic activity, but they provide a pool of circulating precursor for peripheral conversion to more potent androgens (e.g., testosterone, T) and estrogens (e.g., estradiol). The adrenal gland contributes ~1% to the total circulating T in males and up to 30–50% in females, and roughly half of circulating A4 is of adrenal origin; conversely, DHEA and DHEAS derive predominantly from the adrenal. In addition, synthesis of 11OHA and 11β-hydroxytestosterone (11OHT) requires the adrenal specific enzyme 11β-hydroxylase (CYP11B1). Thus, because these steroids are mainly derived from the adrenal, DHEA, DHEAS, 11OHA, and 11OHT are commonly referred to as "adrenal androgens" [1].

Protective steroid hormones such as DHEA decrease with aging. DHEA, and particularly its sulfated derivative, DHEAS, are the most abundant circulating steroid hormones. The plasma concentrations of DHEA and DHEAS progressively decline with age, suggesting that they may be implicated in the aging process and perhaps in cardiovascular aging and in the development of a series of diseases associated with aging. Several epidemiological studies have shown an

M. Caretto · A. Giannini · T. Simoncini (✉)
Division of Obstetrics and Gynecology, Department of Clinical and Experimental Medicine, University of Pisa, Pisa, Italy
e-mail: andrea.giannini@unipi.it; tommaso.simoncini@med.unipi.it

A. R. Genazzani
International School for Gynecological and Reproductive Endocrinology, International Society of Gynecological Endocrinology, Locarno, Switzerland

Division of Obstetrics and Gynecology, Department of Clinical and Experimental Medicine, University of Pisa, Pisa, Italy

© International Society of Gynecological Endocrinology 2019
R. D. Brinton et al. (eds.), *Sex Steroids' Effects on Brain, Heart and Vessels*, ISGE Series, https://doi.org/10.1007/978-3-030-11355-1_5

inverse correlation between DHEA/DHEAS plasma concentrations and mortality, particularly mortality due to cardiovascular disease. The adrenal gland is the second endocrine system whose function declines and that demonstrates an age-related change. Some evidence suggests that DHEAS has a neuromodulatory effect, which might serve to protect certain parts of the prepubertal brain that are more active metabolically [2]. Another theory is that adrenarche supports an evolutionary role of "juvenility," which might have helped human ancestors adapt their body composition to environmental factors during the transition to adulthood. After reaching the intraindividual maximum levels during the third decade of life, DHEAS steadily decline down to 10–20% of its maximum level by around the age of 70 years [3]. This decline has been termed adrenopause, in spite of the fact that cortisol secretion does not significantly change with age. There is a clear sex difference in DHEAS levels with lower concentrations in women compared with men [4]. Adrenopause is independent of menopause and occurs in both sexes as a gradual process at similar age.

5.2 Dehydroepiandrosterone: A Neuroactive Steroid

In the early 1980s, Baulieu' s initial observation was based on experiments measuring DHEA levels in the CNS. It was found that DHEA levels were higher in the CNS than in serum and remained high even after adrenalectomy [5]. Subsequently, experiments documented that the brain was responsible for synthesizing DHEA. This type of steroid was termed "neurosteroid" to differentiate it from steroids produced in the periphery. The major steroids that met the criteria of a neurosteroid included DHEA and pregnenolone, their sulfated derivatives DHEA sulfate (DHEAS) and pregnenolone sulfate, and progesterone, deoxycorticosterone, and their 5 α-reduced metabolites (mainly allopregnanolone, ALLO). In general, they mediate their actions, not through classic steroid hormone nuclear receptors but through ion-gated neurotransmitter receptors. Neurosteroid levels are modified by neurodegenerative conditions (i.e., Alzheimer's and Parkinson's diseases, multiple sclerosis) or in other mental diseases (i.e., depression, schizophrenia) or brain trauma diseases and may have an important role in physiological conditions, as the re/organization of gray and white matter during human intrauterine life, puberty, and adolescence or as a consequence of emotional/cognitive responses.

DHEA has important effects on brain function: this hormone could be considered neuroactive and due to its formation in the brain even designated as a true neurosteroid. In fact there is interest in the therapeutic use of DHEA associated with its function as a neurosteroid [6]. In humans, cross-sectional and longitudinal studies have shown that DHEA might be associated with global measures of well-being and functioning, but positive effects on measures of memory and attention have not been unequivocally found. Studies investigating DHEA and DHEAS levels in patients with dementia have produced controversial results. Short-term experimental studies have not shown significant improvements in global measures of health and functioning in healthy subjects but have revealed preliminary evidence for mood-enhancing and antidepressant effects of DHEA. Moffat et al. [7] determined endogenous levels of DHEAS and related them to quantified cognitive status. Although both DHEAS and cognitive performance declined with age, it seems that a causal relationship is not likely. DHEA modulates endothelial function, reduces inflammation, and improves insulin sensitivity, blood flow, cellular immunity, body composition, bone metabolism, sexual function, and physical strength in frailty, as well as provides neuroprotection, improved cognitive function, and memory enhancement. Biological activities of DHEA and DHEAS include neuroprotection, effects on neurite growth, neuro-neogenesis and neural survival, protection against apoptosis, and antagonistic effects on oxidants and glucocorticoids [8].

There has been great interest in following the levels of DHEAS and their changes in people suffering from psychological and neuropsychological disorders. In general, levels of DHEAS are correlated with indicators of mood, memory, and other mental abilities. Particular attention has been given to changes in DHEAS levels in relation to success in treatment with antidepressants, anti-anxiolytics, and drugs for lowering stress. DHEAS levels have been followed in patients with panic disorders, the drug addicted, anorexics, schizophrenics, and many other patients and compared to levels in healthy people of the same age and sex. Many studies have focused on patients with defects in memory and other mental functions, particularly in those with dementia including Alzheimer's disease [9].

5.3   DHEAS Levels and Cognitive Function

Davis et al. [10] provide the first evidence that cognitively intact women with higher circulating levels of DHEAS exhibit better performance on testing of executive function (FAS test) and that circulating DHEAS is significantly positively associated with higher scores for tests of simple concentration (DSF) and working memory (DSB) in women with at least 12 years of education. There isn't a relation between circulating DHEAS levels and performance on tests of verbal and nonverbal learning and retention or focused attention. The other findings of interest include the favorable independent associations between living with other people, doing crossword puzzles, playing a musical instrument, and cognitive performance.

Cognitive function in elderly women is influenced by a number of other health variables including diabetes, hypertension, and smoking, and longitudinal studies have reported associations between these factors and progression to dementia in elderly individuals [11]. Less is known of the determinants of cognitive function in younger women in the community, well before the onset of cognitive decline. Possible explanations for the correlation between higher endogenous DHEAS levels and executive function, concentration, and working memory include direct actions of DHEA/DHEAS via a putative DHEA receptor, via the androgen receptor, or as neurosteroids and endogenous ligands for σ-1 receptors and/or DHEAS being a marker of overall potential for tissue intracrine androgen and estrogen production in women but not the actual mediator of the effect. DHEAS may be simply a marker of general good health [10]?

5.4   DHEA and Sexual Function

Sexual dysfunction, primarily low libido, is common among women, with prevalences of 8–50% previously reported. The prevalence appears to increase with age from the third decade [12] as well as after oophorectomy. Although multiple psychosocial and health factors contribute to low sexual desire and arousal, it has been proposed that endogenous androgen levels are significant independent determinants of sexual behavior in women. Most studies support a therapeutic benefit of testosterone for women experiencing hypoactive sexual desire disorder. Davis et al. [13] proposed a community-based, cross-sectional study of 1021 women aged 18–75 years, to investigate whether women with low self-reported sexual desire and sexual satisfaction [using the validated Profile of Female Sexual Function (PFSF) [14]] were more likely to have low serum androgen levels than women without self-reported low sexual desire and sexual satisfaction. The PFSF, although validated, had not previously been applied to a large population of women. They observed significant associations between low sexual desire, arousal, and responsiveness in younger women and low responsiveness in older women and low serum DHEAS level relative to age: DHEAS, not free testosterone, seems to be the hormone associated with low self-reported sexual function. This is most likely due to differing circulating levels of these steroids and the complexity of androgen metabolism. DHEA is the most abundant sex steroid in women, and circulating DHEA and its sulfate, DHEAS, provide a large precursor reservoir for the intracellular production of both estrogens and androgens [15]. DHEA and DHEAS are converted in extragonadal target tissues, such as the brain, bone, and adipose, either to androstenedione or testosterone that may then be aromatized to estrone or estradiol or converted by 5-αreductase to dihydrotestosterone in the same cells. Thus androgenic effects vary according to individual variations in the amount and activity of the enzymes 5-αreductase and aromatase and individual differences in the androgen-receptor response. They concluded that the measurement of testosterone is not useful for the diagnosis of the proposed female androgen insufficiency syndrome and the measurement of DHEAS didn't have a diagnostically useful role. This is because despite the increased likelihood that women with low sexual function have a low DHEAS level, the majority of women with a low DHEAS level did not report low sexual function [13].

5.5   DHEA Therapy in Postmenopausal Women: Treatment with a Neurosteroid?

Over the past 15 years, hormone preparations of DHEA have been available over the counter and have been sold as the "fountain of youth." This has raised concerns about the real clinical efficacy and the possible effects of such uncontrolled and widespread hormone self-administration and the lack of quality control in this increasingly financially rewarding business. However, available clinical studies differ in dose and treatment time, the age of women, and the measured function, and some authors state that there is little convincing data to support the use of oral DHEA in healthy postmenopausal women to improve condition evidenced by the aging process, such as reduced sexual function and reduced well-being [16]. The controversial findings from studies investigate the correlation of endogenous DHEAS levels, the aging process, or organ illness versus results coming from studies focusing on the effects of exogenous DHEAS administration on brain function, sexuality or cardiovascular health, and metabolic syndrome. This is also a growing evidence that low DHEAS levels, the most abundant sex steroids in plasma in humans, are negatively correlated with domains of sexual function in pre- and postmenopausal women. Nonetheless, a DHEAS cutoff level for defining androgen deficiency syndrome has not been established. Higher endogenous DHEAS levels are independently and favorably associated with several measures of cognitive function and well-being. As a consequence, DHEA replacement may seem an attractive treatment opportunity. Despite DHEA preparations being available in the market since the 1990s, there are very few definitive reports on the biological functions of this steroid, and mechanism of action of DHEA is unclear. Oral supplementation of DHEA in postmenopausal women results in the formation of significant amounts of 17 β-estradiol and estrone, accompanied by increases in androstenedione, testosterone, and dihydrotestosterone. This, plus the evidence that DHEA can also be converted into estrogens and other androgens within cells, supports the view that many actions of this steroid are indirect and mediated via estrogen and/or androgen receptors. However, the rate of DHEA metabolism into estrogen/testosterone in different tissues, the presence of enzyme regulators, and the effect of the aging process on the intracrinology of DHEA, all require additional investigation. Indeed, DHEA administration in both early and late postmenopausal women directly affects the age-related changes in adrenal enzymatic pathways and steroid synthesis including DHEA and progesterone [17, 18]. Although there is still debate on DHEA receptors, the evidence suggests that DHEA is not just a pre-hormone of the adrenals, but rather a hormone in its own right, and that it modulates a series of biological processes, with a remarkable tropism for the CNS. DHEA is a neurosteroid that acts as a modulator of neurotransmitter receptors, such as GABA-A, N-methyl-D-aspartate, and sigma-1 receptors. In vitro and in vivo documented effects involve neuroprotection, neurite growth, neurogenesis and neuronal survival, apoptosis, catecholamine synthesis and secretion, as well as antioxidant, anti-inflammatory, and anti-glucocorticoid effects. Clinically, the spectrum of women who would benefit from DHEA therapy is not clearly defined and nor is the dosage of hormone treatment. Moreover DHEA supplementation in postmenopausal women (6–12 months) is effective in stimulating the synthesis of neuroactive steroids, in particular ALLO, a 3α-5α-reduced metabolite of progesterone, and some neuropeptides such as β-endorphin, which are crucial in the modulation of mood, memory, and feeling of well-being, during reproductive aging. Whether DHEA therapy could be prescribed as a general antiaging therapy or could be an alternative treatment for women suffering from androgen deficiency syndrome remains uncertain across studies. In particular, among symptomatic women, the spectrum of DHEA-responsive symptoms requires further investigation, to define the type of sexual symptoms (e.g., decreased sexual function or hypoactive sexual desire disorder) and the degree of mood/cognitive symptoms that could be responsive to hormonal treatment. Similarly, the criteria for the choice of starting dosage of DHEA to be prescribed in postmenopausal women need further investigation: the extent of symptoms, baseline DHEAS plasma levels, concomitant estrogen therapy, or the combination of all the previous should be considered.

Several studies had previously demonstrated that 1-year treatment [18, 19], using administration of 10 mg DHEA daily in symptomatic postmenopausal women with lower (5th percentile) baseline DHEAS levels, improved climacteric and sexual symptoms and directly reversed some age-related changes in adrenal enzymatic pathways, including adrenal DHEA and progesterone synthesis. In addition, before drawing definitive conclusions on DHEA replacement therapy, further aspects need to be better investigated, such as the genetics of DHEA intracrinology and adrenal aging as well their relation with climacteric symptoms [20].

Another emerging hormonal therapeutic option for menopausal symptoms is a combination of oral prasterone (DHEA) and acolbifene. Acolbifene is a SERM reported to have ER antagonist activity in the breast and uterus but estrogen agonist effects on bone. The rationale for combining DHEA with acolbifene is to potentially derive a product that combines the benefits of both components. For example, benefits with regard to prevention of osteoporosis may be additive given DHEA's anabolic effects (i.e., stimulation of bone formation) and acolbifene's ability to reduce bone loss.

A phase III multicenter Canadian trial of DHEA/acolbifene in postmenopausal women with moderate-to-severe hot flushes has been completed, but data have not yet been reported. The primary end points of this study were changed from baseline to week 12 in frequency and severity of moderate-to-severe hot flushes. Secondary end points consisted of change from baseline to week 12 in vulvovaginal atrophy (i.e., superficial/parabasal cell counts, pH, atrophy symptoms), as well as sexual function and quality of life (based on questionnaires). Safety/tolerability is also a secondary end point.

Use of DHEA to treat sexual function in postmenopausal women remains controversial due to conflicting results from randomized trials, many of which were small or had other methodologic limitations. Data from initial studies of acolbifene/DHEA are still awaited [21].

All these findings may have far-reaching implications in the debate about the role of DHEAS in the female aging process and might reconcile discordant findings from basic science and clinical studies. The new clinical trials, specifically planned on the biology of symptomatic postmenopausal women and designed for the translation of basic science into clinical practice, are now a required step to move forward in the scientific debate on DHEA [22].

5.6   Conclusion

DHEA demonstrates anabolic properties, whereas DHEAS demonstrates neuroprotective and neuroexcitatory as well as antidepressive and memory-enhancing properties in humans. The biology of the effects of DHEA use on the brain in postmenopausal women is still controversial, although there is need to move forward concerning the lack of evidence for the translation of basic science into clinical practice.

References

1. Turcu A, Smith JM, Auchus R, Rainey WE. Adrenal androgens and androgen precursors: definition, synthesis, regulation and physiologic actions. Compr Physiol. 2014;4(4):1369–81.
2. Campbell B. Adrenarche in comparative perspective. Am J Hum Biol. 2011;23:44–52.
3. Orentreich N, Brind JL, Vogelman JH, Andres R, Baldwin H. Long-term longitudinal measurements of plasma dehydroepiandrosterone sulfate in normal men. J Clin Endocrinol Metab. 1992;75(4):1002–4.
4. Orentreich N, Brind JL, Rizer RL, Vogelman JH. Age changes and sex differences in serum dehydroepiandrosterone sulfate concentrations throughout adulthood. J Clin Endocrinol Metab. 1984;59(3):551–5.
5. Baulieu EE. Neurosteroids: of the nervous system, by the nervous system, for the nervous system. Recent Prog Horm Res. 1997;52:1–32.
6. Friess E, Schiffelholz T, Steckler T, Steiger A. Dehydroepiandrosterone – a neurosteroid. Eur J Clin Investig. 2000;30(Suppl 30):46–50.
7. Moffat SD, Zonderman AB, Harman SM, Blackman MR, Kawas C, Resnick SM. The relationship between longitudinal declines in dehydroepiandrosterone sulfate concentrations and cognitive performance in older men. Arch Intern Med. 2000;160:2193–8.
8. Sherwin BB. Steroid hormones and cognitive functioning in aging men: a mini-review. J Mol Neurosci. 2003;20(3):385–93.
9. Stárka L, Dušková M, Hil M. Dehydroepiandrosterone: a neuroactive steroid. J Steroid Biochem Mol Biol. 2015;145:254–60.
10. Davis SR, Shah SM, McKenzie DP, Kulkarni J, Davison S, Bel RJ. Dehydroepiandrosterone sulfate levels are associated with more favorable cognitive function in women. J Clin Endocrinol Metabol. 2008;93(3):801–8.
11. Barnes DE, Cauley JA, Lui LY, Fink HA, McCulloch C, Stone KL, Yaffe K. Women who maintain optimal cognitive function into old age. J Am Geriatr Soc. 2007;55:259–61.
12. Laumann E, Paik A, Rosen RC. Sexual dysfunction in the United States: prevalence and predictors. JAMA. 1999;281:537–44.
13. Davis S, Davison SL, Donath S, Bell RJ. Circulating androgen levels and self-reported sexual function in women. JAMA. 2005;294(1):91–6.
14. Derogatis L, Rust J, Golombok S, et al. Validation of the Profile of Female Sexual Function (PFSF) in surgically and naturally menopausal women. J Sex Marital Ther. 2004;30:25–36.
15. Labrie F, Luu-The V, Labrie C, et al. Endocrine and intracrine sources of androgens in women: inhibition of breast cancer and other roles of androgens and their precursor dehydroepiandrosterone. Endocr Rev. 2003;24:152–82.
16. Davis SR, Panjari M, Stanczyk FZ. DHEA replacement for postmenopausal women. J Clin Endocrinol Metab. 2011;96:1642–3.
17. Genazzani AR, Pluchino N, Begliuomini S, et al. Long-term low-dose oral administration of dehydroepiandrosterone modulates response to adrenocorticotropic hormone in early and late postmenopausal women. Gynecol Endocrinol. 2006;22:627–35.
18. Pluchino N, Ninni F, Stomati M, et al. One-year therapy with 10 mg/day DHEA alone or in combination with HRT in postmenopausal women: effects on hormonal milieu. Maturitas. 2008;59:293–303.
19. Genazzani AR, Stomati M, Valentino V, et al. Effect of 1-year, low-dose DHEA therapy on climacteric symptoms and female sexuality. Climacteric. 2011;14:661–8.
20. Pluchino N, Genazzani AR. DHEA replacement for postmenopausal women: have we been looking in the right direction? Climacteric. 2015;18:1–3.
21. Genazzani AR, Komm BS, Pickar JH. Emerging hormonal treatments for menopausal symptoms. Expert Opin Emerg Drugs. 2015;20(1):31–46.
22. Pluchino N, Santoro A, Casarosa E, Wenger JM, Genazzani AD, Petignat P, Genazzani AR. Advances in neurosteroids: role in clinical practice. Climacteric. 2013;16(Suppl 1):8–17.

Do Menopausal Symptoms Account for the Declines in Cognitive Function During the Menopausal Transition?

6

Pauline M. Maki and Miriam T. Weber

6.1 Overview of Cognitive Changes at Menopause

Cognitive complaints are frequent in midlife women and increase across the menopausal transition. For example, in a study of US women aged 40–55 years, about 30% of premenopausal women endorse "forgetfulness" compared to 40% of perimenopausal and postmenopausal women [1]. Forgetfulness was the third most frequent symptom endorsed by women in this age range, after neck pain and hot flashes. For perimenopausal women, memory complaints were the second most frequent symptom, after neck pain. Midlife women in Europe and the Middle East show a similar frequency of memory complaints [2]. Cognitive complaints by midlife women are validated in studies showing a significant relationship between the severity of cognitive complaints and the level of performance on neuropsychological tests, particularly in the domains of episodic memory, working memory, and attention [3, 4].

Cognitive symptoms are not typically considered to be a primary symptom of the menopause. Like psychological symptoms (i.e., depression and anxiety), cognitive symptoms were designated by an expert consensus panel from the National Institute of Aging in 2005 as "symptoms *sometimes* associated with menopause [5]." Hot flashes and vaginal dryness/dyspareunia were designated as "classic symptoms of

P. M. Maki (✉)
Department of Psychiatry, University of Illinois at Chicago, Chicago, IL, USA

Department of Psychology, University of Illinois at Chicago, Chicago, IL, USA

Department of Obstetrics and Gynecology, University of Illinois at Chicago, Chicago, IL, USA
e-mail: pmaki@psych.uic.edu

M. T. Weber
Department of Neurology, University of Rochester, Rochester, NY, USA

Department of Obstetrics and Gynecology, University of Rochester, Rochester, NY, USA
e-mail: Miriam_Weber@URMC.Rochester.edu

© International Society of Gynecological Endocrinology 2019
R. D. Brinton et al. (eds.), *Sex Steroids' Effects on Brain, Heart and Vessels*,
ISGE Series, https://doi.org/10.1007/978-3-030-11355-1_6

the menopause." The secondary status of cognitive symptoms was reflected in the view that cognitive and psychological problems emerged secondary to hot flashes and as a consequence of sleep disturbance due to nighttime awakenings. This view of cognitive and psychological symptoms of menopause as not reliably associated with menopause has been challenged by studies showing that these symptoms reliably change across the menopausal transition and are not explained by increasing chronologic age [6, 7]. However, because cognitive symptoms co-occur with hot flashes, psychological symptoms, and sleep disturbance, it is important to evaluate to what extent cognitive symptoms are accounted for by other menopausal symptoms. Additionally, understanding the relationships among depressive symptoms, VMS, and cognitive difficulties is clinically significant because these symptoms affect quality of life, as well as work and relationship quality in midlife women.

The aim of this chapter is to address to what extent cognitive changes in midlife women are due to menopausal symptoms. We will first briefly review the role of sex steroid hormones in cognitive changes during the menopause. Next we will review the three categories of menopausal symptoms that are most often linked to cognition—vasomotor symptoms, psychological symptoms, and sleep. Then we will address the specific issue of whether the cognitive changes that occur during the menopausal transition are accounted for by other menopausal symptoms.

6.2   Sex Steroid Hormones and Cognition

A wealth of studies demonstrate that cognitive performance and cognitive systems in the brain are influenced by sex steroid hormones [8]. Estrogen receptor alpha, estrogen receptor beta, and G protein-coupled estrogen receptor 1 (GPER1) are located in the prefrontal cortex, hippocampus, and other brain regions whose structure and function are key to cognitive performance [8]. These steroid receptors mediate estrogen-induced spinogenesis, synaptogenesis, and excitability, which in turn are associated with improved function. Progesterone and androgens also play a role [9]. In humans, the most direct evidence that estrogen influences cognition comes from randomized, placebo-controlled trials in premenopausal women where performance on tests of verbal memory and working memory decreased following oophorectomy among women randomized to placebo but not among women randomized to estrogen therapy (ET) [10]. Similarly, premenopausal women who undergo oophorectomy show an increased risk of cognitive impairment or dementia compared to age-matched women, but this risk was not seen among those who took ET until the typical age of menopause [11]. Ovariectomized rodents show similar patterns of cognitive dysfunction following surgery, but administration of estradiol in physiological doses improves performance to levels that do not differ from presurgical levels [12]. Notably, the benefits of estradiol are evident when given within a few weeks of surgery but are ineffective if delayed. The nonhuman primate data reveal benefit with cyclical estradiol but not continuous estradiol [8]. Myriad mechanisms underlie these behavioral effects including changes in bioenergetics and neurotransmitter function [8, 13]. Neuroimaging studies in human show benefits of estrogen on hippocampal and prefrontal function and the connectivity of those two regions [14]. Such studies indicate that estrogen plays a direct role in the maintenance of cognitive function by acting on key brain regions.

6.3 Menopausal Symptoms and Cognition

6.3.1 Vasomotor Symptoms

The hormonal changes during menopause provoke symptoms that also can contribute to cognitive dysfunction. The most common symptom, VMS, are reported by about 70% of women during the menopausal transition [15]. For a third of women, they are frequent or severe [16, 17]. Once thought to be isolated to the few years around the final menstrual period, new data indicate that VMS start earlier and last longer than previously thought, lasting on average a decade or more [16, 18]. On questionnaires, the frequency or severity of VMS is often shown to be associated with magnitude of cognitive complaints. In contrast, questionnaire-based reports of VMS are typically unrelated to cognitive test performance.

Studies that measure VMS objectively with ambulatory monitors, however, do suggest that VMS are associated with memory performance. Ambulatory monitors measure the change in skin conductance associated with sweating during a hot flash, a change that has a rapid onset followed by a gradual tapering and that is distinct from the pattern of sweating associated with general physical activity. In studies of women with moderate-to-severe VMS, there is a linear association between the frequency of VMS measured with these monitors and performance on memory tests [19, 20]. As demonstrated in a randomized trial of a hot flash intervention (i.e., stellate ganglion blockade), memory improves in relation to improvement in physiologic VMS but not reported VMS [20]. The clinical significance of studying VMS and memory problems is that VMS appear to be a modifiable risk factor for memory dysfunction in women.

Neuroimaging studies show a relationship between physiologic VMS and adverse alterations in brain structure (i.e., white matter hyperintensities) and brain function (i.e., functional connectivity during the resting state, especially in hippocampus and prefrontal cortex) [21, 22]. Measuring VMS with ambulatory monitors is critical not only because physiologic VMS are more strongly associated with cognitive and brain measures than are questionnaire-based measures [19–22] but also because unlike questionnaires, which may be influenced by subjective factors, physiologic measures provide objective and quantitative data. It is unknown to what extent physiologic hot flashes contribute to the cognitive changes observed across the menopausal transition. To date, such studies have only measured hot flashes on questionnaires.

6.3.2 Depression and Anxiety

Psychological symptoms of the menopause, including depression and anxiety, are also associated with cognitive complaints and compromised cognitive test performance in midlife women. Symptoms of depression and anxiety, as measured by questionnaires, increase as women transition through the menopause [23, 24]. A recent systematic review concluded that major depressive disorder (MDD), as measured by diagnostic psychiatric interviews, is not reliably increased during the menopausal transition, except for the 58% of women with a prior history of MDD who will experience a recurrence during the menopause transition [24]. Cognitive deficits are a key feature of depression. In a recent meta-analysis, small to moderate deficits in executive function, memory and attention were documented not only in individuals with current MDD but also in individuals with rMDD, leading to the conclusion that these deficits occur independently of episodes of low mood in individuals with MDD [25]. It is notable that the KEEPS study demonstrated beneficial effects of HT on depressive and anxiety symptoms in early postmenopausal women with no improvement in cognition. Thus, psychological symptoms and cognitive symptoms are dissociable in midlife women [26].

6.3.3 Sleep

Sleep complaints increase during menopausal transition, especially for women with bothersome VMS [27]. Night sweats can cause nighttime awakenings and lower sleep quality. In menopause studies, sleep quality is typically measured by self-report, which is problematic due to the limited association of self-reported sleep with more objective measures such as actigraphy and polysomnography [28]. In the general population, sleep deprivation and insomnia are associated with disruptions in memory, verbal abilities, executive function, and processing speed [28]. Surprisingly little is known about the relationship between objective measures of sleep quality and cognitive test performance in midlife women as they transition through the menopause.

6.4   Menopausal Symptoms and Cognitive Changes Across the Menopause

Six studies to date examined the association between menopausal stage and cognitive performance, taking into account the potential influence of one or more categories of menopausal symptoms (VMS, depressive symptoms, anxiety symptoms, and sleep; see Table 6.1) [6, 7, 29–32]. To identify those studies, we searched for articles in PubMed using the MeSH terms "menopause," "perimenopause," and "menopause transition" in combination with the terms "cognition" and "memory" with additional limits of "human subjects," "English language," "females," and "adult age 19+." We also conducted a "relevant studies" search on two of the articles [31, 32]. To be included in the review, studies must have included women in at least two different stages of the menopausal transition, utilized a standardized, objective measure of cognitive function, and assessed for the presence or severity of at least one menopausal symptom. We excluded review articles and clinical trials. One author (MW) read each of the abstracts and identified four cross-sectional studies and two longitudinal studies relevant to the topic of this review.

Of the four cross-sectional studies, two found that menopausal stage affected cognitive function, and two found no such effect. Kok et al. [30] found that peri- and

Table 6.1 Studies of the association between menopausal stage and cognition

Study	N	Pre	Early peri	Late peri	Mixed peri	Post	VMS	Sleep	Dep	Anx	Mood	Attn WM	Mem	Exec	Processing speed	Visuospatial
Cross-sectional																
Henderson, 2003	326		X	X	X		C				C		X			
Kok, 2006	1261	X			X	X	C		GHQ28	GHQ28			X			X
Luetters, 2007	1657	X	X	X		X	C	C	CES-D		C	X	X			
Weber, 2013	117	X	X	X		X	WHQ	WHQ	BDI	BAI		X	X	X	X	X
Longitudinal																
Greendale, 2010	1903	X	X	X		X	C	PSQI	CES-D	C		X	X		X	
Epperson, 2013	403	X	X	X		X			CES-D	Zung			X		X	X

C, Symptom checklist or non-standardized questionnaire; GHQ-28, General Health Questionnaire 28; CES-D, Centers for Epidemiologic Studies-Depression; BDI, Beck Depression Inventory; BAI, Beck Anxiety Inventory; PSQI, Pittsburg Sleep Quality Index; ZUNG, Zung Self-Rating Anxiety Scale postmenopausal women performed worse on a timed visual search task compared with premenopausal women of the same age, but found no effect of reproductive stage on a measure of verbal learning. Although higher levels of VMS were associated with worse verbal learning, and psychological symptoms were associated with worse verbal learning and visual search performance, these symptoms did not account for the stage effect on the visual search task. Similarly, Weber et al. [32] found that women in the early postmenopausal stage (<12 months after the final menstrual period) performed significantly worse than pre- and perimenopausal women on measures of attention/working memory, verbal learning, verbal memory, and motor function, after controlling for menopausal symptoms, including VMS, depression, anxiety, and sleep disturbance. In contrast, Luetters et al. [31] found that postmenopausal women performed significantly worse than women in late perimenopause on a verbal memory test and significantly worse than premenopausal and early perimenopausal women on a test of processing speed, but these differences attenuated after adjusting for VMS, sleep disturbance, and depressive symptoms. Finally, Henderson et al. [29] found that verbal memory was negatively associated with mood but unaffected by reproductive stage.

The two longitudinal studies were more consistent in their findings. In the Study of Women's Health Across the Nation (SWAN), Greendale et al. [7] found that premenopausal and early perimenopausal women showed improvements in processing speed with repeated test administrations but that women in the late perimenopause failed to show such improvements. Similarly, premenopausal women showed improvements in a verbal memory task with repeated test administration, but early and late perimenopausal women did not. In a subsequent report [33], they revealed that this lower learning rate was independent of symptoms of anxiety, depression, sleep disturbance, and VMS. In the Penn Ovarian Aging Study, Epperson et al. [6] found that immediate and delayed verbal memory declined as women transitioned from the pre- to postmenopausal stages and that this decline was independent of symptoms of depression and anxiety.

6.5   Summary and Gaps in the Literature

Although it is commonly purported that menopause transition-associated declines in cognition are due to menopausal symptoms such as depression, anxiety, sleep disturbance, and VMS, the existing data do not support this claim. The majority of published studies that address this question reveal that reproductive aging affects cognition independent of symptoms. However, there are several limitations to the existing literature. There are few studies addressing this question, and only two of them utilize a large sample size and longitudinal follow-up. Many of the studies have used non-standardized assessments of symptoms, and the relationship between these questionnaires and validated measures of these constructs of interest is uncertain. In particular, better measures of anxiety are needed, as current understanding is based largely on a few self-report questionnaires. Finally, all of the studies rely on self-report of symptoms.

To more definitively characterize the natural history of cognitive changes across the menopausal transition and the factors that contribute to those changes, appropriately powered, longitudinal studies with validated approaches for defining menopausal stage and with assessments of multiple cognitive domains are needed. Such studies should not only include validated self-report measures of VMS, depression, anxiety, and sleep but also objectively defined measures of VMS and sleep, as well as standardized psychiatric inventories to determine the role of psychiatric diagnoses. The use of actigraphy to measure sleep and skin conductance monitors to measure VMS is particularly important given discrepancies between self-reported and objectively measured symptoms [34, 35] and their interrelationships [36, 37]. The inclusion of such measures will help to better differentiate the effects of reproductive aging and menopausal symptoms on cognitive function in midlife women.

Such studies would be needed to identify the patterns and predictors of cognitive changes during the menopausal transition. It is unlikely that there is one universal pattern of cognitive change across the menopause. Some women may experience cognitive changes related to sleep disturbance and nighttime awakenings due to hot flashes. Others, with elevated depressive symptoms but minimal VMS, may show a different pattern of change. Those with multiple, co-occurring menopause symptoms may show yet another pattern of change. Whether those cognitive effects persist into aging after menopausal symptoms have subsided is another key question. We do not know, for example, whether women with persistent VMS are at risk for accelerated cognitive aging. Continued research in this area will help to identify and personalize interventions for improving at cognition at midlife and beyond.

References

1. Gold EB, Sternfeld B, Kelsey JL, Brown C, Mouton C, Reame N, et al. Relation of demographic and lifestyle factors to symptoms in a multi-racial/ethnic population of women 40–55 years of age. Am J Epidemiol. 2000;152(5):463–73.
2. Obermeyer CM, Reher D, Saliba M. Symptoms, menopause status, and country differences: a comparative analysis from DAMES. Menopause. 2007;14(4):788–97.
3. Drogos LL, Rubin LH, Geller SE, Banuvar S, Shulman LP, Maki PM. Objective cognitive performance is related to subjective memory complaints in midlife women with moderate to severe vasomotor symptoms. Menopause. 2013;20(12):1236–42.
4. Weber MT, Mapstone M, Staskiewicz J, Maki PM. Reconciling subjective memory complaints with objective memory performance in the menopausal transition. Menopause. 2012;19(7):735–41.
5. National Institutes of Health. State-of-the-Science Conference statement: management of menopause-related symptoms. Ann Intern Med. 2005;142(12 Pt 1):1003–13.
6. Epperson CN, Sammel MD, Freeman EW. Menopause effects on verbal memory: findings from a longitudinal community cohort. J Clin Endocrinol Metab. 2013;98(9):3829–38.
7. Greendale GA, Huang MH, Wight RG, Seeman T, Luetters C, Avis NE, et al. Effects of the menopause transition and hormone use on cognitive performance in midlife women. Neurology. 2009;72(21):1850–7.
8. Hara Y, Waters EM, McEwen BS, Morrison JH. Estrogen effects on cognitive and synaptic health over the lifecourse. Physiol Rev. 2015;95(3):785–807.

9. Genazzani AR, Bernardi F, Pluchino N, Begliuomini S, Lenzi E, Casarosa E, et al. Endocrinology of menopausal transition and its brain implications. CNS Spectr. 2005;10(6):449–57.
10. Sherwin BB. Estrogen and/or androgen replacement therapy and cognitive functioning in surgically menopausal women. Psychoneuroendocrinology. 1988;13(4):345–57.
11. Rocca WA, Bower JH, Maraganore DM, Ahlskog JE, Grossardt BR, de Andrade M, et al. Increased risk of cognitive impairment or dementia in women who underwent oophorectomy before menopause. Neurology. 2007;69(11):1074–83.
12. Gibbs RB. Long-term treatment with estrogen and progesterone enhances acquisition of a spatial memory task by ovariectomized aged rats. Neurobiol Aging. 2000;21(1):107–16.
13. Brinton RD, Yao J, Yin F, Mack WJ, Cadenas E. Perimenopause as a neurological transition state. Nat Rev Endocrinol. 2015;11(7):393–405.
14. Maki PM, Dumas J. Mechanisms of action of estrogen in the brain: insights from human neuroimaging and psychopharmacologic studies. Semin Reprod Med. 2009;27(3):250–9.
15. Gold EB, Colvin A, Avis N, Bromberger J, Greendale GA, Powell L, et al. Longitudinal analysis of the association between vasomotor symptoms and race/ethnicity across the menopausal transition: study of women's health across the nation. Am J Public Health. 2006;96(7):1226–35.
16. Avis NE, Crawford SL, Greendale G, Bromberger JT, Everson-Rose SA, Gold EB, et al. Duration of menopausal vasomotor symptoms over the menopause transition. JAMA Intern Med. 2015;175(4):531–9.
17. Freeman EW, Sammel MD, Sanders RJ. Risk of long-term hot flashes after natural menopause: evidence from the Penn Ovarian Aging Study cohort. Menopause. 2014;21(9):924–32.
18. Freeman EW, Sammel MD, Lin H, Liu Z, Gracia CR. Duration of menopausal hot flushes and associated risk factors. Obstet Gynecol. 2011;117(5):1095–104.
19. Maki PM, Drogos LL, Rubin LH, Banuvar S, Shulman LP, Geller SE. Objective hot flashes are negatively related to verbal memory performance in midlife women. Menopause. 2008;15(5):848–56.
20. Maki PM, Rubin LH, Savarese A, Drogos L, Shulman LP, Banuvar S, et al. Stellate ganglion blockade and verbal memory in midlife women: evidence from a randomized trial. Maturitas. 2016;92:123–9.
21. Thurston RC, Aizenstein HJ, Derby CA, Sejdic E, Maki PM. Menopausal hot flashes and white matter hyperintensities. Menopause. 2016;23(1):27–32.
22. Thurston RC, Maki PM, Derby CA, Sejdic E, Aizenstein HJ. Menopausal hot flashes and the default mode network. Fertil Steril. 2015;103(6):1572–8.e1.
23. Bromberger JT, Kravitz HM, Chang Y, Randolph JF Jr, Avis NE, Gold EB, et al. Does risk for anxiety increase during the menopausal transition? Study of women's health across the nation. Menopause. 2013;20(5):488–95.
24. Maki PM, Kornstein SG, Joffe H, Bromberger JT, Freeman EW, Athappilly G, et al. Guidelines for the evaluation and treatment of perimenopausal depression: summary and recommendations. Menopause. 2018;25(10):1069–85.
25. Rock PL, Roiser JP, Riedel WJ, Blackwell AD. Cognitive impairment in depression: a systematic review and meta-analysis. Psychol Med. 2014;44(10):2029–40.
26. Gleason CE, Dowling NM, Wharton W, Manson JE, Miller VM, Atwood CS, et al. Effects of hormone therapy on cognition and mood in recently postmenopausal women: findings from the randomized, controlled KEEPS-cognitive and affective study. PLoS Med. 2015;12(6):e1001833; discussion e1001833.
27. Kravitz HM, Ganz PA, Bromberger J, Powell LH, Sutton-Tyrrell K, Meyer PM. Sleep difficulty in women at midlife: a community survey of sleep and the menopausal transition. Menopause. 2003;10(1):19–28.
28. Luik AI, Zuurbier LA, Hofman A, Van Someren EJ, Ikram MA, Tiemeier H. Associations of the 24-h activity rhythm and sleep with cognition: a population-based study of middle-aged and elderly persons. Sleep Med. 2015;16(7):850–5.
29. Henderson V, Guthrie J, Dudley E, Burger H, Dennerstein L. Estrogen exposures and memory at midlife: a population-based study of women. Neurology. 2003;60:1369–71.

30. Kok HS, Kuh D, Cooper R, van der Schouw YT, Grobbee DE, Wadsworth ME, et al. Cognitive function across the life course and the menopausal transition in a British birth cohort. Menopause. 2006;13(1):19–27.
31. Luetters C, Huang MH, Seeman T, Buckwalter G, Meyer PM, Avis NE, et al. Menopause transition stage and endogenous estradiol and follicle-stimulating hormone levels are not related to cognitive performance: cross-sectional results from the study of women's health across the nation (SWAN). J Womens Health (Larchmt). 2007;16(3):331–44.
32. Weber MT, Rubin LH, Maki PM. Cognition in perimenopause: the effect of transition stage. Menopause. 2013;20(5):511–7.
33. Greendale GA, Wight RG, Huang MH, Avis N, Gold EB, Joffe H, et al. Menopause-associated symptoms and cognitive performance: results from the study of women's health across the nation. Am J Epidemiol. 2010;171(11):1214–24.
34. Carpenter JS, Monahan PO, Azzouz F. Accuracy of subjective hot flush reports compared with continuous sternal skin conductance monitoring. Obstet Gynecol. 2004;104(6):1322–6.
35. Sievert LL, Freedman RR, Garcia JZ, Foster JW, del Carmen Romano Soriano M, Longcope C, et al. Measurement of hot flashes by sternal skin conductance and subjective hot flash report in Puebla, Mexico. Menopause. 2002;9(5):367–76.
36. Thurston RC, Santoro N, Matthews KA. Are vasomotor symptoms associated with sleep characteristics among symptomatic midlife women? Comparisons of self-report and objective measures. Menopause. 2012;19(7):742–8.
37. Joffe H, White DP, Crawford SL, McCurnin KE, Economou N, Connors S, et al. Adverse effects of induced hot flashes on objectively recorded and subjectively reported sleep: results of a gonadotropin-releasing hormone agonist experimental protocol. Menopause. 2013;20(9):905–14.

Allopregnanolone as a Therapeutic to Regenerate the Degenerated Brain

Gerson D. Hernandez and Roberta Diaz Brinton

7.1　Introduction

Allopregnanolone (3α-hydroxy-5α-pregnan-20-one; Fig. 7.1) is an endogenous pregnane neurosteroid and a reduced metabolite of progesterone [1, 2]. Steroidogenesis takes place in the brain and peripheral glands, with biosynthetic pathways that are very similar. Neurosteroids are synthesized de novo in the brain by glial cells and principal neurons from their precursor steroids. In the case of allopregnanolone (Allo), progesterone undergoes a 5α reduction to yield 5α-dihydroprogesterone which is further reduced via 3ßHSD (Fig. 7.2). Unlike its precursor, Allo is inactive at nuclear progesterone receptors and instead mediates its effects modulating GABA_A receptors [1–3].

As an endogenous metabolite of progesterone, men and women are exposed to Allo throughout their lifetime. Early in development, both progesterone and Allo are synthesized in the central nervous system in the pluripotential progenitor cells. During reproductive years, women are chronically exposed to Allo concentrations ranging from less than 1 nmol/l (0.32 ng/ml) to over 4 nmol/l (1.27 ng/ml) during the luteal phase [4]. During pregnancy, blood production rate of Allo can reach 100 mg per day and reach their highest concentrations during the third trimester of pregnancy at levels up to 157 nmol/l (50 ng/ml), which are not associated with adverse effects for either mother or fetus [1, 5–7]. In contrast, in the aged and degenerated brain, Allo content is diminished, and both the pool of neural stem cells and proliferative capacity are markedly reduced [1, 8, 9].

G. D. Hernandez · R. D. Brinton (✉)
Center for Innovation in Brain Science, College of Medicine, University of Arizona, Tucson, AZ, USA
e-mail: gersonhe@email.arizona.edu; rbrinton@email.arizona.edu

© International Society of Gynecological Endocrinology 2019
R. D. Brinton et al. (eds.), *Sex Steroids' Effects on Brain, Heart and Vessels*,
ISGE Series, https://doi.org/10.1007/978-3-030-11355-1_7

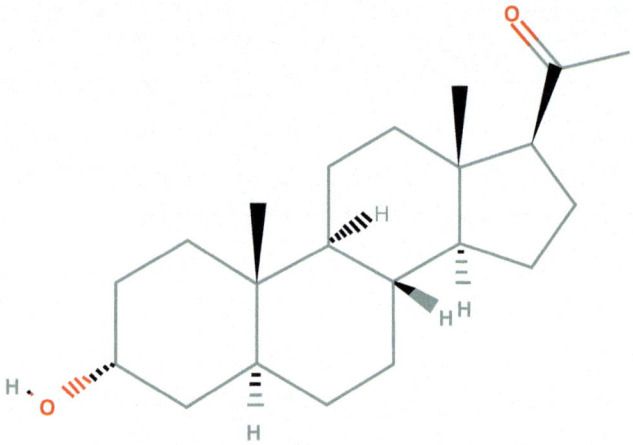

Fig. 7.1 Allopregnanolone chemical structure ($C_{21}H_{34}O_2$)

Neurons have the ability to change in form or function in response to different environmental stimuli. This adaptive response is known as neuroplasticity and involves the formation of new cells in specific parts of the brain such as the subgranular zone of the hippocampal dentate gyrus and subventricular zone [10].

7.1.1 The Degenerating Brain and Regeneration in Aging

Regeneration is a developmental process that has obligatory temporal and spatial requirements. The regenerative potential of neural stem cells diminishes with age and is accelerated in age-associated neurodegenerative disease like Alzheimer's disease (AD) [11–13]. However, the regenerative system of the aging and diseased brain remains viable until late in life and even responsive to interventions [12, 14, 15]. With age, a decline in regenerative factors in the neurogenic compartment leads to increasing numbers of neural stem cells transitioning from an actively dividing population to a dormant state rather than a decline in their absolute number [15–17]. Among the regenerative factors that are declining in the brain is the neurosteroid Allo. In the human brain with AD, significant deficits in Allo content correlate with the burden of pathology [18]. Findings in the 3×TgAD mice are consistent, exhibiting significantly lower brain Allo relative to wild-type suggesting either impairment of Allo generation in the brain or accelerated Allo degradation [14]. Comparative analyses of plasma vs. cortex levels of Allo indicate that reduced Allo is a central problem and not a problem in peripheral sources of Allo.

Regenerative medicine and therapeutics hold the promise of self-renewal and repair. The challenge is to access the innate regenerative potential of the brain to halt or even reverse the trajectory of degeneration. To achieve this feat, it is critical to activate the regenerative system of the brain while simultaneously addressing the etiology underlying degeneration.

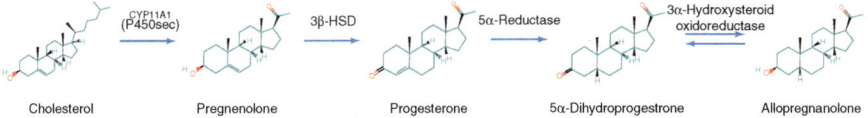

Fig. 7.2 Biosynthetic pathway of allopregnanolone

The regenerative system affected by Allo is tightly regulated with closely guarded thresholds for both activation and magnitude of proliferation. Allo significantly increases both the number of newly generated cells and their survival, restoring the regenerative potential of the brain to normal, but not exceeding what is normal [12, 14]. In addition, the regenerative effect of Allo is dose-dependent and exhibits a classic inverted U-shaped dose-response curve [1, 14], simply demonstrating that more is not better.

7.1.2 Allopregnanolone: Regenerative Mechanism of Action

In the central nervous system, Allo is a proliferative factor for both neural stem cells and pre-progenitor oligodendrocytes [1, 14, 19, 20]. It induced mitosis in cultures of hippocampal neurons of rodents and human neural stem cells [1]. In vitro, the proliferation of rodent-derived neural stem cells treated with Allo ranged from 20% to 30%, whereas a greater magnitude of proliferation was observed in human-derived neural stem cells (37–49%) [1]. In vivo, Allo significantly increased neurogenesis which reversed neurogenic deficits in both regenerative zones of the brain in 3×TgAD mice. Allo induced neurogenesis and restored regenerative potential in the 3×TgAD mice brain to a magnitude comparable to age-matched wild-type mice.

Proposed mechanisms by which Allo promotes neurogenesis are:

1. *GABA receptor activation.* At nanomolar concentrations, Allo potentiates the natural affinity of GABA for the GABA type A (GABA$_A$) receptor, whereas at micromolar concentrations, it directly activates GABA$_A$ to initiate the efflux of chloride ions (Cl−) from neural progenitor and neural stem cells (Fig. 7.3). Extrusion of Cl− from the intracellular compartment leads to membrane depolarization and activation of the voltage-dependent L-type calcium channel. The intracellular calcium (Ca++) rise activates Ca++-dependent kinases that ultimately lead to regulation of gene expression and protein synthesis of cell cycle proteins. Allo upregulates the expression of cell cycle genes that promote mitosis while simultaneously downregulating genes that repress cell division. The mechanism of Allo-induced neurogenesis takes advantage of the developmentally regulated direction of Cl− flux to induce neurogenesis in those cells that are phenotypically competent to divide while not activating those mechanisms in mature neurons [1, 21]. The direct effect of Allo on GABA$_A$ receptors produces sedative, anxiolytic, and anticonvulsant effects [22].

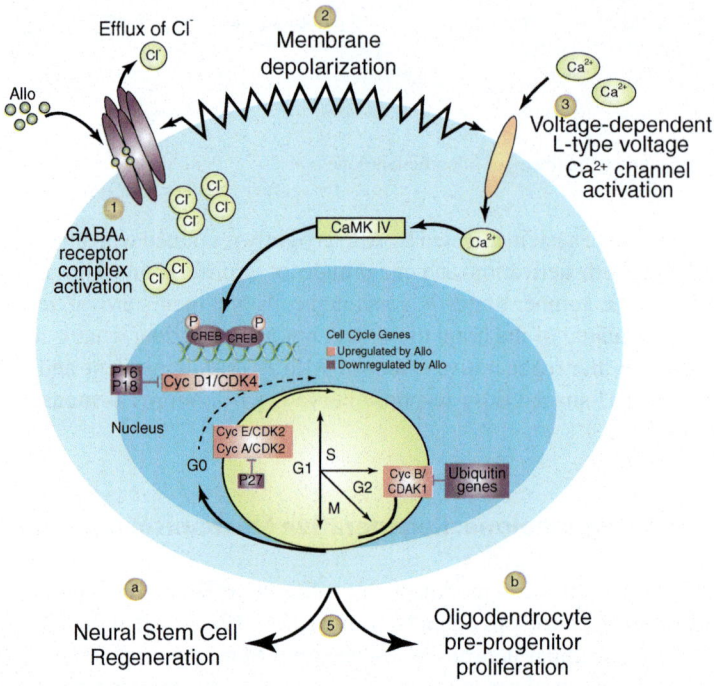

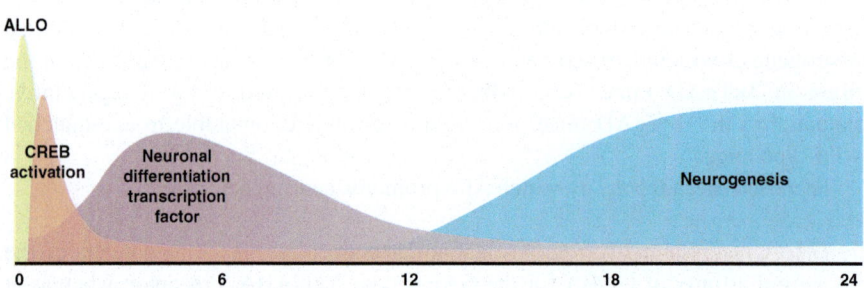

Fig. 7.3 Allopregnanolone GABA receptor activation. Allo promotes regeneration through a well-characterized pathway in neural stem cells to increase neurogenesis and oligo-genesis for both gray and white matter generation. Allo binds to sites within the transmembrane domains of the GABAA receptor chloride (Cl−) channel complex (GBRC) to both potentiate and directly activate the GRBC. The time course for Allo regenerative action is evident across a 24-h period

2. *Cholesterol trafficking.* Myelin generation is dependent upon high levels of cholesterol, which requires the expression of the enzyme HMG-CoA reductase for
   its synthesis [23]. Increasing evidence indicates that altered cholesterol metabolism is linked to AD pathology [24, 25]. In both normal and 3×TgAD mice, Allo
   significantly increased HMG-CoA-R expression necessary to address the demand
   for cholesterol required for myelin membrane growth [23, 26]. It has been proposed that Allo regulates cholesterol homeostasis via the LXR and PXR system

[27, 28] and dysregulation of cholesterol homeostasis is associated with the generation of Aβ [29]. Mechanistic analyses indicated that 1/week Allo begun prior to extraneuronal accumulation of Aβ increased expression of LXR, PXR, and HMG-CoA reductase, three proteins that regulate cholesterol homeostasis. LXR, a nuclear hormone receptor abundant in the brain [30], acts as a molecular sensor of cholesterol levels and initiates cholesterol clearance [29]. LXR activation increases cholesterol efflux through upregulating ABCA1 and ApoE expression and prevents the hyper-activation of γ-secretase and overproduction of Aβ [29, 31, 32]. LXR activation has been demonstrated to improve cognitive function in multiple mouse models of amyloidogenesis [29, 33–37].

LXR ligands frequently activate PXR [38]. Results from previous analyses indicated that in parallel with an APα-induced increase in LXR expression in the pre-pathology condition, APα also increased PXR expression in the pre-pathology 3×TgAD mouse brain. PXR activation induces CYP3A enzymes including CYP3A4 and CYP3A13 and leads to cholesterol hydroxylation and activation of organic anion transporters for cholesterol extrusion [39]. The increase in brain LXR and PXR induced by Allo leads to increased cholesterol efflux, thereby reducing γ-secretase activation by cholesterol-laden lipid rafts. Increased cholesterol efflux provides a plausible mechanism to explain how Allo decreased the generation of both 27 and 56 kDa intraneuronal Aβ oligomers [26].

7.2   Allopregnanolone Restores Cognitive Function

A strong relationship between neurogenesis and some hippocampal-dependent cognitive functions has been well described for many years [40–42]. Associative learning and memory across time appears to be dependent upon the generation of new neurons in the dentate gyrus. In order to test the functional impact of Allo on neurogenesis, a unique and regenerative system appropriate treatment paradigm was developed to treat mice. At time zero, mice were treated with Allo or vehicle followed by BrdU-labeling for proliferating cells. Mice were then returned to their cage for 7 days to allow neurogenesis, phenotypic differentiation, and early integration events to occur. Mice were then followed by 5 days of associative learning trials. After the learning phase of the cognitive assessment, mice were once again returned to their cage for another 9 days and then submitted to more memory function testing. Lastly, 22 days after the Allo treatment, they were sacrificed for detection of surviving BrdU-positive cells (Fig. 7.4a). This experiment demonstrated that functionally, Allo restored associative learning and memory function in 3×TgAD mice to the level of age-matched norms [12, 43] (Fig. 7.4c). Moreover, Allo-induced survival of neural progenitors was significantly correlated with Allo-induced memory performance [12, 43]. Learning and memory function in Allo-treated 3×TgAD mice was 100% greater in magnitude compared to the age-matched vehicle-treated group and in general was comparable to the maximal age-matched normal nonTg mouse performance. As with the regenerative response, the effect of Allo on cognitive function was a restoration of learning and memory to age-appropriate normal performance not supranormal. Results obtained

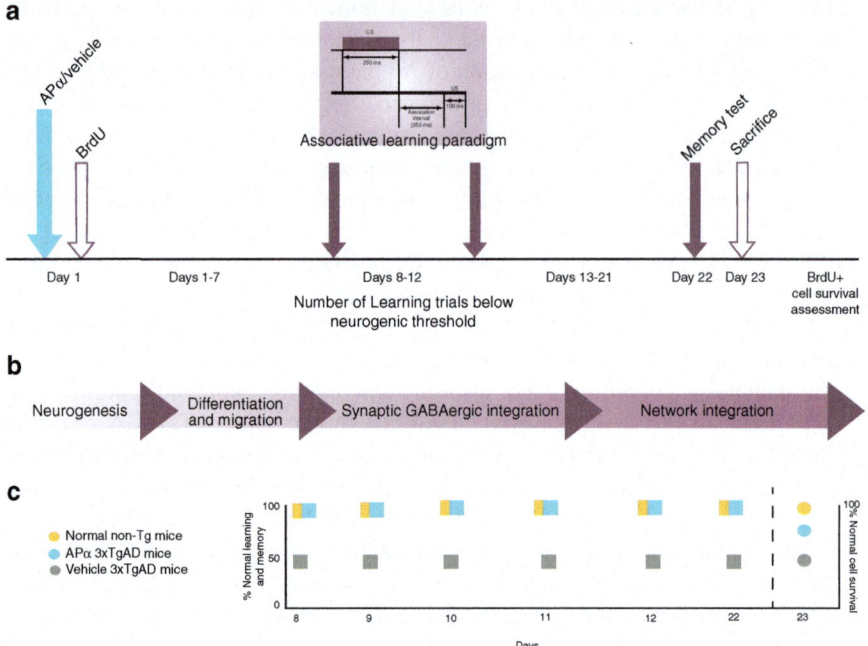

Fig. 7.4 Single treatment of allopregnanolone restores learning and memory function and new neuron survival in aged 3×TgAD and normal wild-type mice. Restoration of cognitive function aligns with the time course of proliferation, migration, and network integration

from this particular treatment design and behavioral analyses make it unlikely that the restoration of cognition after a single administration of Allo is due to mechanisms other than the generation and survival of new neurons.

To better understand how a single exposure of Allo could impact learning and memory function in subsequent weeks after its administration, one must take a close look at the process of neurogenesis and the circuit integration phase in the dentate gyrus. Newly arrived neurons have a reduced threshold for induction of long-term potentiation coupled with increased synaptic plasticity, which is a critical phenotype for neural network formation. This early period of residence within the dentate gyrus corresponds to a critical period when activity and experience can modify survival and network integration of these newly arrived neurons [41]. Disruption of this critical period can result in reduced integration and survival of newly generated neurons and be associated with deficits in long-term memory [40]. Based on the timeline for generation and integration of newly generated neurons, neurogenesis induced by Allo after its administration (day 1) would have generated neurons arriving in the dentate gyrus the following week (Fig. 7.4b). During the associative learning phase, these neurons would have received GABAergic inputs and increased synaptic plasticity, which would be manifested as increased learning. By day 21 these neurons would have received glutamatergic inputs and integrated into dentate and CA3 neural circuits, which would be manifested as memory of the learned association. Allo-induced neurogenesis, survival of newly generated neurons, and behavioral outcomes are consistent with a conceptual framework that links the unique properties of immature neurons to associative learning across time and with the memory functions of the hippocampal circuit [41].

In humans, Allo seemingly improved cognition and partially alleviated some aspects of neurodegeneration in patients with fragile X-associated tremor/ataxia syndrome [44]. Currently clinical trials are underway to evaluate the effect of Allo in patients with early AD.

7.3   Allopregnanolone Reduces Alzheimer's Pathology Burden

A major challenge for regenerative strategies for AD is that the burden of pathology progressively increases with age and duration of disease. Thus, regenerative therapeutic regimens, while principally targeting the regenerative system of the brain, must also address pathological burden of the disease. Such is the case with Allo, whose regenerative effect co-varies with age and AD pathology burden. In the 3×TgAD mice model, Allo was neurogenically active in mice aged 3–9 months but was no longer effective in 12-month-old mice, which were heavily burdened with extraneuronal ß-amyloid plaques [13, 45]. Chronically Allo-treated 3×TgAD mice once per week for 6 months reduced the burden of AD pathology compared to vehicle (Fig. 7.4) [46]. Allo significantly reduced the generation of intracellular Aß oligomers and, in particular, the oligomeric form associated with synaptic dysfunction, Aß*56 [47]. Consistent with the decrease of Aß oligomers, the mitochondrial protein Aß-binding alcohol dehydrogenase (ABAD) was also significantly reduced [46]. The mechanisms underlying Allo-induced reduction of Aß generation involve both the glial-associated liver X receptor (LXR) and the neuron-associated pregnane X receptor (PXR) transcription factors which together activate systems of responses required for cholesterol transport, metabolism, and efflux [46, 48]. LXR functions as a cholesterol sensor to protect against elevated cholesterol by increasing transcription of cholesterol trafficking and efflux pathways, specifically the ABC transporters ABCA1 and ABCG1, which facilitate transfer of cholesterol to ApoE for transport between glial and neuronal compartments or across the blood-brain barrier for efflux to the periphery [24, 49, 50]. Activation of the LXR pathway is associated with significant reduction in Aß generation and recovery of cognitive function in multiple preclinical models of AD [35, 48, 50, 51]. In parallel, PXR provides a neuronal protective mechanism against cholesterol oxidation products [28] principally generated by free radicals that produce lipid peroxides. Once activated, PXR regulates the expression of cytochrome P450, conjugating enzymes, and transporters required for detoxification and clearance [52]. Within brain, PXR transcriptionally regulates P450 enzymes including CYP3A4 [27], CYP3A11, and CYP3A13. The latter two, CYP3A11 and CYP3A13, are highly expressed in hippocampal pyramidal and granule neurons [53]. Together, LXR and PXR act synergistically to regulate clearance of both enzymatic and nonenzymatic cholesterol-derived oxysterols from the brain thereby reducing Aß generation and neurotoxicity. Because the mechanisms underlying Allo reduction of Aß are upstream to γ-secretase activation and do not target physical sequestration and removal of Aß, Allo should not encounter the clinical pitfalls of γ-secretase/notch inhibitors or antibodies against Aß.

Inflammation is a feature of neurodegenerative diseases in general and in particular of AD [54]. Consistent with increased clearance of cholesterol and reduction in Aß generation, Allo significantly reduced microglia activation in the 3×TgAD brain, particularly hippocampus [46] (Fig. 7.5). These findings from our translational analyses are consistent with observations in multiple preclinical models of neurodegenerative disease, Niemann-Pick type C disease [28, 55], traumatic brain and spinal cord injury [56], and multiple sclerosis [57], in which Allo reduced inflammatory microglial activation and pro-inflammatory cytokine gene expression. The exact mechanisms of Allo anti-inflammatory effects are not known. One possibility is that Allo directly activates anti-inflammatory pathways. Alternatively, the reduction in pathology may be driving the decline in inflammatory markers.

7.4   Allopregnanolone Regenerative Treatment Regimen

Therapeutics and regimens of treatment that promote endogenous regeneration and are temporally aligned with renewal processes in vivo have the potential to translate from preclinical to clinical efficacy. Results of preclinical translational

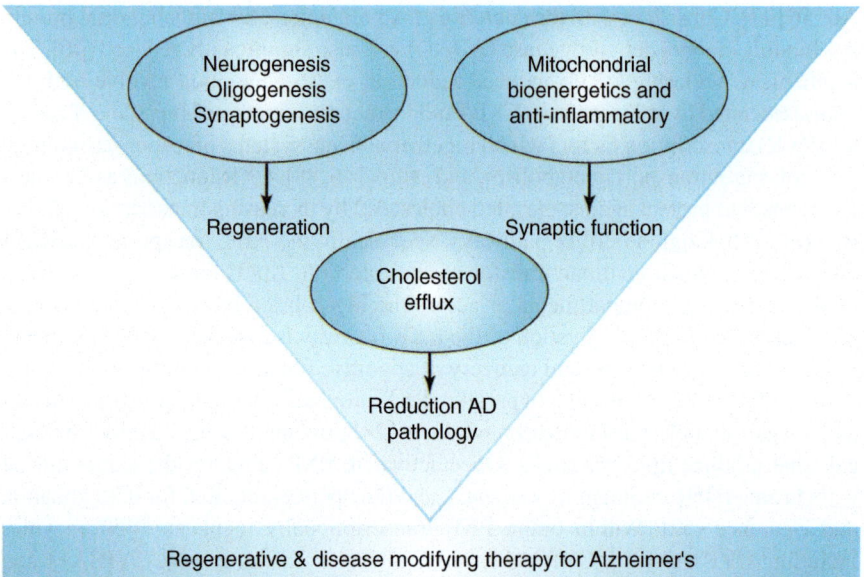

Fig. 7.5 Allopregnanolone is a systems biology therapeutic that simultaneously promotes regeneration, mitochondrial function, cholesterol efflux, and reduction in burden of AD pathology

analyses indicate that an optimal treatment regimen of Allo is one that is administered once per week over the course of months [46] (Fig. 7.6). Using such treatment regimen, Allo significantly increased survival of newly generated neurons; simultaneously reduced Aß generation in the hippocampus, cortex, and amygdala; and reduced microglial activation. The strategy is to activate the systems and let them proceed to recruit all members and functions of the system under their innate time course. Ceasing activation to avoid repression mechanisms is just as important as starting the process. Multiple neurodegenerative preclinical models indicate that episodic and intermittent Allo treatment regimens are optimally efficacious for regeneration, increased survival, and restoration of function (Fig. 7.5) [11, 12, 19, 43, 58–60].

Previous analyses have documented that more Allo for longer periods of time is not better [48] (Fig. 7.6). Continuous infusion of Allo for 30–90 days at high doses can worsen pathology in a preclinical amyloid model of AD. Further, administering sedative hypnotic doses of Allo can induce modest memory impairments immediately after infusion [61–63]. The reported impairment was based on a word recall task but no effect occurred on either semantic or working memory test [63]. This finding in humans coupled with preclinical dose-response analyses indicate that, as with many therapeutics, dose and duration of exposure matter [48]. For Allo, more for longer is not better.

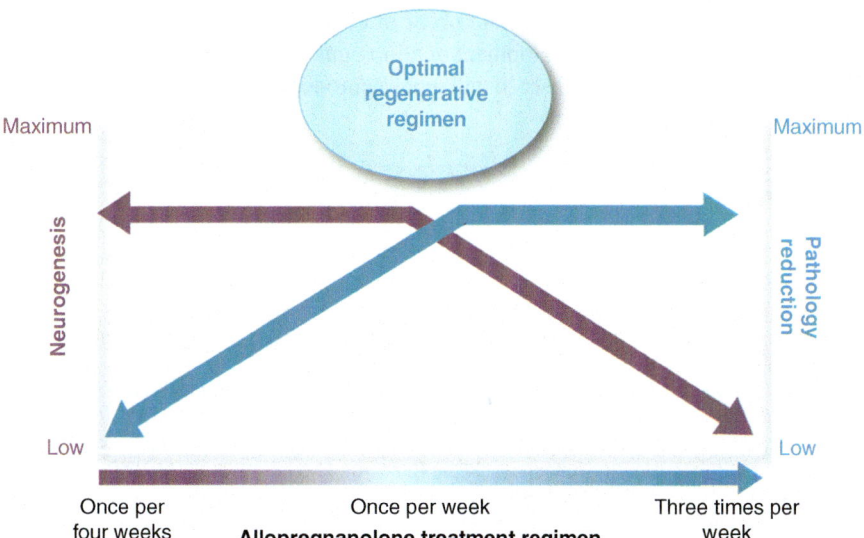

Fig. 7.6 Allopregnanolone optimal regenerative treatment regimen. A once per week treatment regimen of Allo was optimal to maximally promote neurogenesis while also activating systems that reduced AD pathology. By contrast, a single exposure to Allo induced neurogenesis and behavioral recovery but had no effect on pathology, whereas a treatment regimen of three times per week for 3 months suppressed neurogenesis but greatly reduced AD pathology

The first clinical study investigating the safety, tolerability, and pharmacokinetics of Allo in AD patients has recently been concluded (ClinicalTrials.gov Identifier: NCT02221622).

7.5   Conclusions

Regenerative medicine and therapeutics hold the promise of self-renewal and repair. The challenge is to access the innate regenerative potential of the brain in order to halt or even reverse the downward path of degeneration. To accomplish this mission, it is critical to activate the regenerative system while simultaneously addressing the etiology underlying degeneration.

As we enter the era of precision medicine, we are exploring new ways to evolve the drug development process so that treatment advances can be matched to specific diseases and specific patients. In the twenty-first century, there is no therapeutics to cure any of the neurodegenerative diseases. Allo is an innovative therapeutic for Alzheimer's disease that has the potential to regenerate the degenerated brain by targeting the regenerative system of the brain while simultaneously activating systems to reduce AD pathology burden [1, 11, 12, 26, 64, 65]. Identifying the subset of the population that is likely to respond to Allo and targeting them with the precise dosing regimen for regeneration and repair in the human brain will improve the probability of clinical efficacy.

The extensive efficacious preclinical studies and previous human safety data [44, 66], coupled with a recent safety and proof of concept clinical trial, are all strong foundation for the clinical development of allopregnanolone as the first regenerative therapeutic for Alzheimer's disease and other neurodegenerative diseases.

References

1. Wang JM, Johnston PB, Ball BG, Brinton RD. The neurosteroid allopregnanolone promotes proliferation of rodent and human neural progenitor cells and regulates cell-cycle gene and protein expression. J Neurosci. 2005;25(19):4706–18.
2. Mellon SH. Neurosteroid regulation of central nervous system development. Pharmacol Ther. 2007;116(1):107–24.
3. Majewska MD, Harrison NL, Schwartz RD, Barker JL, Paul SM. Steroid hormone metabolites are barbiturate-like modulators of the GABA receptor. Science. 1986;232(4753):1004–7.
4. Genazzani AR, Petraglia F, Bernardi F, et al. Circulating levels of allopregnanolone in humans: gender, age, and endocrine influences. J Clin Endocrinol Metab. 1998;83(6):2099–103.
5. Dombroski RA, Casey ML, MacDonald PC. 5-Alpha-dihydroprogesterone formation in human placenta from 5alpha-pregnan-3beta/alpha-ol-20-ones and 5-pregnan-3beta-yl-20-one sulfate. J Steroid Biochem Mol Biol. 1997;63(1-3):155–63.
6. Luisi S, Petraglia F, Benedetto C, et al. Serum allopregnanolone levels in pregnant women: changes during pregnancy, at delivery, and in hypertensive patients. J Clin Endocrinol Metab. 2000;85(7):2429–33.
7. Gago N, El-Etr M, Sananes N, et al. 3α, 5α-tetrahydroprogesterone (allopregnanolone) and γ-aminobutyric acid: autocrine/paracrine interactions in the control of neonatal PSA-NCAM+ progenitor proliferation. J Neurosci Res. 2004;78(6):770–83.

8. Bernardi F, Salvestroni C, Casarosa E, et al. Aging is associated with changes in allopreg-nanolone concentrations in brain, endocrine glands and serum in male rats. Eur J Endocrinol. 1998;138(3):316–21.

9. Weill-Engerer S, David JP, Sazdovitch V, et al. Neurosteroid quantification in human brain regions: comparison between Alzheimer's and nondemented patients. J Clin Endocrinol Metab. 2002;87(11):5138–43.

10. Lledo PM, Alonso M, Grubb MS. Adult neurogenesis and functional plasticity in neuronal circuits. Nat Rev Neurosci. 2006;7(3):179–93.

11. Brinton RD. Neurosteroids as regenerative agents in the brain: therapeutic implications. Nat Rev Endocrinol. 2013;9(4):241–50.

12. Singh C, Liu L, Wang JM, et al. Allopregnanolone restores hippocampal-dependent learning and memory and neural progenitor survival in aging 3×TgAD and nonTg mice. Neurobiol Aging. 2012;33(8):1493–506.

13. Kuhn HG, Dickinson-Anson H, Gage FH. Neurogenesis in the dentate gyrus of the adult rat: age-related decrease of neuronal progenitor proliferation. J Neurosci. 1996;16(6):2027–33.

14. Wang JM, Singh C, Liu L, et al. Allopregnanolone reverses neurogenic and cognitive deficits in mouse model of Alzheimer's disease. Proc Natl Acad Sci. 2010;107(14):6498–503.

15. Lazarov O, Mattson MP, Peterson DA, Pimplikar SW, van Praag H. When neurogenesis encounters aging and disease. Trends Neurosci. 2010;33(12):569–79.

16. Hattiangady B, Shetty AK. Aging does not alter the number or phenotype of putative stem/progenitor cells in the neurogenic region of the hippocampus. Neurobiol Aging. 2008;29(1):129–47.

17. Lugert S, Basak O, Knuckles P, et al. Quiescent and active hippocampal neural stem cells with distinct morphologies respond selectively to physiological and pathological stimuli and aging. Cell Stem Cell. 2010;6(5):445–56.

18. Marx CE, Trost WT, Shampine LJ, et al. The neurosteroid allopregnanolone is reduced in prefrontal cortex in Alzheimer's disease. Biol Psychiatry. 2006;60(12):1287–94.

19. Sun C, Ou X, Farley JM, et al. Allopregnanolone increases the number of dopaminergic neurons in substantia nigra of a triple transgenic mouse model of Alzheimer's disease. Curr Alzheimer Res. 2012;9(4):473–80.

20. Schumacher M, Hussain R, Gago N, Oudinet JP, Mattern C, Ghoumari AM. Progesterone synthesis in the nervous system: implications for myelination and myelin repair. Front Neurosci. 2012;6:10.

21. Brinton RD, Wang JM. Therapeutic potential of neurogenesis for prevention and recovery from Alzheimer's disease: allopregnanolone as a proof of concept neurogenic agent. Curr Alzheimer Res. 2006;3(3):185–90.

22. Carver CM, Reddy DS. Neurosteroid interactions with synaptic and extrasynaptic GABA(A) receptors: regulation of subunit plasticity, phasic and tonic inhibition, and neuronal network excitability. Psychopharmacology. 2013;230(2):151–88.

23. Saher G, Brugger B, Lappe-Siefke C, et al. High cholesterol level is essential for myelin membrane growth. Nat Neurosci. 2005;8(4):468–75.

24. Repa JJ, Li H, Frank-Cannon TC, et al. Liver X receptor activation enhances cholesterol loss from the brain, decreases neuroinflammation, and increases survival of the NPC1 mouse. J Neurosci. 2007;27(52):14470–80.

25. Leduc V, Jasmin-Belanger S, Poirier J. APOE and cholesterol homeostasis in Alzheimer's disease. Trends Mol Med. 2010;16(10):469–77.

26. Chen S, Wang JM, Irwin RW, Yao J, Liu L, Brinton RD. Allopregnanolone promotes regeneration and reduces β-amyloid burden in a preclinical model of Alzheimer's disease. PLoS One. 2011;6(8):e24293.

27. Lamba V, Yasuda K, Lamba JK, et al. PXR (NR1I2): splice variants in human tissues, including brain, and identification of neurosteroids and nicotine as PXR activators. Toxicol Appl Pharmacol. 2004;199(3):251–65.

28. Langmade SJ, Gale SE, Frolov A, et al. Pregnane X receptor (PXR) activation: a mechanism for neuroprotection in a mouse model of Niemann-Pick C disease. Proc Natl Acad Sci U S A. 2006;103(37):13807–12.

29. Koldamova RP, Lefterov IM, Staufenbiel M, et al. The liver X receptor ligand T0901317 decreases amyloid beta production in vitro and in a mouse model of Alzheimer's disease. J Biol Chem. 2005;280(6):4079–88.

30. Whitney KD, Watson MA, Collins JL, et al. Regulation of cholesterol homeostasis by the liver X receptors in the central nervous system. Mol Endocrinol. 2002;16(6):1378–85.

31. Schultz JR, Tu H, Luk A, et al. Role of LXRs in control of lipogenesis. Genes Dev. 2000;14(22):2831–8.

32. Xiong H, Callaghan D, Jones A, et al. Cholesterol retention in Alzheimer's brain is responsible for high beta- and gamma-secretase activities and Abeta production. Neurobiol Dis. 2008;29(3):422–37.

33. Sun Y, Yao J, Kim TW, Tall AR. Expression of liver X receptor target genes decreases cellular amyloid beta peptide secretion. J Biol Chem. 2003;278(30):27688–94.

34. Yang Y, Varvel NH, Lamb BT, Herrup K. Ectopic cell cycle events link human Alzheimer's disease and amyloid precursor protein transgenic mouse models. J Neurosci. 2006;26(3):775–84.

35. Riddell DR, Zhou H, Comery TA, et al. The LXR agonist TO901317 selectively lowers hippocampal Abeta42 and improves memory in the Tg2576 mouse model of Alzheimer's disease. Mol Cell Neurosci. 2007;34(4):621–8.

36. Jiang Q, Lee CY, Mandrekar S, et al. ApoE promotes the proteolytic degradation of Abeta. Neuron. 2008;58(5):681–93.

37. Donkin JJ, Stukas S, Hirsch-Reinshagen V, et al. ATP-binding cassette transporter A1 mediates the beneficial effects of the liver-X-receptor agonist GW3965 on object recognition memory and amyloid burden in APP/PS1 mice. J Biol Chem. 2010;285(44):34144–54.

38. Shenoy SD, Spencer TA, Mercer-Haines NA, et al. CYP3A induction by liver x receptor ligands in primary cultured rat and mouse hepatocytes is mediated by the pregnane X receptor. Drug Metab Dispos. 2004;32(1):66–71.

39. Sonoda J, Xie W, Rosenfeld JM, Barwick JL, Guzelian PS, Evans RM. Regulation of a xenobiotic sulfonation cascade by nuclear pregnane X receptor (PXR). Proc Natl Acad Sci U S A. 2002;99(21):13801–6.

40. Shors TJ, Townsend DA, Zhao M, Kozorovitskiy Y, Gould E. Neurogenesis may relate to some but not all types of hippocampal-dependent learning. Hippocampus. 2002;12(5):578–84.

41. Deng W, Aimone JB, Gage FH. New neurons and new memories: how does adult hippocampal neurogenesis affect learning and memory? Nat Rev Neurosci. 2010;11(5):339–50.

42. Aimone JB, Deng W, Gage FH. Resolving new memories: a critical look at the dentate gyrus, adult neurogenesis, and pattern separation. Neuron. 2011;70(4):589–96.

43. Wang JM, Singh C, Liu L, et al. Allopregnanolone reverses neurogenic and cognitive deficits in mouse model of Alzheimer's disease. Proc Natl Acad Sci U S A. 2010;107(14):6498–503.

44. Wang JY, Trivedi AM, Carrillo NR, et al. Open-label allopregnanolone treatment of men with fragile X-associated tremor/ataxia syndrome. Neurotherapeutics. 2017;14(4):1073–83.

45. Haughey NJ, Liu D, Nath A, Borchard AC, Mattson MP. Disruption of neurogenesis in the subventricular zone of adult mice, and in human cortical neuronal precursor cells in culture, by amyloid beta-peptide: implications for the pathogenesis of Alzheimer's disease. NeuroMolecular Med. 2002;1(2):125–35.

46. Chen S, Wang JM, Irwin RW, Yao J, Liu L, Brinton RD. Allopregnanolone promotes regeneration and reduces beta-amyloid burden in a preclinical model of Alzheimer's disease. PLoS One. 2011;6(8):e24293.

47. Lesne S, Koh MT, Kotilinek L, et al. A specific amyloid-beta protein assembly in the brain impairs memory. Nature. 2006;440(7082):352–7.

48. Irwin RW, Wang JM, Chen S, Brinton RD. Neuroregenerative mechanisms of allopregnanolone in Alzheimer's disease. Front Endocrinol. 2011;2:117.

49. Kang J, Rivest S. Lipid metabolism and neuroinflammation in Alzheimer's disease: a role for liver X receptors. Endocr Rev. 2012;33(5):715–46.

50. Mandrekar-Colucci S, Karlo JC, Landreth GE. Mechanisms underlying the rapid peroxisome proliferator-activated receptor-gamma-mediated amyloid clearance and reversal of cognitive deficits in a murine model of Alzheimer's disease. J Neurosci. 2012;32(30):10117–28.
51. Cramer PE, Cirrito JR, Wesson DW, et al. ApoE-directed therapeutics rapidly clear beta-amyloid and reverse deficits in AD mouse models. Science. 2012;335(6075):1503–6.
52. Willson TM, Kliewer SA. PXR, CAR and drug metabolism. Nat Rev Drug Discov. 2002;1(4):259–66.
53. Hagemeyer CE, Rosenbrock H, Ditter M, Knoth R, Volk B. Predominantly neuronal expression of cytochrome P450 isoforms CYP3A11 and CYP3A13 in mouse brain. Neuroscience. 2003;117(3):521–9.
54. Skovronsky DM, Lee VM, Trojanowski JQ. Neurodegenerative diseases: new concepts of pathogenesis and their therapeutic implications. Annu Rev Pathol. 2006;1:151–70.
55. Zampieri S, Mellon SH, Butters TD, et al. Oxidative stress in NPC1 deficient cells: protective effect of allopregnanolone. J Cell Mol Med. 2009;13(9B):3786–96.
56. He J, Evans CO, Hoffman SW, Oyesiku NM, Stein DG. Progesterone and allopregnanolone reduce inflammatory cytokines after traumatic brain injury. Exp Neurol. 2004;189(2):404–12.
57. Noorbakhsh F, Ellestad KK, Maingat F, et al. Impaired neurosteroid synthesis in multiple sclerosis. Brain. 2011;134(Pt 9):2703–21.
58. Griffin LD, Gong W, Verot L, Mellon SH. Niemann-Pick type C disease involves disrupted neurosteroidogenesis and responds to allopregnanolone. Nat Med. 2004;10(7):704–11.
59. Melcangi RC, Giatti S, Pesaresi M, et al. Role of neuroactive steroids in the peripheral nervous system. Front Endocrinol. 2011;2:104.
60. Adeosun SO, Hou X, Jiao Y, et al. Allopregnanolone reinstates tyrosine hydroxylase immunoreactive neurons and motor performance in an MPTP-lesioned mouse model of Parkinson's disease. PLoS One. 2012;7(11):e50040.
61. Lan NC, Gee KW. Neuroactive steroid actions at the GABAA receptor. Horm Behav. 1994;28(4):537–44.
62. Reddy DS, Rogawski MA. Neurosteroid replacement therapy for catamenial epilepsy. Neurotherapeutics. 2009;6(2):392–401.
63. Kask K, Backstrom T, Nilsson LG, Sundstrom-Poromaa I. Allopregnanolone impairs episodic memory in healthy women. Psychopharmacology. 2008;199(2):161–8.
64. Irwin RW, Brinton RD. Allopregnanolone as regenerative therapeutic for Alzheimer's disease: translational development and clinical promise. Prog Neurobiol. 2014;113:40–55.
65. Irwin RW, Solinsky CM, Brinton RD. Frontiers in therapeutic development of allopregnanolone for Alzheimer's disease and other neurological disorders. Front Cell Neurosci. 2014;8:203.
66. van Broekhoven F, Backstrom T, van Luijtelaar G, Buitelaar JK, Smits P, Verkes RJ. Effects of allopregnanolone on sedation in men, and in women on oral contraceptives. Psychoneuroendocrinology. 2007;32(5):555–64.

Reproductive Depression and the Response to Hormone Therapy

8

John W. Studd, Mike Savvas, and Neale Watson

Many cases of depression in women are due to endocrine factors and inappropriate treatment by antidepressants or mood-stabilizing drugs such as lithium. The syndrome reproductive depression includes premenstrual depression (PMDD), postnatal depression (PND) and climacteric depression which is more severe in the transitional phase 2 or 3 years before the periods cease rather than in the years after the menopause. Such patients are usually free of depression during pregnancy. The diagnosis cannot be made by measuring hormone levels but by a careful history relating depression to monthly cycles and the postnatal state. The range and aetiology of depression in women is different than in men and cannot be understood without knowledge of the effect that oestrogen, progesterone and androgens have upon mood. These frequent problems are usually treated badly by psychiatrists who have little knowledge and less interest in the effect of hormones on mood. Treatment should be by oestrogens preferably by the transdermal route possibly with the addition of testosterone and if necessary the addition of progesterone to protect the endometrium.

It is probable that the first quantitative account of the different incidence of depression in women and men came from Charles Dickens [1] who studied the records of St Luke's hospital for the insane reporting in his journal *Household Words* the increase of admission for depression in women. He claimed that this increase in depression occurred particularly in "women of the servant class", thus indicating the effect of both gender and social deprivation on mental illness. The excess of depression in women compared with men can be the result of social and

J. W. Studd (✉)
London PMS and Menopause Centre, London, UK
e-mail: laptop@studd.co.uk

M. Savvas
King's College Hospital, London, UK
e-mail: mike.savvas@nhs.net

N. Watson
Hillingdon Hospital, Middlesex, UK
e-mail: nrwatson@mac.com

© International Society of Gynecological Endocrinology 2019
R. D. Brinton et al. (eds.), *Sex Steroids' Effects on Brain, Heart and Vessels*,
ISGE Series, https://doi.org/10.1007/978-3-030-11355-1_8

environmental factors, but most convincingly it occurs at times of hormonal fluctuation and is a result of these endocrine changes.

8.1   Reproductive Depression and Ovarian Hormones

Depression in women commonly occurs at times of hormonal changes [2], most commonly seen with depression in the premenstrual days. There is also a peak of depression in the postnatal months, often following a pregnancy characterised by a good mood with less depression. Later in life depression occurs at its most severe in the 2 or 3 years before the periods cease in the menopausal transition. Together these three components of premenstrual depression, postnatal depression and climacteric depression with its probable endocrine aetiology mostly influenced by changes in ovarian hormones are best termed "reproductive depression" [3]. This name gives emphasis to the fact that it is a hormone-mediated mood change, wider than the name PMMD would suggest and which may well be most effectively treated by correction of these hormonal changes [4].

These peaks of depression often occur in the same woman. The typical story is one who has mild to moderate PMS as a teenager which may become worse with age with fewer good days per month. When pregnancy occurs they are normally in a good mood throughout pregnancy in spite of possible common problems such as nausea, pre-eclampsia or other obstetric complications. After delivery they develop postnatal depression for many months, and it is at this point that women often have their first "nervous breakdown". They are treated with various antidepressants which are barely effective. When the periods return, the depression becomes cyclical and more severe but improves with subsequent pregnancies. They still have cyclical depression in their 40s, and the depression becomes worse in the 2 or 3 years of the menopause transition [5]. If they develop vasomotor symptoms of flushes and sweats, they may be given oestrogens which will cure these symptoms and usually often help the depression.

With this history in mind, it is important to realise that hormone-responsive depression cannot be diagnosed by any blood test. Too frequently women who believe that their depression is related to her hormone visit their family doctor, their gynaecologist or psychiatrist who measures their hormone levels which are normal and the association with hormonal changes is dismissed. These are all premenopausal women who will have normal FSH and oestradiol levels which may not be optimal for the individual but are normal. It is a huge mistake to exclude hormone-responsive depression because of normal blood levels [2]. The clue to the diagnosis is in the history, and even then psychiatrists will often regard the association of depression with periods and postpartum changes as irrelevant, and the role of hormones for the treatment of depression in women requires further study [6].

8.2   Premenstrual Depression

Most women will be aware of physical and mood changes a day or two before the periods which indicates that they are premenstrual, but this is not a severe abnormality. Perhaps 10% of women suffer severe premenstrual syndrome for 10–14 days a month with severe depression, behavioural changes, anxiety, aggression, loss of energy, loss of libido and somatic symptoms of headaches, abdominal bloating and mastalgia.

The American Association of Psychiatrists in their DSM IV publication has termed this premenstrual dysphoric disorder. The word dysphoric strongly indicates a psychiatric origin of a condition we can now view as incorrect. The motive behind this renaming by psychiatrists is one done for a reason of territory and of course reimbursement in the American system. "Ovarian cycle syndrome" would be a better name as it clearly establishes the cyclical and hormonal aetiology of the condition and the fact that the ovary is the architect of these changes, but this has not found favour with psychiatrists involved in the treatment of "PMDD", and gynaecologist will continue to refer to the disorder as premenstrual syndrome—PMS. A working party of many experts both psychiatrists and gynecologists was set up to clarify nomenclature diagnosis and treatment has had four meetings with conclusions as confused as at the outset [7].

This most common component of reproductive depression is an endocrine problem due to the hormonal changes that occur following ovulation, and it is logical that effective treatment should be one which suppresses ovulation and suppresses the ovarian hormonal changes (whatever they are) that produce the cyclical symptoms of the premenstrual syndrome. In our view the most logical and easiest way to suppress ovulation is the birth control pill, but the combined contraceptive pill is associated with an increase in depression [8] because these women are usually progesterone/progestogen intolerant [9], and hence the birth control pill even when taken "back to back" will suppress cycles and even suppress bleeding, but they may have depressive and somatic symptoms most of the time without having the usual 10–14 good days a month that even the most severe cases enjoy. The progestogen-only pill or Depot-Provera usually produces increasing depression.

Suppression of ovulation by transdermal oestradiol in the form of oestradiol patch 200 μg twice weekly has been shown to be effective [10] and transdermal oestrogen in the form of oestradiol gels, Oestrogel two measures daily or Sandrena 2 g/day, will also be effective. It is necessary to give cyclical progestogen by some route to prevent endometrial hyperplasia, but it is common for the PMS symptoms to recur during these days; hence a minimum duration of progestogen is recommended for the first 7–10 days of each calendar month with a withdrawal bleeding occurring on about day 10–13 of each calendar month. Alternatively a Mirena IUS is usually very effective although perhaps 10% of women do have absorption of the d-norgestrel and suffer almost continuous PMS symptoms [11]. These symptoms disappear within 24 h of the removal of the Mirena IUS.

Alternatively ablation of ovulation by the use of GnRH analogues is the most effective [12] and indeed is a useful diagnostic tool if a hysterectomy and bilateral salpingo-oophorectomy are contemplated. There is a risk of distressing menopausal symptoms and even osteopenia, so add-back HRT is essential if prolonged treatment is required. This will usually be in the form of transdermal oestradiol and cyclical oral progestogen [12–14] which may produce a return of PMS symptoms or the insertion of a Mirena IUS. Using tibolone as add-back is an effective way of avoiding bleeding and progestogenic side effects [15].

Women with severe PMS who respond partially to treatment because of progestogenic side effects or bleeding problems should be offered a hysterectomy and bilateral salpingo-oophorectomy. A hysterectomy alone is not effective because the ovaries will still produce the cyclical hormonal changes and the cyclical symptoms although menstruation has been abolished the cyclical symptoms have not.

There are now many studies showing the very beneficial effect of surgery and long-term replacement therapy for the most severe PMS [16, 17]. This is a further example to indicate that the condition is endocrine and not psychiatric.

The great danger to women with severe PMS who do not respond to antidepressants is that they are given a higher dose and then a second or third antidepressant which also does not work. They are then diagnosed as the DSMV favourites "borderline personality disorder" and "treatment resistant depression" and are then they are labelled as bipolar disorder and the scene is set for mood stabilising drugs, antidepressants hospitalisation and even electroconvulsive therapy. After 10 or more years of this therapy, it is difficult but not impossible to wean off these psychotropic drugs by transdermal oestradiol which they should have had in the first place. The clues of course are in the history.

There are eight vital questions to diagnose PMS and to exclude bipolar disorder [18].

1. Relating depressive episodes to the menstrual cycle.
2. The relief of depressive symptoms during pregnancy.
3. The recurrence of depression postpartum.
4. Premenstrual depression on menstruation recurs after delivery.
5. The premenstrual depression becoming worse with age blending into the menopausal transition.
6. Often the coexistence of somatic symptoms such as menstrual migraine, abdominal bloating or cyclical mastalgia.
7. These patients usually have seven to 10 good days per month.
8. Although depression can be cyclical, they rarely have highs.

Another useful observation is that women who breast-feed for a long time have little depression during lactation, but when they stop after a year or so, ovulation returns as do the cycles and the depression which is often as severe as it is unexpected.

The place of antidepressants and oral contraception for PMDD has been recently reviewed and supported by a psychiatrist [19] giving no support to the use of transdermal oestrogens.

8.3   Postnatal Depression

The seriousness of this condition cannot be overstated as both the mother and the child can be in great danger. It occurs in 10% of healthy women and can last for months or years. It is not the "baby blues" occurring in the week after delivery. It is usually treated with varying success with antidepressant drugs, psychotherapy or admission to mother and baby units, but once again the association with profound, abrupt hormone changes after childbirth should point to a hormonal aetiology. Prolonged breast-feeding which is associated with lower oestradiol levels often produces more severe and prolonged depression.

Depression has been reproduced experimentally in women with a history of post-natal depression by creating a pseudopregnancy with excess doses of oestradiol and progesterone which is then suddenly discontinued [20]. Depression occurred in women with a history of postnatal depression but not in the women in the study without a previous history of postnatal problems. Transdermal oestradiol is effective in the treatment of postnatal depression even in those women who have inadequately responded to antidepressants [21]. Unfortunately psychiatrists rarely use this ther-apy preferring antidepressants, psychotherapy or admission to mother and baby units. Formerly progesterone and progestogen have been recommended, but there is no evidence that they are effective. On the contrary, studies have shown them to be ineffective, and the Cochrane report has agreed that oestrogen improves mood and postnatal depression and norethisterone makes depression worse [22].

8.4   Climacteric Depression

There are many reasons why women become depressed around the time of meno-pause. Hot flushes and sweats produce insomnia and social embarrassment, head-aches are troublesome and the vaginal atrophy producing dyspareunia and recurrent cystitis together with loss of libido is enough to cause some depression. These typi-cal symptoms of oestrogen deficiency can easily be treated with routine HRT, and the low mood associated with these problems of sexuality and sleep is improved [2]. However there is another type of depression not associated with characteristic menopausal symptoms in the 3 or 4 years before the periods cease, the so-called menopausal transition [23]. This is the depression that occurs usually in the absence of vasomotor symptoms or vaginal dryness and has been shown in many studies to be responsive to oestrogens, both oral oestrogens and transdermal oestrogens [24, 25]. In fact, the evidence for the benefit of oestrogens on perimenopausal depression is more convincing than the beneficial effects in the depression of the postmeno-pausal woman [26]. This treatment is best done by transdermal oestrogens in the form of gels or patches continuously with cyclical progestogen if the woman has a uterus [2]. Gynaecologists are aware that depression occurring in *most* perimeno-pausal women responds well to oestrogens given for the depression or associated symptoms although most psychiatrists are unaware of this because they do not use oestrogens. Antidepressants would be their first choice therapy. Recently a debate on this issue was strongly supported by one side [27], but the psychiatrist was of the view that more evidence from trials were required [28].

8.5   Hysterectomy

It may seem odd to include a section of hysterectomy, but there is much evidence from psychiatrists that depression is less common after hysterectomy [29]. In spite of this, virtually all newspaper and magazine articles on this subject stress the belief that hysterectomy causes profound depression, loss of sexuality and marital break-up. The reverse is true. In younger women having persistent cyclical depression as well as other cyclical problems of bleeding, pain and cyclical headaches and hysterectomy with bilateral oophorectomy will usually cure these problems. In the specific case of premenstrual depression in those women with progestogen intolerance, hysterectomy with bilateral oophorectomy and replacement of oestradiol and testosterone have been shown in all studies to be beneficial [30]. Thus a well conducted hysterectomy for the correct indication should be seen as a life enhancing procedure, will remove the need for progestogen and avoid the 4% of women who die of cancer of the ovary, cervix and uterus should be seen as a life saving as well as a life enhancing procedure [31]. This should not be seen as a radical last choice—or never choice option.

8.6   General Principles of Hormone Therapy for Reproductive Depression

The use of transdermal oestrogens is recommended to suppress ovulation in women with premenstrual syndrome or in correcting the profound oestrogen decrease with postpartum depression. It should be the first choice therapy in perimenopausal women with depression whether they have associated vasomotor symptoms or not. But such therapy does not exclude the combined therapy with antidepressants [32]. Most studies looking at hormone-responsive depression have used transdermal patches or implants, but there is no reason why oral oestrogen should not be effective although the appropriate studies have yet to be published. However, transdermal oestrogens are preferable because they do not invoke hepatic coagulation factors and are not associated with the higher rates of venous thromboembolism of oral oestrogens. The preferred regimen would be oestradiol patches 200 μg twice weekly or oestradiol gels 2–4 g daily throughout the month. Cyclical progestogen in women with a uterus should be used for the first 7 days of each calendar month which would produce a scanty withdrawal bleed on approximately day 10 of each calendar month.

The monthly progestogen duration has been reduced from the orthodox 14 days as these women with depression are usually progestogen intolerant and, there is now mounting evidence that the major side effects of HRT are related to the progestogen component.

For the women with libido and energy problems which often coexist with depression and treatment by antidepressants, testosterone can be added in the form of testosterone gel in the appropriate dose. This would be approximately 10% of the average male dose which in practical terms would be one quarter of a sachet of Testogel alternate days or a quarter of a tube of Testim alternate days. One hundred milligram testosterone pellets would be ideal, but at the time of writing they are no longer available.

The cornerstone of our treatment of many types of depression in women is based on the above principles following a detailed history to reveal any current or past association of the depression with menstruation, the postnatal state, the menopausal transition or the postmenopausal state. An audit of the success or otherwise of this practice has been published [33].

An email survey of patients attending the clinic produced 238 patients whose principal presenting symptom was depression. Seventy-seven percent claimed to have had severe or moderate depression, 17% had had at least one psychotic episode and 14% had attempted suicide. Fifty-eight percent had seen a psychiatrist. Seventy-one percent had received antidepressants, and 17% had received mood stabilising drugs such as lithium.

Twelve percent had been admitted to a psychiatric hospital, and 3.8% had received electroconvulsive therapy. Sixty-eight percent had premenstrual syndrome as a teenager, and 145 women (89%) out of 165 women who had been pregnant had no depression during pregnancy, but 110 (66%) developed postnatal depression.

Ninety-seven women (58%) who had been pregnant had suffered both premenstrual depression and postnatal depression.

All were treated with transdermal oestrogens, and 93% also had transdermal testosterone. One hundred and seventy-one patients had a uterus and received cyclical progestogen to protect the endometrium, and 63% of these developed the premenstrual syndrome-type symptoms of progesterone intolerance during the progestogen days. Thirty-five percent of patients claimed to be cured, and 55% had a considerable improvement with oestrogen therapy. Only 3.7% reported that there was no improvement.

For 94%, the hormone therapy was a life-changing event for the better. None were worse. Forty patients had hysterectomy and bilateral oophorectomy for progesterone intolerance or heavy uterine bleeding, and 38 replied that it was life changing for the better with less or no depression.

It is concluded that premenstrual and postnatal depressions appear in the same vulnerable women. These women are typically well during pregnancy and are a subgroup of reproductive depression which also develops climacteric depression in the transition phase. These types of depression are the product of hormonal changes and respond well to transdermal hormone therapy which in our view should be first choice therapy.

8.7 Teaching Points

1. The syndrome of reproductive depression consists of postnatal depression, premenstrual depression and climacteric depression.
2. This depression is caused or aggravated by a fall and fluctuations of oestradiol.
3. These women are often progesterone/progestogen intolerant.
4. This depression cannot be diagnosed or excluded by measuring hormone levels.
5. This depression usually responds to oestrogen therapy.
6. Transdermal oestradiol by gel patch or implant is preferable and safer than oral oestrogens.

References

1. Dickens C. Household words, vol. 95. New York, NY: D. Appleton; 1852. p. 385–9.
2. Studd J. A guide to hormone therapy for the treatment of depression in women. Climacteric. 2011;14:637–42.
3. Studd J, Nappi RE. Reproductive Depression. Gynecol Endocrinol. 2012;28(Suppl 1):42–5.
4. Nappi RE, Tonani S, Santamaria V, Ornati A, Albani F, Pisani C, Polatti F. Luteal phase dysphoric disorder and premenstrual syndrome. It J Psych. 2009;28:27–33.
5. Burger HG, Hale GE, Robertson DN, Dennerstein L. A review of hormonal changes during the menopausal transition. Hum Reprod Update. 2007;13:559–65.
6. Craig MC. Should psychiatrist be prescribing oestrogen therapy to their patients? Br J Psychiatry. 2013;202(1):9–13.
7. Ismaili E, Walsh S, O'Brien PMS, et al. Fourth consensus of the international society of premenstrual disorders (ISPMD): auditable standards for the diagnosis and management of premenstrual disorder. Arch Womens Ment Health. 2016;19(6):953–8.
8. Wessel Skovlund C, Steinrud Morch L, Vedel Kessing L, Liddegaard O. Association of hormonal contraception with depression. JAMA Psychiat. 2016;73(11):1154–62.
9. Panay N, Studd J. Progestogen intolerance and compliance with hormone replacement therapy in menopausal women. Hum Reprod Update. 1997;3:159–71.
10. Watson NR, Studd JWW, Savvas M, Garnett T, Baber RJ. Treatment of severe premenstrual syndrome with oestradiol patches and cyclical oral norethisterone. Lancet. 1989;8665:730–2.
11. Elovainio M, Teperi J, Aalto AM. Depressive symptoms as predictors of discontinuation of levonorgestrel releasing intrauterine system. Int J Behav Med. 2007;14:70–5.
12. Leather AT, Studd JW, Watson NR, Holland EF. The treatment of severe premenstrual syndrome with goserelin with and without 'add-back' estrogen therapy: a placebo-controlled study. Gynecol Endocrinol. 1999;13:48–55.
13. Leather AT, Studd JWW, Watson NR, Holland EFN. The prevention of bone loss in young women treated with GnRh analogues with 'add back' oestrogen therapy. Obstet Gynecol. 1993;81:104–7.
14. Wyatt KM, Dimmock PW, Ismail KM, Jones PW, O'Brien PM. The effectiveness of GnRH analogue with and without "addback" therapy in treating premenstrual syndrome: a meta analysis. BJOG. 2004;111:585–93.
15. Di Carlo C, Palomba S, GAm T, et al. Use of leuprolide acetate plus tibolone in the treatment of severe premenstrual syndrome. Fertil Steril. 2001;76:850–2.
16. Casson P, Hahn PM, Van Vugt DA, Reed RL. Lasting response to ovariectomy in severe intractable premenstrual syndrome. Am Obstet Gynecol. 1990;162:99–105.
17. Cronje WH, Vashisht A, Studd JW. Hysterectomy and bilateral oophorectomy for severe premenstrual syndrome. Hum Reprod. 2004;19:2152–5.
18. Studd J. Severe premenstrual syndrome and bipolar disorder; a frequent tragic confusion. Menopause Int. 2012;18:65–7.
19. Yonkers KA, Simoni MK. Premenstrual disorders. Am J Obstet Gynecol. 2018;1:68–74.
20. Bloch M, Schmidt PJ, Danaceau M, Murphy J, Nieman L, Rubinow DR. Effects of gonadal steroids in women with a history of postpartum depression. Am J Psychiatry. 2000;157:924–30.
21. Gregoire AJ, Kumar R, Everitt B, Henderson AF, Studd JW. Transdermal estrogen for the treatment of severe post-natal depression. Lancet. 1996;347:930–3.
22. Dennis CL, Ross LE, Herxheimer A. Oestrogens and progestins for preventing and treating postpartum depression. Cochrane Database Syst Rev. 2008;4:CD001690.
23. Dennerstein L, Lehert P, Burger H, et al. Mood and the menopausal transition. J Nerv Ment Dis. 1999;187:685–91.
24. Brincat M, Magos A, Studd JW, et al. Subcutaneous hormone implants for the control of climacteric symptoms. A prospective study. Lancet. 1984;1:16–8.

25. Soares CN, Almeida JH, Cohen LS. Efficacy of estradiol for the treatment of depressive disorders in perimenopausal women: a double-blind, randomized, placebo-controlled trial. Arch Gen Psychiatry. 2001;58:529–34.
26. Montgomery JC, Brincat M, Tapp A, et al. Effect of oestrogen and testosterone implants on psychological disorders in the climacteric. Lancet. 1987;1:297–9.
27. Studd J. HRT should be considered as first line therapy for perimenopausal depression: FOR: estrogens are the first line treatment for perimenopausal women. BJOG. 2016;123:1011.
28. Craig MC. HRT should be considered as first line therapy for perimenopausal depression: against: more clinical trials are needed. BJOG. 2016;123:1011.
29. Gath D, Rose N, Bond A, et al. Hysterectomy and psychiatric disorder. Psychol Med. 1995;25:277–83.
30. Khastgir G, Studd J. Patient's outlook experience and satisfaction with hysterectomy bilateral oophorectomy and subsequent hormone replacement therapy. Am J Obstet Gynecol. 2000;183:1427–33.
31. Studd J. Hysterectomy A life saving as well life enhancing operation. Menopause Int. 2009;15:2–3.
32. Graziottin A, Serafini A. Depression and the menopause: why antidepressants are not enough? Menopause Int. 2009;15:76–81.
33. Studd J. Hormone therapy for reproductive depression in women. Post Reprod Health. 2014;20(4):132–7.

Sex, Gender, and the Decline of Dementia

9

Walter A. Rocca

9.1 Sex, Gender, and Dimorphic Neurology

9.1.1 Introduction

As we have originally discussed elsewhere [1], two important conceptual trends in the last 20 years will contribute to our future understanding of the risk of developing dementia or Alzheimer's disease (AD). First, there has been an increasing attention to differences between men and women in the causes, manifestations, responses to treatment, and outcomes of neurological diseases (dimorphic neurology) [2–6]. These differences in brain structure and function between men and women manifest throughout the entire life course (intrauterine life, early childhood development, adult life, and aging) [3, 4, 7, 8]. Second, there has been an increasing recognition of the distinction between sex and gender. Sex is biology and refers to chromosomal, hormonal, or reproductive differences between men and women [1, 2, 5, 6]. By contrast, gender refers to psychological, social, political, and cultural differences between men and women [1, 5, 6, 9]. These two conceptual trends are now confronted with a growing body of evidence suggesting that the risk of dementia has declined in North America and Western Europe in the last 25 years and that the decline is different in men and women [10]. We can now use concepts of dimorphic neurology to help explain these time trends [10].

W. A. Rocca (✉)
Division of Epidemiology, Department of Health Sciences Research, Mayo Clinic, Rochester, MN, USA

Department of Neurology, Mayo Clinic, Rochester, MN, USA
e-mail: rocca@mayo.edu

© International Society of Gynecological Endocrinology 2019
R. D. Brinton et al. (eds.), *Sex Steroids' Effects on Brain, Heart and Vessels*,
ISGE Series, https://doi.org/10.1007/978-3-030-11355-1_9

9.1.2 Sex Versus Gender

It is important to distinguish sex and gender for the understanding of risk and protective mechanisms of disease. The US Institute of Medicine clarified the difference between sex and gender in a 2010 report: "Sex" refers to the classification of living things as male or female according to their reproductive organs and functions assigned by chromosomal complement, and "gender" refers to a person's self-representation as male or female or to how that person is responded to by social institutions on the basis of that presentation [6]. Thus, sex refers to biological characteristics of men and women, such as chromosomal differences (e.g., XX vs. XY chromosomes), hormonal differences (e.g., effects of estrogen, progesterone, or testosterone), or reproductive differences (e.g., pregnancy or menopause) [1, 2, 5, 6].

In contrast to sex, gender includes both a subjective component of self-representation (or sexual identity) and societal components related to the social, cultural, and legal contexts in which men and women live. For example, a woman may rate herself higher or lower on a masculinity vs. femininity personality scale [11]. However, her right to drive a car, vote for political elections, or own property will depend on the legal system of the country in which the woman lives at a given point in history (e.g., Sweden vs. Saudi Arabia or the United States early 1900s vs. early 2000s). The personal aspects of gender (e.g., psychology, personality, or behavior) are linked with the social and political aspects (e.g., legal system, religious practices, or local traditions), and it is sometimes difficult to determine to which extent the self-representation of gender is the determinant or the consequence of cultural, political, or religious norms. Thus, sex and gender are tightly related and interdependent; however, they are not the same. Each variable should be studied independently [1, 11, 12].

9.1.3 Sex, Gender, and Time (History)

Gender-related factors have also varied over history. For example, women in the United States were not allowed to vote until the passage of the 19th Amendment to the United States Constitution in 1920 (Women's Suffrage). Similarly, women in the United States have been less likely than men to smoke cigarettes during most of the twentieth century. The gap in smoking behavior is now narrowing [13, 14]. Finally, in most countries, including the United States, men have historically had more access to advanced education than women. This pattern is now undergoing a complete reversal [15]. These historical transformations may have impacted the cognitive life of men and women differently and may explain in part the observed trends in risk of dementia.

9.2 The Risk of Dementia Is Declining

9.2.1 Evidence of a Decline

We were among the first authors who suggested that the incidence of dementia may be declining. At the time of our publication in 2011, we were uncertain about the data and somewhat surprised about the trend [16]. However, in the following years, similar trends were reported from several other studies in Western Europe. Some additional confirmations came from Canada in 2015, and from two US studies and one UK study in 2016. Following the report of declining incidence rates of dementia in the Framingham study in early 2016 (Framingham, Massachusetts) [17], another study reported a declining trend in incidence rates in the United Kingdom [18], and a third study confirmed a declining trend in the prevalence of dementia in a sample representative of the entire United States [19]. A more extensive analysis of the declining trend in Canada was published in 2017 [20], and a study of trends by birth cohorts in a US population was published in 2017 [21].

As of today, we have a sizeable body of epidemiologic evidence indicating a decline in the incidence or prevalence of dementia in high-income countries in the past 25 years. Several experts from different countries have written commentaries or reviews on these declining trends and have discussed the possible role of vascular risk factors, education, wealth, and other personal or social factors [22–28]. Of particular interest is the commentary by Jones and Greene, two experts on the history of medicine, who have framed the declining trend for dementia within the broader context of trends for cardiovascular diseases [22]. In this chapter, I restrict my consideration to countries with higher income, primarily from Europe and North America, because the time trends of neurological diseases, and of dementia in particular, may be different in other parts of the world with different demographic, social, cultural, and economic characteristics [29–32].

9.2.2 Evidence of Sex and Gender Differences

The trends for dementia incidence or prevalence may vary by sex. The decline in the incidence of dementia in the Framingham study, in Germany, and in Canada was more pronounced in women than men [17, 20, 33]. As an example, Fig. 9.1 shows the decline in the incidence of dementia in the Framingham study. The decline started earlier and was more pronounced in women than men. By contrast, the decline in the incidence of dementia was almost completely restricted to men in a UK study and was greater for men in Spain [18, 34]. The declining trends of dementia for men and women may vary across countries and across time periods because of the interaction of sex and gender factors with a changing physical, social, and cultural environment (e.g., interaction of sex and gender with "living conditions").

9.2.3 Explanations for the Decline

The trends in dementia incidence or prevalence remain partly unexplained. For example, in the study by Langa et al., the prevalence of dementia declined even though the cardiovascular risk profile worsened (e.g., increased prevalence of hypertension, diabetes, and obesity over time) [19]. These findings suggest that the

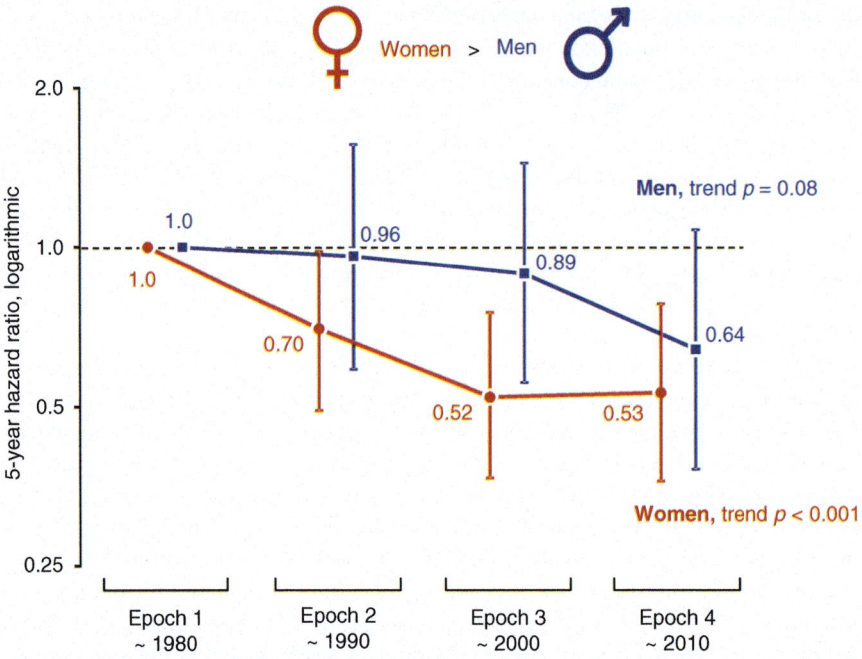

Fig. 9.1 Hazard ratios (HR) contrasting the incidence of dementia across four epochs. The epoch around 1980 served as the reference (HR = 1.0). The incidence declined earlier and more sizably in women (red line) than men (blue line). Figure drawn from the original data reported by Satizabal et al. [17]

increase in prevalence of cardiovascular risk factors was probably counterbalanced by an improvement in treatment (better treatment of hypertension and diabetes). The increasing trends in late-life obesity and overweight in relation to dementia risk need further study. It is possible that overweight and obesity in late life may protect against dementia rather than increase the risk.

Langa et al. conducted a series of analyses to explore whether the known risk factors for dementia can explain completely the time trends (mediation analyses). Comparing the prevalence in 2012 to the prevalence in 2000, they obtained an odds ratio of 0.69 (31% reduction). The odds ratio only increased to 0.82 after accounting for all of the factors considered (age, sex, race/ethnicity, education, net worth, cardiovascular risk factors and diseases, and body mass index). Therefore, a large segment of the decline remained to be explained by yet unknown factors (18% of the decline in risk was unexplained) [19]. Similarly, Derby et al. reported a decline in the incidence of dementia within age groups over several sequential birth cohorts (decades of years of birth) in an urban US population (New York City). These declines were not explained by trends in putative risk factors such as education, racial composition, or cardiovascular risk factors [21].

9.2.4 Broader Historical Context

The trends for dementia incidence and prevalence have occurred within the context of large-scale historical events. Important dynamic interactions between sex, gender, socioeconomic factors, and cultural factors have occurred over historical epochs of the last century. For example, the people who have developed dementia in the last 20–30 years in Western Europe and North America have lived through World War I (1914–1918), the Spanish flu pandemic (1918–1920), the Great Depression (1929–1937), Word War II (1939–1945), the polio epidemic (1949), the Korean War (1950–1953), the Vietnam War (1955–1975), political protest movements in the 1960s, the end of the Cold War (1991), and the more recent conflicts in the Middle East. Some of these events have caused food restriction or famine, massive migrations, incarceration, persecution, violence, and stress. Patients with dementia have also lived through natural catastrophes, such as earthquakes and floods.

These patients have lived through changes in access to information, changes in the physical environment, changes in food availability and diet, and changes in life habits. Examples of changes are widespread use of radios and televisions, of telephones, and more recently of the Internet, increase in urbanization and population density, mechanization of agriculture and increased use of herbicides and pesticides, increase in air and water pollution, introduction of frozen food, distant transportation of fruit and vegetables, reduced time spent in preparing food, use of food additives to increase shelf life, the initial increase and later decrease in cigarette smoking, and the increase in sedentary lifestyle. Finally, they have lived through changes in medical care (e.g., introduction of antibiotics, antihypertensive drugs, diabetes drugs, dyslipidemia drugs, anticoagulant drugs, and psychiatric drugs). As I have previously discussed in an invited review, the impact of these large-scale historical events on the health and diseases of men and women remains poorly understood [10]. The effects may be particularly sizeable for diseases such as cognitive decline and dementia that involve higher cortical functions.

The dramatic historical changes that occurred in the last century have impacted women differently from men. For example, men went to war in 1939–1945, whereas women stayed home with the elderly and children and took on new roles to support the war efforts (many women started working in industry or agriculture). Men started to smoke cigarettes earlier than women, men reached much higher percentages of use, and men experienced a steeper decline in smoking in more recent decades. Attention to sex-related factors (chromosomal, endocrine, and reproductive factors) or to gender-related factors (social and cultural factors) may help us to interpret the time trends. These sex and gender factors may be part of the missing explanation of the decline in the incidence or prevalence of dementia. We and others have recommended looking at risk and protective factors for dementia separately in men and women [1, 13, 35].

9.3   The Role of Sex and Gender

9.3.1   Three Examples

I discuss three examples of sex- and gender-related risk factors that may have influenced the time trends: (1) one risk factor is equally common in men and women but has a stronger effect in one sex or gender group (*APOE* genotype), (2) one risk factor is believed to have a similar effect in men and women but has been historically more common in one sex or gender group because of cultural reasons (education), and (3) one risk factor is restricted to one sex (oophorectomy). Figure 9.2 provides a schematic representation of the three examples.

9.3.2   *APOE* Genotype and Alzheimer's Disease

As we reported in greater details elsewhere [1, 13], the E4 allele of the apolipoprotein E gene (*APOE*) is the strongest known genetic susceptibility variant for AD [36, 37]. There are three major isoforms of the ApoE protein (ApoE2, ApoE3, and ApoE4) that are encoded by three alleles of the *APOE* gene (E2, E3, and E4). Carriers of one E4 allele are three to four times more likely to develop AD than noncarriers. Carriers of the E4 allele also have an earlier age at onset of AD that can be visualized in cumulative incidence curves. Carriers of two E4 alleles have an even higher risk of AD than carriers of one allele (trend by genetic dose). The majority of studies, and a large meta-analysis published by Farrer et al. in 1997, showed higher age-specific odds ratios of AD in women compared with men both for carriers of one E4 allele and for carriers of two E4 alleles (Fig. 9.2) [36].

Among E4 allele carriers, women showed greater hippocampal atrophy, more changes in the default mode connectivity, more cortical atrophy, and worse memory performance compared with men [38–40]. In addition, a large autopsy study showed a higher burden of amyloid plaques and neurofibrillary tangles in the brains of women who were carriers of an E4 allele than in the brains of men who were carriers [41]. Finally, a recent study suggested that the greater risk of AD in women compared with men who carry one *APOE* E4 allele may be mediated by tau pathology [42].

The stronger effect of the *APOE* E4 allele in women compared with men offers an excellent example of a completely biological factor (a genetic variant) interacting with other biological factors (e.g., hormones produced by the ovaries or other genes hosted on chromosomes X or Y) or with gender-related factors (e.g., education, physical activity, behavioral preferences, type of occupation). We will first describe possible interactions between *APOE* E4 and sex mediated by hormonal mechanisms.

It has been postulated that the estrogen produced by the ovaries in a woman before the onset of menopause has an important neuroprotective effect on the brain [43, 44]. In addition, it has been hypothesized that the apolipoprotein E (ApoE: the protein coded by the *APOE* gene) may be a critical factor in the neuroprotective actions of estrogen [45, 46]. There is increasing evidence from both in vivo (mice)

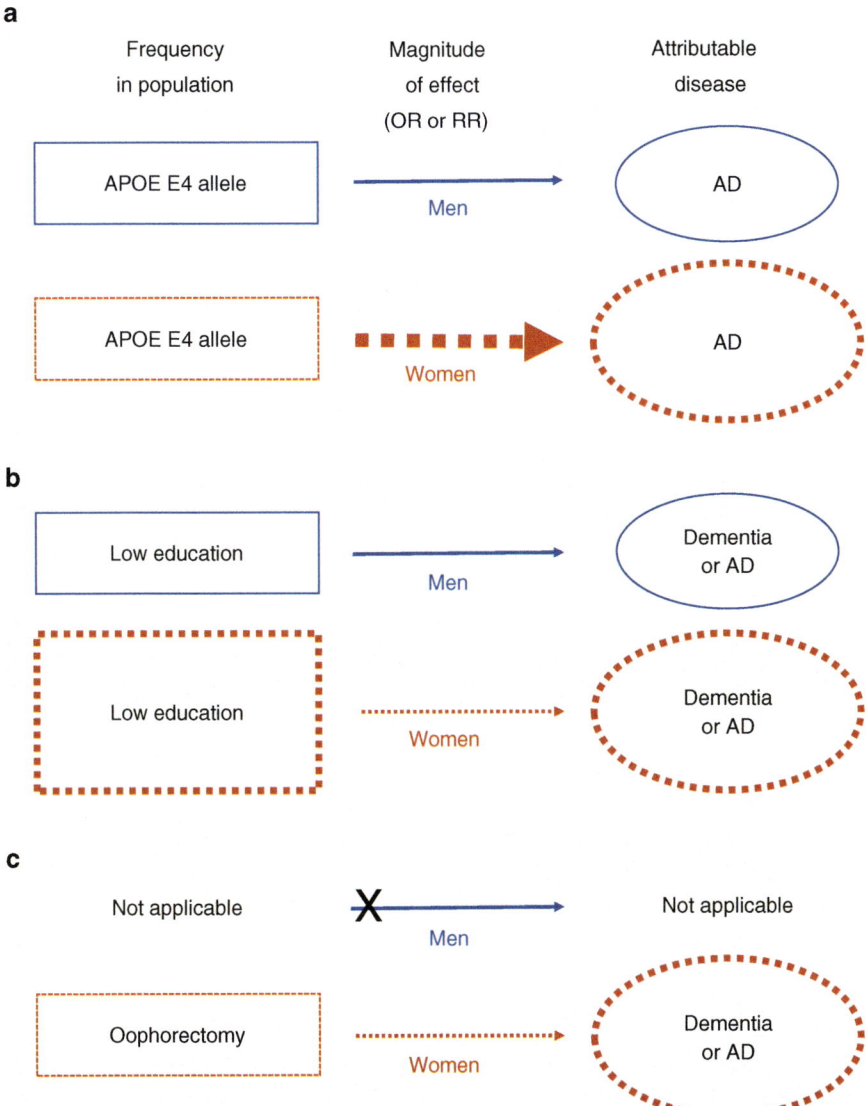

Fig. 9.2 Schematic representation of three examples of sex and gender differences related to the risk of dementia or Alzheimer's disease (AD) that may have contributed to the decline in incidence over time. Men are represented by blue boxes, arrows, and ovals and women by red-dashed boxes, arrows, and ovals. In all three examples, women experienced a higher risk of dementia or AD attributable to the specific risk factors (bigger red oval on the right). Panel **a**: *APOE* E4 allele is equally frequent in men and women (equal boxes on the left) but has a stronger effect in women (thicker red arrow). Panel **b**: low education has the same effect on the risk of dementia or AD in both men and women (equal thickness of the blue and red arrow). However, low education has been historically more common in women than men in many countries (bigger red box in women on the left). Panel **c**: oophorectomy increases the risk of dementia or AD in women but is not applicable to men. *OR* odds ratio, *RR* relative risk, *APOE* apolipoprotein E, *AD* Alzheimer's disease. Modified from the original figure reported by Rocca et al. [1]

and in vitro (cell cultures) studies that estrogen may modulate the ApoE protein and its receptor, namely, the low-density lipoprotein receptor-related protein [46, 47]. A number of studies have shown that the ApoE protein is a critical intermediary for the beneficial effects of estrogen on neuronal protection and repair [46, 48–50]. The hypothesis that the neuroprotective effects of estrogen may be modified by the *APOE* genotype is also supported by some epidemiologic studies in women [51–54].

Another line of reasoning for the differences between men and women focuses on possible interactions between *APOE* genotype and more conventional risk or protective factors for dementia or AD. *APOE* E4 genotype may interact synergistically with alcohol intake, cigarette smoking, physical inactivity, and high intake of saturated fat with the diet [55, 56]. These interactions may explain the increased risk of dementia and AD in *APOE* carriers in general. These interactions may also explain the differential effects of *APOE* genotype in men and women because men and women differ in their exposure to cigarette smoking, alcohol drinking, dietary preferences, and willingness to engage in physical activity. It remains unclear whether these behavioral factors are completely gender-related or whether they are partly biologically driven (sex-related). It has also been suggested that higher education may reduce the harmful effects of *APOE* E4. Indeed, women who carried an *APOE* E4 allele had reduced risk of developing dementia if they obtained a higher level of education early in life [57]. Dietary habits, lifestyle behaviors, the consumption of addictive substances, and education have changed over history in men and women and may have contributed to the decline in risk of dementia.

9.3.3   Education and Dementia

Lower education is recognized as one of the most established risk factors for dementia and AD. Some studies suggested that the effect of lower education may be even stronger than the effect of the *APOE* E4 genotype [58]. It remains unknown how education may prevent dementia and AD, and current data suggest that the impact of education on the risk of dementia or AD is similar in men and women (Fig. 9.2) [59–63]. It may be strategic to consider education within a broader concept of intellectual enrichment that includes other protective activities or behaviors. For example, it has been shown that subjects who are involved in mentally stimulating activities at work (e.g., occupations requiring complex interactions with data and people) may reduce their initial risk related to lower education [64]. Therefore, education, primary occupation in earlier life, and cognitively stimulating leisure activities in midlife or later life have been combined into the concept of lifetime intellectual enrichment. It has been hypothesized that lifetime intellectual enrichment may provide an important brain reserve mechanism to delay the onset of cognitive decline and dementia [62, 63].

Education in earlier life (through schooling or formal training), mental stimulation as part of a job, and stimulating leisure activities later in life are three examples of factors that are primarily gender-related and historically contingent. As I discussed earlier, in some countries, men had historically more access to advanced education than women; this pattern has now reversed. For example, at the most recent US Census, the educational attainment in women was higher than in men [15]. Similarly, cognitively demanding jobs used to be restricted to men (e.g., directing public or private institutions, serving in high-ranking political roles, holding high academic ranks, etc.); the pattern is changing in some countries [13].

The dimorphic effects of education, occupation, and leisure activities on the risk of dementia and AD should be further investigated and may be leveraged in developing preventive interventions [62, 63]. The dramatic changes in social and cultural attitudes and norms about gender that have occurred in many western countries in recent decades may explain part of the observed decline in the risk of dementia [10].

9.3.4   Oophorectomy and Dementia

Oophorectomy and other gynecological surgeries are examples of factors restricted to one sex because of anatomical differences (Fig. 9.2). The neuroprotective effect of estrogen may be lost in women who experience premature menopause (before age 40 years) or early menopause (between age 40 and 45 years) either naturally or because of medical or surgical interventions (more commonly, bilateral oophorectomy) [44, 65]. In 2007, the Mayo Clinic Cohort Study of Oophorectomy and Aging showed that women who underwent bilateral oophorectomy before the onset of menopause experienced a long-term increased risk of cognitive impairment or dementia [43, 44, 65–67]. The risk increased with younger age at oophorectomy, did not vary by indication for the oophorectomy, and was attenuated by estrogen therapy initiated after the surgery and continued up to age 50 years or longer. In most of the women, the bilateral oophorectomy was performed at the time of a hysterectomy. Most of these bilateral oophorectomies were performed under the belief that removal of the ovaries was a preventive measure against ovarian cancer and would not have any major systemic long-term effects.

The findings from the Mayo Clinic study were first replicated 3 years later, in 2010, by a Danish nationwide study [67, 68]. In 2014, Bove et al. reported the results of a cohort study on the association between surgical menopause and cognitive decline and AD pathology conducted in an urban US population (Chicago, IL) [69]. Earlier age at surgical menopause was associated with faster decline in global cognition, and specifically in episodic memory and semantic memory. Earlier age at surgical menopause was also associated with increased AD neuropathology, in particular neuritic plaques. Estrogen therapy that was initiated within 5 years of the surgery and that was continued for at least 10 years was associated with a slower decline in global cognition. None of these associations were observed for women who underwent natural menopause.

It has been suggested that bilateral oophorectomy causes an abrupt decline in the levels of circulating estrogen and that this decline may trigger a chain of biological events leading to degenerative and vascular lesions in the brain. These brain lesions may manifest as cognitive impairment or dementia several decades after the oophorectomy. The role of other ovarian hormones (e.g., progesterone) and of other etiologic mechanisms (e.g., disruption of the hypothalamus-pituitary-ovarian axis) remains uncertain [43, 44]. The incidence rate of bilateral oophorectomy more than doubled between 1950–1954 and 1995–1999 and declined thereafter [70]. In addition, treatment with estrogen replacement therapy after the oophorectomy also changed dramatically over the last half a century. Therefore, the impact of bilateral oophorectomy with or without estrogen replacement on the trends for dementia risk in women remains unknown.

9.3.5 Risk Factors Restricted to Men

Bilateral oophorectomy is an example of a sex-specific condition restricted to women. Similar sex-specific conditions have been investigated less frequently in men. For example, it remains unclear whether men who are treated for prostate hypertrophy or prostate cancer with testosterone antagonists have an increased risk of dementia.

9.4 Conclusions

The incidence rate of dementia and AD has declined in high-income countries in the past 25 years. The decline has varied in men and women, and the sex pattern has varied across different countries. This decline has been explained in part by better treatments for some cardiovascular risk factors and by improvements in education and wealth. However, a sizeable segment of the decline remains unexplained.

At this point in the history of research on the etiology of dementia or AD, we need new concepts, new theories, and new points of view rather than simply additional data. An impressive number of individual papers, monographs, books, literature reviews, and meta-analyses on the etiology of dementia or AD have been written [1, 13]. It may be time to take some distance from the existing literature and see whether there are new lines of investigation to be explored. The partly unexplained decline observed in the incidence rate of dementia provides an additional stimulus to consider new risk and protective factors for dementia and to develop a broader approach to causal explanations.

I hope that this chapter will stimulate other groups of investigators to further explore the impact of sex- and gender-related factors on cognitive aging [13, 43, 44, 65, 71]. Consideration of risk and protective factors in men and women separately may accelerate etiologic research in neurological diseases in general and for dementia and AD in particular [3, 4, 13, 43, 71]. Finally, a dimorphic approach may be essential in trying to understand the decline in the risk of dementia observed over the last 25 years and in developing preventive strategies to accelerate the decline.

References

1. Rocca WA, Mielke MM, Vemuri P, Miller VM. Sex and gender differences in the causes of dementia: a narrative review. Maturitas. 2014;79:196–201. https://doi.org/10.1016/j.maturitas.2014.05.008.
2. Institute of Medicine. Exploring the biological contributions to human health: does sex matter? Washington, DC: The National Academies Press; 2001.
3. Carter CL, Resnick EM, Mallampalli M, Kalbarczyk A. Sex and gender differences in Alzheimer's disease: recommendations for future research. J Womens Health (Larchmt). 2012;21:1018–23. https://doi.org/10.1089/jwh.2012.3789.
4. Cahill L. A half-truth is a whole lie: on the necessity of investigating sex influences on the brain. Endocrinology. 2012;153:2541–3. https://doi.org/10.1210/en.2011-2167.
5. Woods NF, Tsui AO. Editorial: Epidemiologic approaches to women's health. Epidemiol Rev. 2014;36:1–4. https://doi.org/10.1093/epirev/mxt013.
6. Women's Health Research. Progress, pitfalls, and promise. Washington, DC: The National Academies Press; 2010.
7. Nugent BM, Tobet SA, Lara HE, Lucion AB, Wilson ME, Recabarren SE, et al. Hormonal programming across the lifespan. Horm Metab Res. 2012;44:577–86. https://doi.org/10.1055/s-0032-1312593.
8. Ingalhalikar M, Smith A, Parker D, Satterthwaite TD, Elliott MA, Ruparel K, et al. Sex differences in the structural connectome of the human brain. Proc Natl Acad Sci U S A. 2014;111:823–8. https://doi.org/10.1073/pnas.1316909110.
9. Krieger N. Epidemiology and the peoples health theory and context. New York, NY: Oxford University Press, Inc; 2011.
10. Rocca WA. Time, sex, gender, history, and dementia. Alzheimer Dis Assoc Disord. 2017;31:76–9. https://doi.org/10.1097/WAD.0000000000000187.
11. Ristvedt SL. The evolution of gender. JAMA Psychiat. 2014;71:13–4. https://doi.org/10.1001/jamapsychiatry.2013.3199.
12. Miller VM. Why are sex and gender important to basic physiology and translational and individualized medicine? Am J Physiol Heart Circ Physiol. 2014;306:H781–8. https://doi.org/10.1152/ajpheart.00994.2013.
13. Mielke MM, Vemuri P, Rocca WA. Clinical epidemiology of Alzheimer's disease: assessing sex and gender differences. Clin Epidemiol. 2014;6:37–48. https://doi.org/10.2147/CLEP.S37929.
14. American Lung Association. Research and Program Services, Epidemiology and Statistics Unit. Trends in tobacco use. Washington, DC: Research and Program Services EaSU; 2011. http://www.lung.org/finding-cures/our-research/trend-reports/Tobacco-Trend-Report.pdf. Accessed 7 Apr 2014.
15. Ryan CL, Siebens J. Educational attainment in the United States: 2009. Current population reports. Washington, DC: US Department of Commerce, US Census Bureau; 2012. http://www.census.gov/prod/2012pubs/p20-566.pdf. Accessed 31 Mar 2014.
16. Rocca WA, Petersen RC, Knopman DS, Hebert LE, Evans DA, Hall KS, et al. Trends in the incidence and prevalence of Alzheimer's disease, dementia, and cognitive impairment in the United States. Alzheimers Dement. 2011;7:80–93. https://doi.org/10.1016/j.jalz.2010.11.002.
17. Satizabal CL, Beiser AS, Chouraki V, Chene G, Dufouil C, Seshadri S. Incidence of dementia over three decades in the Framingham Heart Study. N Engl J Med. 2016;374:523–32. https://doi.org/10.1056/NEJMoa1504327.
18. Matthews FE, Stephan BC, Robinson L, Jagger C, Barnes LE, Arthur A, et al. A two decade dementia incidence comparison from the cognitive function and ageing studies I and II. Nat Commun. 2016;7:11398. https://doi.org/10.1038/ncomms11398.
19. Langa KM, Larson EB, Crimmins EM, Faul JD, Levine DA, Kabeto MU, et al. A comparison of the prevalence of dementia in the United States in 2000 and 2012. JAMA Intern Med. 2016. doi: https://doi.org/10.1001/jamainternmed.2016.6807.

20. Cerasuolo JO, Cipriano LE, Sposato LA, Kapral MK, Fang J, Gill SS, et al. Population-based stroke and dementia incidence trends: age and sex variations. Alzheimers Dement. 2017. doi: https://doi.org/10.1016/j.jalz.2017.02.010.
21. Derby CA, Katz MJ, Lipton RB, Hall CB. Trends in dementia incidence in a birth cohort analysis of the Einstein Aging Study. JAMA Neurol. 2017;74:1345–51. https://doi.org/10.1001/jamaneurol.2017.1964.
22. Jones DS, Greene JA. Is dementia in decline? Historical trends and future trajectories. New Engl J Med. 2016;374:507–9.
23. Langa KM. Is the risk of Alzheimer's disease and dementia declining? Alzheimers Res Ther. 2015;7:34. https://doi.org/10.1186/s13195-015-0118-1.
24. Larson EB, Yaffe K, Langa KM. New insights into the dementia epidemic. N Engl J Med. 2013;369:2275–7. https://doi.org/10.1056/NEJMp1311405.
25. Banerjee S. Good news on dementia prevalence—we can make a difference. Lancet. 2013;382:1384–6. https://doi.org/10.1016/S0140-6736(13)61579-2.
26. Skoog I. Dementia: dementia incidence – the times, they are a-changing. Nat Rev Neurol. 2016;12:316–8. https://doi.org/10.1038/nrneurol.2016.55.
27. Okonkwo OC, Asthana S. Dementia trends in the United States: read up and weigh in. JAMA Intern Med. 2016. doi: https://doi.org/10.1001/jamainternmed.2016.7073.
28. Wu YT, Fratiglioni L, Matthews FE, Lobo A, Breteler MM, Skoog I, et al. Dementia in Western Europe: epidemiological evidence and implications for policy making. Lancet Neurol. 2016;15:116–24. https://doi.org/10.1016/S1474-4422(15)00092-7.
29. Gao S, Ogunniyi A, Hall KS, Baiyewu O, Unverzagt FW, Lane KA, et al. Dementia incidence declined in African-Americans but not in Yoruba. Alzheimers Dement. 2016;12:244–51. https://doi.org/10.1016/j.jalz.2015.06.1894.
30. GBD 2015 Mortality and Causes of Death Collaborators. Global, regional, and national life expectancy, all-cause mortality, and cause-specific mortality for 249 causes of death, 1980–2015: a systematic analysis for the Global Burden of Disease Study 2015. Lancet. 2016;388:1459–544. https://doi.org/10.1016/S0140-6736(16)31012-1.
31. Sekita A, Ninomiya T, Tanizaki Y, Doi Y, Hata J, Yonemoto K, et al. Trends in prevalence of Alzheimer's disease and vascular dementia in a Japanese community: the Hisayama Study. Acta Psychiatr Scand. 2010;122:319–25. https://doi.org/10.1111/j.1600-0447.2010.01587.x.
32. Honda H, Sasaki K, Hamasaki H, Shijo M, Koyama S, Ohara T, et al. Trends in autopsy-verified dementia prevalence over 29 years of the Hisayama study. Neuropathology. 2016;36:383–7. https://doi.org/10.1111/neup.12298.
33. Doblhammer G, Fink A, Zylla S, Willekens F. Compression or expansion of dementia in Germany? An observational study of short-term trends in incidence and death rates of dementia between 2006/07 and 2009/10 based on German health insurance data. Alzheimers Res Ther. 2015;7:66. https://doi.org/10.1186/s13195-015-0146-x.
34. Lobo A, Saz P, Marcos G, Dia JL, De-la-Camara C, Ventura T, et al. Prevalence of dementia in a southern European population in two different time periods: the ZARADEMP Project. Acta Psychiatr Scand. 2007;116:299–307. https://doi.org/10.1111/j.1600-0447.2007.01006.x.
35. Snyder HM, Asthana S, Bain L, Brinton R, Craft S, Dubal DB, et al. Sex biology contributions to vulnerability to Alzheimer's disease: a think tank convened by the Women's Alzheimer's Research Initiative. Alzheimers Dement. 2016;12:1186–96. https://doi.org/10.1016/j.jalz.2016.08.004.
36. Farrer LA, Cupples LA, Haines JL, Hyman B, Kukull WA, Mayeux R, et al. Effects of age, sex, and ethnicity on the association between apolipoprotein E genotype and Alzheimer disease. A meta-analysis. APOE and Alzheimer Disease Meta Analysis Consortium. JAMA. 1997;278:1349–56. https://doi.org/10.1001/jama.278.16.1349.
37. Jorm AF, Mather KA, Butterworth P, Anstey KJ, Christensen H, Easteal S. APOE genotype and cognitive functioning in a large age-stratified population sample. Neuropsychology. 2007;21:1–8.

38. Liu Y, Paajanen T, Westman E, Wahlund LO, Simmons A, Tunnard C, et al. Effect of APOE epsilon4 allele on cortical thicknesses and volumes: the AddNeuroMed study. J Alzheimers Dis. 2010;21:947–66. https://doi.org/10.3233/JAD-2010-100201.
39. Damoiseaux JS, Seeley WW, Zhou J, Shirer WR, Coppola G, Karydas A, et al. Gender modulates the APOE epsilon4 effect in healthy older adults: convergent evidence from functional brain connectivity and spinal fluid tau levels. J Neuroscie Res. 2012;32:8254–62. https://doi.org/10.1523/JNEUROSCI.0305-12.2012.
40. Fleisher A, Grundman M, Jack CR Jr, Petersen RC, Taylor C, Kim HT, et al. Sex, apolipoprotein E epsilon 4 status, and hippocampal volume in mild cognitive impairment. Arch Neurol. 2005;62:953–7. https://doi.org/10.1001/archneur.62.6.953.
41. Corder EH, Ghebremedhin E, Taylor MG, Thal DR, Ohm TG, Braak H. The biphasic relationship between regional brain senile plaque and neurofibrillary tangle distributions: modification by age, sex, and APOE polymorphism. Ann N Y Acad Sci. 2004;1019:24–8. https://doi.org/10.1196/annals.1297.005.
42. Altmann A, Tian L, Henderson VW, Greicius MD. Sex modifies the APOE-related risk of developing Alzheimer's disease. Ann Neurol. 2014. doi: https://doi.org/10.1002/ana.24135.
43. Rocca WA, Henderson VW. Is there a link between gynecologic surgeries and Alzheimer disease? Neurology. 2014;82:196–7. https://doi.org/10.1212/WNL.0000000000000043.
44. Rocca WA, Grossardt BR, Shuster LT. Oophorectomy, estrogen, and dementia: a 2014 update. Mol Cell Endocrinol. 2014;389:7–12. https://doi.org/10.1016/j.mce.2014.01.020.
45. McAsey ME, Cady C, Jackson LM, Li M, Randall S, Nathan BP, et al. Time course of response to estradiol replacement in ovariectomized mice: brain apolipoprotein E and synaptophysin transiently increase and glial fibrillary acidic protein is suppressed. Exp Neurol. 2006;197:197–205.
46. Struble RG, Cady C, Nathan BP, McAsey M. Apolipoprotein E may be a critical factor in hormone therapy neuroprotection. Front Biosci. 2008;13:5387–405.
47. Cheng X, McAsey ME, Li M, Randall S, Cady C, Nathan BP, et al. Estradiol replacement increases the low-density lipoprotein receptor related protein (LRP) in the mouse brain. Neurosci Lett. 2007;417:50–4.
48. Stone DJ, Rozovsky I, Morgan TE, Anderson CP, Finch CE. Increased synaptic sprouting in response to estrogen via an apolipoprotein E-dependent mechanism: implications for Alzheimer's disease. J Neurosci. 1998;18:3180–5.
49. Horsburgh K, Macrae IM, Carswell H. Estrogen is neuroprotective via an apolipoprotein E-dependent mechanism in a mouse model of global ischemia. J Cereb Blood Flow Metab. 2002;22:1189–95.
50. Nathan BP, Barsukova AG, Shen F, McAsey M, Struble RG. Estrogen facilitates neurite extension via apolipoprotein E in cultured adult mouse cortical neurons. Endocrinology. 2004;145:3065–73.
51. Mattila KM, Axelman K, Rinne JO, Blomberg M, Lehtimaki T, Laippala P, et al. Interaction between estrogen receptor 1 and the epsilon4 allele of apolipoprotein E increases the risk of familial Alzheimer's disease in women. Neurosci Lett. 2000;282:45–8.
52. Yaffe K, Haan M, Byers A, Tangen C, Kuller L. Estrogen use, APOE, and cognitive decline: evidence of gene-environment interaction. Neurology. 2000;54:1949–54.
53. Burkhardt MS, Foster JK, Laws SM, Baker LD, Craft S, Gandy SE, et al. Oestrogen replacement therapy may improve memory functioning in the absence of APOE epsilon4. J Alzheimers Dis. 2004;6:221–8.
54. Rippon GA, Tang MX, Lee JH, Lantigua R, Medrano M, Mayeux R. Familial Alzheimer disease in Latinos: interaction between APOE, stroke, and estrogen replacement. Neurology. 2006;66:35–40.
55. Mangialasche F, Kivipelto M, Solomon A, Fratiglioni L. Dementia prevention: current epidemiological evidence and future perspective. Alzheimers Res Ther. 2012;4:6. https://doi.org/10.1186/alzrt104.

56. Solomon A, Kivipelto M, Soininen H. Prevention of Alzheimer's disease: moving backward through the lifespan. J Alzheimers Dis. 2013;33(Suppl 1):S465–9. https://doi.org/10.3233/JAD-2012-129021.

57. Wang HX, Gustafson DR, Kivipelto M, Pedersen NL, Skoog I, Windblad B, et al. Education halves the risk of dementia due to apolipoprotein epsilon4 allele: a collaborative study from the Swedish Brain Power initiative. Neurobiol Aging. 2012;33:1007 e1–7. https://doi.org/10.1016/j.neurobiolaging.2011.10.003.

58. Kivipelto M, Ngandu T, Laatikainen T, Winblad B, Soininen H, Tuomilehto J. Risk score for the prediction of dementia risk in 20 years among middle aged people: a longitudinal, population-based study. Lancet Neurol. 2006;5:735–41. https://doi.org/10.1016/S1474-4422(06)70537-3.

59. Letenneur L, Gilleron V, Commenges D, Helmer C, Orgogozo JM, Dartigues JF. Are sex and educational level independent predictors of dementia and Alzheimer's disease? Incidence data from the PAQUID project. J Neurol Neurosurg Psychiatry. 1999;66:177–83.

60. Cobb JL, Wolf PA, Au R, White R, D'Agostino RB. The effect of education on the incidence of dementia and Alzheimer's disease in the Framingham Study. Neurology. 1995;45:1707–12.

61. Stern Y, Gurland B, Tatemichi TK, Tang MX, Wilder D, Mayeux R. Influence of education and occupation on the incidence of Alzheimer's disease. JAMA. 1994;271:1004–10.

62. Vemuri P, Lesnick TG, Przybelski SA, Knopman DS, Roberts RO, Lowe VJ, et al. Effect of lifestyle activities on Alzheimer disease biomarkers and cognition. Ann Neurol. 2012;72:730–8. https://doi.org/10.1002/ana.23665.

63. Vemuri P, Lesnick TG, Przybelski SA, Machulda MM, Knopman DS, Mielke MM, et al. Association of lifetime intellectual enrichment with cognitive decline in the older population. JAMA Neurol. 2014;71:1017–24. https://doi.org/10.1001/jamaneurol.2014.963.

64. Karp A, Andel R, Parker MG, Wang HX, Winblad B, Fratiglioni L. Mentally stimulating activities at work during midlife and dementia risk after age 75: follow-up study from the Kungsholmen Project. Am J Geriatr Psychiatry. 2009;17:227–36. https://doi.org/10.1097/JGP.0b013e318190b691.

65. Rocca WA, Grossardt BR, Shuster LT. Oophorectomy, menopause, estrogen treatment, and cognitive aging: clinical evidence for a window of opportunity. Brain Res. 2011;1379:188–98. https://doi.org/10.1016/j.brainres.2010.10.031.

66. Rocca WA, Bower JH, Maraganore DM, Ahlskog JE, Grossardt BR, de Andrade M, et al. Increased risk of cognitive impairment or dementia in women who underwent oophorectomy before menopause. Neurology. 2007;69:1074–83. https://doi.org/10.1212/01.wnl.0000276984.19542.e6.

67. Rocca WA, Grossardt BR, Shuster LT, Stewart EA. Hysterectomy, oophorectomy, estrogen, and the risk of dementia. Neurodegener Dis. 2012;10:175–8. https://doi.org/10.1159/000334764.

68. Phung TK, Waltoft BL, Laursen TM, Settnes A, Kessing LV, Mortensen PB, et al. Hysterectomy, oophorectomy and risk of dementia: a nationwide historical cohort study. Dement Geriatr Cogn Disord. 2010;30:43–50. https://doi.org/10.1159/000314681.

69. Bove R, Secor E, Chibnik LB, Barnes LL, Schneider JA, Bennett DA, et al. Age at surgical menopause influences cognitive decline and Alzheimer pathology in older women. Neurology. 2014;82:222–9.

70. Laughlin-Tommaso SK, Stewart EA, Grossardt BR, Gazzuola Rocca L, Rocca WA. Incidence, time trends, laterality, indications, and pathological findings of unilateral oophorectomy before menopause. Menopause. 2014;21:442–9. https://doi.org/10.1097/GME.0b013e3182a3ff45.

71. Miller VM, Garovic VD, Kantarci K, Barnes JN, Jayachandran M, Mielke MM, et al. Sex-specific risk of cardiovascular disease and cognitive decline: pregnancy and menopause. Biol Sex Differ. 2013;4:6. https://doi.org/10.1186/2042-6410-4-6.

Obstetric History and Cardiovascular Disease (CVD) Risk

10

Eleni Armeni, Evangelia Karopoulou, and Irene Lambrinoudaki

10.1 Introduction

While overall cardiovascular disease (CVD) mortality has decreased in the prior decade, mostly due to the advances in primary and secondary preventive methods, CVD remains the leading cause of morbidity and mortality worldwide with more people dying from CVD than from any other reason every year. As reported by the World Health Organization (WHO), CVD caused 17.7 million deaths in 2015, accounting for 31% of all global deaths. Coronary heart disease and stroke were the most common CVD events causing 7.4 million and 6.7 million deaths, respectively. CVD is also responsible for the 37% of the 17 million premature deaths due to non-communicable diseases in 2015. Furthermore, more than four million deaths from CVD are reported annually in Europe, representing the 45% of all deaths. The number of deaths from CVD is expected to increase even more by 2030 [1, 2].

For many years, heart disease was considered a "man's disease." However, it is more usually seen in women than in men, accounting for 40% of all deaths in men and 49% of all deaths in women across Europe [1–3]. This impact of CVD is mainly attributed to traditional risk factors which apply to both women and men, namely, hypertension, hypercholesterolemia, smoking, obesity, diabetes, and sedentary lifestyle. In addition, most women tent to present with atypical symptoms or no symptoms at all resulting in delayed diagnosis and treatment. In the past years, many attempts have been made to develop a women-specific preventive model for CVD; however diagnosis and risk assessment of heart disease in women are still challenging [4, 5].

As stated in recent scientific data, it is now well established that the pathophysiology, the symptoms, and the response to treatment of CDV differ between genders. This diversity in the clinical features of the disease between women and men makes

E. Armeni · E. Karopoulou · I. Lambrinoudaki (✉)
2nd Department of Obstetrics and Gynecology, Medical School, National and Kapodistrian University of Athens, Athens, Greece
e-mail: ilambrinoudaki@aretaieio.uoa.gr

© International Society of Gynecological Endocrinology 2019
R. D. Brinton et al. (eds.), *Sex Steroids' Effects on Brain, Heart and Vessels*,
ISGE Series, https://doi.org/10.1007/978-3-030-11355-1_10

the need for searching and studying women-specific CVD risk factors urgent. Along this same line of improving CVD prevention in women, researchers turned their attention to novel risk factors that are met exclusively in women such as adverse pregnancy outcome (APO) [6]. Hypertensive disorders of pregnancy (HDP) (pregnancy-induced hypertension, preeclampsia, eclampsia) and gestational diabetes mellitus are the most common complications of pregnancy that are associated with future CVD events for both mother and child. Moreover, these conditions represent the failure of the pregnant woman to adapt to the physiological alterations of pregnancy, which is expressed with elevated blood pressure, impaired lipid metabolism, and glucose intolerance and has a predictive role in future CVD. In particular, women who experience HDP and gestational diabetes mellitus (GDM) double their risk of developing CVD later in life [6, 7].

The causal pathway that relates APO with future disease as well as specific characteristics of women who experience pregnancy complications is the new subject of current research. The identification of women at risk early during their pregnancy and their involvement in preventive programs would contribute to the reduction of burden of CVD in women [8].

10.2   Hemodynamic Changes of Normal Pregnancy

Normal pregnancy induces a series of physiological changes in the maternal hemodynamic and cardiovascular system, which begin early in gestation. These changes are triggered by the systemic vascular vasodilation and reflect on plasma volume, red cell mass, heart rate, blood pressure, cardiac output, and coagulation system [9].

The vasodilation starts at the fifth week of gestation and serves the generation of placenta and the development of uteroplacental vascular system. The plasma volume increases throughout pregnancy with its major part being contained in the uterus and the uteroplacental circulation. It expands by 10–15% between the 6th and the 12th weeks of gestation, reaching 30–50% over the nonpregnant level by the 34th week. Given that there is a greater increase in the plasma volume compared to the red cell mass, red blood count and hemoglobin concentration fall resulting in physiological anemia of pregnancy [6, 10, 11].

Cardiac output rises to 30–50% above baseline during pregnancy in order to serve the exclusive needs of both mother and fetus. This alteration in cardiac output is stimulated by the expand in blood volume and the increase in heart rate [6]. Maternal heart rate increases gradually by 10–15 beats per minute by the 32nd week of gestation and turns back to normal at term [12]. Moreover, the size of the uterus and position of the mother at the time of measurement can affect the cardiac output rates [11].

During pregnancy, systematic vascular resistance decreases gradually to 35–40% of baseline due to systematic vasodilation by the middle of the second trimester. It increases to nonpregnant levels postpartum [13]. This systematic vasodilation causes an underfilled vascular system with slightly increased renin activity and slightly reduced atrial natriuretic peptide levels.

Blood pressure (BP), in pregnant state, has a falling course, with the most pronounced drop typically occurring between 16 and 20 weeks. During the second half of the third trimester, BP gradually increases to prepregnancy levels. These changes concern both systolic BP (SBP) and diastolic BP (DBP) [14, 15].

There are also alterations in the coagulation system that provoke a physiological hypercoagulable state. Plasma concentrations of clotting factors VII, VIII, IX, X, and von Willebrand increase progressively with the advancement of gestation. Fibrinogen is also increased, while fibrinolytic activity is decreased. The natural anticoagulants are affected as well. Levels of protein S decrease as gestation progresses and acquired resistance to activated protein C appears. While this hypercoagulability has a supporting role in case of hemorrhage during labor, it exposes the pregnant women to increased risk of venous thrombosis. In particular, women are 4–5 times more likely to develop venous thromboembolism during pregnancy than in the nonpregnant state. In addition, venous stasis in the lower limbs occurs due to compression of the inferior vena cava by the uterus and is more obvious in the left limb [6, 16]. Therefore, thromboembolic events are more common in the left leg; there are many recent scientific data about the May-Thurner syndrome in pregnancy where the left common iliac vein is occluded by the right common iliac artery [17].

10.3   Metabolic Changes of Normal Pregnancy

During normal pregnancy, a set of metabolic adaptations occur in order to meet the increased demands of the growing fetus.

10.3.1 Glucose Metabolism

The state of pregnancy is considered to be diabetogenic, and the changes in glucose metabolism allow glucose supply to the fetus to ensure its growing and development. Pancreatic beta-cells undergo proliferation leading to increased insulin secretion and increased insulin sensitivity and subsequently progressive insulin resistance.

Insulin resistance begins in the second trimester and gradually increases peaking in the third trimester. Moreover, secretion of diabetogenic hormones such as placental hormones, progesterone, growth factors, and cortisol affects insulin sensitivity. The etiologic relationship between these hormones and insulin sensitivity is confirmed postpartum when insulin resistance declines abruptly. Gestational diabetes develops when pancreatic function is impaired and fails to overcome the insulin resistance [18].

10.3.2 Lipid Metabolism

During pregnancy, profound changes occur in lipid metabolism as well. Total serum cholesterol and triglycerides levels increase markedly, beginning at the first trimester and peaking during the second trimester. This is considered to be the result of increased estrogen concentrations and insulin resistance of pregnancy.

Triglyceride levels increase mainly due to increased hepatic synthesis and decreased lipoprotein lipase activity. Furthermore, there is a progressive increase in low-density lipoprotein (LDL) up to 50% above nonpregnant levels as well as in high-density lipoprotein (HDL). HDL rises in the first trimester and then falls in the third trimester afterward, remaining however above baseline.

Maternal hypertriglyceridemia accommodates the adequate fetal growth and development and serves as maternal fatty acid store. The placenta uses cholesterol for steroidogenesis and fatty acids for oxidation and formation of placental membranes. The mother uses fat as the main energy source, while she preserves glucose and amino acids for fetal metabolism [11, 18].

10.4 Hypertensive Disorders of Pregnancy and Cardiovascular Implications

Hypertensive disorders are common complications encountered during pregnancy [19]. The National High Blood Pressure Education Program Working Group on High Blood Pressure in Pregnancy classified hypertensive disorders into the following categories, namely, preeclampsia/eclampsia, chronic hypertension, preeclampsia superimposed on chronic hypertension, and gestational hypertension [19]. Gestational hypertension is the new onset of hypertension after 20 weeks of gestation. Moreover, the diagnosis may be done retrospectively provided blood pressure readings return to normal by the 12th week after delivery and the patient does not develop preeclampsia [20]. Preeclampsia is the multiorgan process defined by hypertension and proteinuria, occurring after the 20th week of gestation. Eclampsia is the development of convulsions presenting unexpectedly in a pregnant women with mildly elevated blood pressure and no prevalent proteinuria or in a pregnancy previously complicated by preeclampsia [19]. The prevalence of hypertensive disorders of pregnancy has been estimated as 5.2–8.2%, and preeclampsia is evident in 0.2–9.2% of pregnancies, while gestational hypertension is identified in 1.8–4.4% of pregnancies [21].

A previous history of HDP is emerging as a risk factor of future hypertension. A recent meta-analysis of 6904 women reported that the risk of hypertension increases in women with a history of HDP from the age of 45 years onward, with 1 in 5 women suffering from hypertension at 15 years postpartum [22]. Similarly, the cumulative incidence of chronic hypertension observed in women with previous HDP was modified by body mass index (BMI) [23]. More specifically, the risk of chronic hypertension increased stepwise with increasing BMI category, with a hazard ratio (HR) of 2.13, 3.54, 5.92, and 8.66 corresponding to women with BMI of 22.5–24.9 kg/m^2 vs. 25.0–29.9 kg/m^2 vs. 30.0–34.9 kg/m^2 vs. ≥35.0 kg/m^2, for women aged 32–39 years [23]. Moreover, a recent retrospective cohort study of 1261 women with a previous history of gestational diabetes described that the risk of subsequent hypertension up to 5 years post-delivery was predicted by a history of

HDP, weight increase higher than 7 kg throughout pregnancy, and elevated prepregnancy BMI [24]. Interestingly, women with a history of HDP have a higher risk of cardiomyopathy in later life, which corresponds to 2.22 times higher risk in women with severe preeclampsia and 2.25 times higher risk in women with gestational hypertension, for the occurrence of cardiomyopathy more than 5 years after last delivery [25].

Women with gestational hypertension have also been associated with a higher risk of maternal hypertension in the future. The prevalence of modifiable cardiometabolic risk factors and the risk of future hypertension are higher in women with gestational hypertension compared with women presenting with preeclampsia [26, 27]. Kestenbaum et al. (2003) evaluated 31,239 hypertensive pregnancies and described that the risk of cardiovascular events is up to 2.8-fold higher in women with a personal history of gestational hypertension (95% CI: 1.6–4.8) [28]. Women with a previous history of gestational hypertension without proteinuria have been linked with a 1.9-fold higher risk of incident ischemic heart disease in the future, as reported by a Swedish cross-sectional population-based study [29]. Finally, gestational hypertension has been linked with higher odds of admission for future disease when compared with preeclampsia only, namely, OR of 4.08 vs. 3.06 for chronic hypertension, OR of 3.19 vs. 2.67 for ischemic heart disease, OR of 0.57 vs. 2.03 for stroke, and OR of 3.45 vs. 4.72 for renal disease [30].

Preeclampsia has been related with a higher prevalence of cardiometabolic risk factors of the mother. An adverse cardiovascular risk profile has been described in 611 women with a previous history of mild or moderate preeclampsia, with results describing a more atherogenic lipid profile, higher insulin resistance, higher BMI, and elevated readings of blood pressure, 11 years after pregnancy [31]. The Preeclampsia Risk Evaluation in FEMales study (PREVFEM) evaluated the prevalence of hypertension within 10 years post-delivery in women exposed to preeclampsia compared to non-exposed women [32]. This study recognized that women with a personal history of preeclampsia have an 3.59 higher prevalence of hypertension compared to non-exposed women at 10 years postexposure [32]. The risk of chronic hypertension in the future has been estimated as up to sevenfold higher in women with recurrent preeclampsia when compared with women having a single episode of preeclampsia [33]. The impact of early-onset preeclampsia on cardiovascular risk factors seems to persist up until middle age, as described in a recent prospective observational study, in which women with early-onset preeclampsia had higher readings of blood pressure, more insulin resistance, greater BMI, and albuminuria in comparison with control women, when assessed in their fifth decade of life [34].

A personal history of preeclamptic pregnancies has been also been shown to predict future cardiovascular risk, whereas the subclinical cardiovascular involvement during preeclampsia does not resolve following delivery. A recent meta-analysis reported that women having experienced preeclampsia had a 2.01 times higher risk of CVD diagnosis, a 2.89 times higher risk of a fatal CVD event, and an up to 1.77 times higher risk of cerebrovascular event in later life [35]. Moreover, preeclampsia has been linked with a fourfold higher risk of heart failure and twofold higher risk of coronary heart disease in later life [36]. Similarly, an up to 2.3-fold greater risk of thromboembolic events has been identified in women with a personal history of severe preeclampsia [28]. Additionally, evidence of subclinical vascular disease has been observed in women with history of preeclampsia, who had higher carotid artery intima-media thickness compared to controls (IMT, median values, 0.80 mm vs. 0.73 mm, p-value = 0.004). Furthermore, insight with respect to the long-term impact of preeclampsia on the cardiovascular system of middle-aged women (45–55 years of age) will be provided following the completion of the CREw-IMAGO (Cardiovascular Risk profilE-Imaging and gender-specific disOrders) multicenter cohort study [37]. This study will assess indices of subclinical atherosclerosis like coronary artery calcium scoring, carotid calcium scoring, as well as arterial stiffness [37].

10.5   Gestational Diabetes Mellitus and Cardiovascular Risk

The prevalence of GDM among pregnancies in the USA has been described as 6–7% [38]. The equivalent European prevalence of GDM, diagnosed using the International Association of the Diabetes and Pregnancy Study Groups (IADPSG)/ WHO 2013 criteria, corresponds to rates up to 39% in obese women, with no significant differences in prevalence across counties [39]. GDM is a well-documented risk factor for the future development of type 2 diabetes mellitus (T2DM), with the risk of future maternal T2DM being estimated as more than sevenfold, according to the results of a meta-analysis [40]. In addition, a diagnosis of GDM confers an additional adverse effect on the actual cardiometabolic risk, with the number of previous GDM diagnosis associating with abnormal postpartum glucose metabolism in a dose-response pattern [41]. In fact, women experiencing a single episode of GDM had an up to 2.9 times higher relative risk of dysglycemia within the first 5 years after delivery (95% CI: 1.7–4.7), whereas women with recurrent diagnosis of GDM had an almost four times higher relative risk of postpartum dysglycemia (95% CI: 2.1–6.8) [41].

Available evidence from cohort studies which addressed the potential impact of GDM with respect to future maternal cardiovascular outcomes indicated a higher risk for CVD, CHD, and stroke in women experiencing glycemic dysregulation during pregnancy [38]. In fact, Retnakaran et al. [42] observed a large cohort of 1,450,097 women without baseline T2DM for a duration of 10 years [42]. The results of this study indicated that women with a previous history of GDM had an up to 1.3 times (95% CI: 1.07–1.59) as well as an up to 1.41 times higher CHD risk (95% CI: 1.11–1.80), compared to women who did not develop GDM during pregnancy [42]. Similarly, Tobias et al. observed the development of cardiovascular complications in a total of 89,479 women, participants of the Nurses' Health Study II, during an average duration of 25.7 years [43]. This study showed that women with GDM when compared with non-GDM women had an up to 1.53 higher risk of myocardial infarction in the future (95% CI: 1.16–2.17), an up to 1.22 times higher risk of stroke (95% CI: 0.83–1.78), as well as an up to 1.43 higher risk of overall cardiovascular events (95% CI: 1.12–1.81) [43]. Moreover, as reported following the results of a French nationwide population-based study, GDM was associated with higher risk for CVD (OR 1.25, 95% CI: 1.09–1.43), angina pectoris (OR 1.68, 95% CI: 1.29–2.20), myocardial infarction (OR 1.92, 95% CI: 1.36–2.71), and hypertension (OR 2.72, 95% CI: 2.58–2.88), but not with stroke, even within the first 7 years after delivery [44]. Shah et al. [45] assessed matched cohorts of 8191 women with GDM and 81,262 women without GDM for an average duration of 11.5 years following delivery. Accordingly, women with a history of GDM had higher risk for cardiovascular events (HR 1.13, 95% CI: 0.67–1.89), adjusting for subsequent type 2 diabetes [45].

A growing body of evidence tried to address the potential link between GDM and noninvasive indices of subclinical structural vascular disease. As reported by a systemic review and meta-analysis of 15 studies with 2247 women, GDM was linked with higher carotid IMT values compared to women without GDM (weighted mean difference 0.05, 95% CI: 0.03–0.07, p-value < 0.001) [46]. This association was characterized with significant heterogeneity, mainly attributed to values of body mass index [47]. Moreover, higher epicardial fat thickness and carotid was identified in women with a previous history of GDM when compared with age- and sex-matched controls, further supporting the predisposition of women with previous GDM to develop atherosclerosis [48]. In addition, the Coronary Artery Risk Development in Young Adults study evaluated evidence of subclinical atherosclerosis in a total of 898 apparently healthy parous women [49]. This study identified higher common carotid IMT values in GDM vs. no-GDM women [49]. These results were observed only in participants who did not develop subsequent diabetes or metabolic syndrome, indicating evidence of subclinical vascular disease in patients with GDM independent of prepregnancy obesity [49].

A few studies evaluated the link between subclinical arterial dysfunction and a personal history of GDM. Moreover, GDM-complicated vs. normoglycemic pregnancies presented as significant risk factor predicting higher arterial stiffness, which was evaluated according to measures of pulse wave velocity (PWV), in women up to 5 years following pregnancy [50]. Similarly, a hospital-based cohort study evaluated 120 women with a personal history of GDM and 120 women serving as controls, describing higher values of PWV in women with GDM vs. normoglycemic pregnancies, up to 3.7 years after delivery [51]. Finally, women with a personal history of GMD were found to have higher levels of PWV and augmentation index, indicating more extensive arterial stiffens, compared to women with normoglycemia during pregnancy, after a median follow-up time of 6 years [52].

Accumulating data tried to elucidate pathophysiological mechanisms potentially contributing to the development of subclinical vascular disease in patients with a personal history of GDM. A small study of 39 pregnant women with GDM and 40 healthy pregnant women serving as controls observed a disturbance of antioxidative mechanisms in women with GDM [53]. Accordingly, GDM women had significantly higher levels of lipid hydroperoxide and significantly lower levels of antioxidative parameters like paraoxonase activity as well as free sulfhydryl groups [53]. In addition, higher levels of inflammatory and proatherogenic markers were observed in a smaller cross-sectional study of pregnant women with GMD vs. pregnant women serving as controls, like high-sensitivity C-reactive protein and tumor necrosis factor (TNF) alpha as well as plasminogen activator inhibitor-1 [54]. Higher levels of tissue inhibitor of metalloproteinase-1 (TIMP-1) indicative of low-grade inflammation were observed in women with a previous history of GDM, further contributing to the development of atherosclerosis [51]. Moreover, impaired profile of regulatory T cells and natural killer cells, possibly linked with the development of inflammation and insulin resistance, has been evidenced in a smaller case-control study of 27 glucose-tolerant controls and 31 GDM overweight pregnant women [55].

10.6   Breastfeeding and Cardiovascular Disease in Later Life

The pregnancy-related metabolic alterations may exhibit a more prolonged effect on maternal cardiovascular risk. This link is likely affected by parity and presence of additional cardiovascular risk factors. On the other hand, a growing amount of evidence has described that breastfeeding is reversing some of the pregnancy-related proatherogenic implications toward the female cardiovascular system and thus may potentially reduce the amount of the additional cardiovascular risk conferred by pregnancy [56]. In fact, results of the Study of Women's Health Across the Nation (SWAN) study suggested an up to 21% lower risk of metabolic syndrome in women who lactated in the past versus women who never lactated, while cumulative duration of lactation is associated with lower prevalence of the metabolic syndrome in midlife [57]. Moreover, lower prevalence of diabetes, hyperlipidemia, and hypertension was associated with the longer cumulative duration of lifetime lactation, as reported in the Women's Health Initiative, indicating a dose-response association [58].

Preliminary data evaluated the impact of lactation on vascular characteristics, supporting an overall beneficial association. The Coronary Artery Risk Development in Young Adults (CARDIA) study evaluated prospectively a total of 846 women during a follow-up period of 20 years [59]. The results of this study showed a graded inverse association between a personal history of lactation and mean values of common carotid intima-media thickness in middle-aged women, with the association being modestly attenuated after controlling for traditional cardiovascular risk factors [59]. Parous women who never breastfed exhibited a 0.13 mm larger lumen diameter and 0.12 mm larger adventitial diameter of carotid arteries compared to women who breastfed for at least 3 months after every birth, independently of traditional risk factors or health-related behavior, as reported in 607 premenopausal women of the Women and Infants Study of Healthy Hearts study [60]. In a cross-sectional evaluation of 297 women enrolled in the SWAN study [61], mothers who had not breastfed exhibited 5.26 times higher risk of aortic calcification (95% CI: 1.47–20.0) compared to women who breastfed, independently of traditional cardiovascular risk factors, socioeconomic status as well as lifestyle and family history variables, and body mass index. Data on the link between a personal history of lactation and arterial stiffness remains sparse. One available study could not confirm a link between arterial stiffness and a personal history of lactation in premenopausal women [60].

In addition, a history of lactation has been linked with lower risk of developing hypertension in later life. The beneficial effects of breastfeeding on blood pressure readings become evident even from the first month postnatal, as described in non-overweight women [62]. A personal history of breastfeeding was associated with lower risk of hypertension in midlife, as described in a cohort of 3119 non-smoking postmenopausal women participating in the Korea National Health and Nutrition Examination Survey [63]. In fact, the population attributable fraction of hypertension in women who breastfeed for less than 5 years was estimated as 6.5%, while the protective impact of lactation on the risk of maternal hypertension was attenuated by greater insulin resistance and obesity [63]. In addition, women who breastfed at least 3 months per child had lower odds of developing hypertension in midlife when compared with parous women who never breastfed, as described in the 45 and Up Study, which evaluated a sample of 74,785 Australian women [64].

Moreover, breastfeeding has been associated with lower incidence of cardiovascular or coronary heart disease in later life. A recent sub-analysis of the European Prospective Investigation into Cancer and Nutrition (EPI-CVD) prospective case-cohort study assessed the development of coronary events overtime in a total of 17,640 participants from ten countries [65]. This study described that the risk of coronary events was lower among women who breastfed when compared with women who did not breastfeed (adjusted HR, 0.71; 95% CI: 0.52–0.98). The additional CHD risk conferred by pregnancy was confirmed based on the results of this study, which reported a higher risk of coronary events among parous versus nulliparous women (adjusted HR 1.19; 95% CI: 1.01–1.41) [65]. A similar prospective study performed among 300,000 Chinese women [66] indicated a significantly lower risk of CVD in women with a personal history of breastfeeding when compared with women who never breastfed (adjusted HR for CHD 0.91; 95% CI%, 0.84–0.99; for stroke 0.92; 95% CI, 0.85–0.99). More specifically, an up to 18% lower risk of CHD and up to 17% lower risk of stroke was observed in women who breastfed for at least 24 months [66]. In addition, women who had never breastfed had higher risk of experiencing a fatal cardiovascular event when compared to women with a personal history of breastfeeding, after adjustment for parity, sociodemographic and traditional cardiovascular risk factors (HR 2.53, 95% CI: 1.39 to 4.99), as reported by the results of the HUNT2 study [67]. This effect was attenuated with increasing age and thus was evident in women older than 65 years.

10.7   Conclusion

Hypertensive disorders of pregnancy and diabetes mellitus are associated with a significant adverse effect on the maternal cardiovascular system as well as on the accumulation of cardiometabolic risk factors. Implications become prevalent soon after delivery and seem to last up until middle age. Breastfeeding on the other hand may reverse these adverse changes to some extent, improving the cardiovascular profile of the mother.

References

1. WHO. Cardiovascular disease key facts. Geneva: WHO. www.who.int/mediacentre/factsheets/fs317/en/. Accessed 27 Feb 2018.
2. Townsend N, et al. Cardiovascular disease in Europe: epidemiological update 2016. Eur Heart J. 2016;37(42):3232–45.
3. Appelman Y, et al. Sex differences in cardiovascular risk factors and disease prevention. Atherosclerosis. 2015;241(1):211–8.
4. Park K, et al. Adverse pregnancy conditions, infertility, and future cardiovascular risk: implications for mother and child. Cardiovasc Drugs Ther. 2015;29(4):391–401.
5. Mosca L, et al. Effectiveness-based guidelines for the prevention of cardiovascular disease in women—2011 update: a guideline from the american heart association. Circulation. 2011;123(11):1243–62.
6. Gongora MC, Wenger NK. Cardiovascular complications of pregnancy. Int J Mol Sci. 2015;16(10):23905–28.
7. Lind JM, Hennessy A, McLean M. Cardiovascular disease in women: the significance of hypertension and gestational diabetes during pregnancy. Curr Opin Cardiol. 2014;29(5):447–53.
8. Smith GN. The maternal health clinic: improving women's cardiovascular health. Semin Perinatol. 2015;39(4):316–9.
9. Thornburg KL, et al. Hemodynamic changes in pregnancy. Semin Perinatol. 2000;24(1):11–4.
10. Bernstein IM, Ziegler W, Badger GJ. Plasma volume expansion in early pregnancy. Obstet Gynecol. 2001;97(5 Pt 1):669–72.
11. Ouzounian JG, Elkayam U. Physiologic changes during normal pregnancy and delivery. Cardiol Clin. 2012;30(3):317–29.
12. Creasy RK, Resnik R. Maternal-fetal medicine. Philadelphia, PA: Saunders; 1999.
13. Tiralongo GM, et al. Assessment of total vascular resistance and total body water in normotensive women during the first trimester of pregnancy. A key for the prevention of preeclampsia. Pregnancy Hypertens. 2015;5(2):193–7.
14. Ayala DE, et al. Blood pressure variability during gestation in healthy and complicated pregnancies. Hypertension. 1997;30(3 Pt 2):611–8.
15. Grindheim G, et al. Changes in blood pressure during healthy pregnancy: a longitudinal cohort study. J Hypertens. 2012;30(2):342–50.
16. James AH. Pregnancy-associated thrombosis. Hematology Am Soc Hematol Educ Program. 2009;2009:277.
17. DeStephano CC, et al. Diagnosis and management of iliac vein thrombosis in pregnancy resulting from May-Thurner syndrome. J Perinatol. 2014;34(7):566–8.
18. Butte NF. Carbohydrate and lipid metabolism in pregnancy: normal compared with gestational diabetes mellitus. Am J Clin Nutr. 2000;71(5 Suppl):1256S–61S.
19. Mammaro A, et al. Hypertensive disorders of pregnancy. J Prenat Med. 2009;3(1):1–5.
20. National High Blood Pressure Education Program Working Group on High Blood Pressure in Pregnancy. Report of the National High Blood Pressure Education Program Working Group on High Blood Pressure in Pregnancy. Am J Obstet Gynecol. 2000;183(1):S1–S22.
21. Umesawa M, Kobashi G. Epidemiology of hypertensive disorders in pregnancy: prevalence, risk factors, predictors and prognosis. Hypertens Res. 2017;40(3):213–20.
22. Groenhof TKJ, et al. Preventing cardiovascular disease after hypertensive disorders of pregnancy: searching for the how and when. Eur J Prev Cardiol. 2017;24(16):1735–45.
23. Timpka S, et al. Lifestyle in progression from hypertensive disorders of pregnancy to chronic hypertension in Nurses' Health Study II: observational cohort study. BMJ. 2017;358:j3024.
24. Wang L, et al. Association between hypertensive disorders of pregnancy and the risk of postpartum hypertension: a cohort study in women with gestational diabetes. J Hum Hypertens. 2017;31(11):725–30.
25. Behrens I, et al. Association between hypertensive disorders of pregnancy and later risk of cardiomyopathy. JAMA. 2016;315(10):1026–33.

26. Veerbeek JH, et al. Cardiovascular disease risk factors after early-onset preeclampsia, late-onset preeclampsia, and pregnancy-induced hypertension. Hypertension. 2015;65(3):600–6.
27. Andersgaard AB, et al. Recurrence and long-term maternal health risks of hypertensive disorders of pregnancy: a population-based study. Am J Obstet Gynecol. 2012;206(2):6.
28. Kestenbaum B, et al. Cardiovascular and thromboembolic events following hypertensive pregnancy. Am J Kidney Dis. 2003;42(5):982–9.
29. Wikstrom AK, et al. The risk of maternal ischaemic heart disease after gestational hypertensive disease. BJOG. 2005;112(11):1486–91.
30. Tooher J, et al. All hypertensive disorders of pregnancy increase the risk of future cardiovascular disease. Hypertension. 2017;70(4):798–803.
31. Alsnes IV, et al. A population-based study of associations between preeclampsia and later cardiovascular risk factors. Am J Obstet Gynecol. 2014;211(6):17.
32. Drost JT, et al. Cardiovascular risk factors in women 10 years post early preeclampsia: the Preeclampsia Risk EValuation in FEMales study (PREVFEM). Eur J Prev Cardiol. 2012;19(5):1138–44.
33. Sibai BM, el-Nazer A, Gonzalez-Ruiz A. Severe preeclampsia-eclampsia in young primigravid women: subsequent pregnancy outcome and remote prognosis. Am J Obstet Gynecol. 1986;155(5):1011–6.
34. Bokslag A, et al. Effect of early-onset preeclampsia on cardiovascular risk in the fifth decade of life. Am J Obstet Gynecol. 2017;216(5):14.
35. Brown MC, et al. Cardiovascular disease risk in women with pre-eclampsia: systematic review and meta-analysis. Eur J Epidemiol. 2013;28(1):1–19.
36. Wu P, et al. Preeclampsia and future cardiovascular health: a systematic review and meta-analysis. Circ Cardiovasc Qual Outcomes. 2017;10(2):22.
37. Zoet GA, et al. Cardiovascular RiskprofilE – IMaging and gender-specific disOrders (CREw-IMAGO): rationale and design of a multicenter cohort study. BMC Womens Health. 2017;17:60.
38. Hauspurg A, et al. Adverse pregnancy outcomes and future maternal cardiovascular disease. Clin Cardiol. 2018;15(10):22887.
39. Egan AM, et al. Epidemiology of gestational diabetes mellitus according to IADPSG/WHO 2013 criteria among obese pregnant women in Europe. Diabetologia. 2017;60(10):1913–21.
40. Buchanan TA, Xiang AH, Page KA. Gestational diabetes mellitus: risks and management during and after pregnancy. Nat Rev Endocrinol. 2012;8(11):639–49.
41. Li LJ, et al. Effect of gestational diabetes and hypertensive disorders of pregnancy on postpartum cardiometabolic risk. Endocr Connect. 2018;14:17–0359.
42. Retnakaran R, Shah BR. Mild glucose intolerance in pregnancy and risk of cardiovascular disease: a population-based cohort study. CMAJ. 2009;181(6–7):371–6.
43. Tobias DK, et al. Association of history of gestational diabetes with long-term cardiovascular disease risk in a large prospective cohort of US women. JAMA Intern Med. 2017;177(12):1735–42.
44. Goueslard K, et al. Early cardiovascular events in women with a history of gestational diabetes mellitus. Cardiovasc Diabetol. 2016;15(15):016–0338.
45. Shah BR, Retnakaran R, Booth GL. Increased risk of cardiovascular disease in young women following gestational diabetes mellitus. Diabetes Care. 2008;31(8):1668–9.
46. Li J-W, et al. Association of gestational diabetes mellitus (GDM) with subclinical atherosclerosis: a systemic review and meta-analysis. BMC Cardiovasc Disord. 2014;14:132.
47. Li JW, et al. Association of gestational diabetes mellitus (GDM) with subclinical atherosclerosis: a systemic review and meta-analysis. BMC Cardiovasc Disord. 2014;14(132):1471–2261.
48. Caliskan M, et al. Does gestational diabetes history increase epicardial fat and carotid intima media thickness? Echocardiography. 2014;31(10):1182–7.
49. Gunderson EP, et al. History of gestational diabetes mellitus and future risk of atherosclerosis in mid-life: the coronary artery risk development in young adults study. J Am Heart Assoc. 2014;3(2):000490.

50. Lekva T, et al. Aortic stiffness and cardiovascular risk in women with previous gestational diabetes mellitus. PLoS One. 2015;10(8):e0136892.
51. Vilmi-Kerala T, et al. Subclinical inflammation associated with prolonged TIMP-1 upregulation and arterial stiffness after gestational diabetes mellitus: a hospital-based cohort study. Cardiovasc Diabetol. 2017;16(1):017–0530.
52. Tam WH, et al. PP103. Arterial stiffness in women with previous GDM – a follow up of Chinese HAPO study cohort. Pregnancy Hypertens. 2012;2(3):13.
53. Vural M, et al. Evaluation of the future atherosclerotic heart disease with oxidative stress and carotid artery intima media thickness in gestational diabetes mellitus. Endocr Res. 2012;37(3):145–53.
54. Salmi AA, et al. Arterial stiffness, inflammatory and pro-atherogenic markers in gestational diabetes mellitus. Vasa. 2012;41(2):96–104.
55. Lobo TF, et al. Impaired Treg and NK cells profile in overweight women with gestational diabetes mellitus. Am J Reprod Immunol. 2018;79(3):5.
56. Perrine CG, et al. Lactation and maternal cardio-metabolic health. Annu Rev Nutr. 2016;36:627–45.
57. Ram KT, et al. Duration of lactation is associated with lower prevalence of the metabolic syndrome in midlife—SWAN, the study of women's health across the nation. Am J Obstet Gynecol. 2008;198(3):268.e1–6.
58. Schwarz EB, et al. Duration of lactation and risk factors for maternal cardiovascular disease. Obstet Gynecol. 2009;113(5):974–82.
59. Gunderson EP, et al. Lactation duration and midlife atherosclerosis. Obstet Gynecol. 2015;126(2):381–90.
60. McClure CK, et al. Lactation and maternal subclinical cardiovascular disease among premenopausal women. Am J Obstet Gynecol. 2012;207(1):2.
61. Schwarz EB, et al. Lactation and maternal measures of subclinical cardiovascular disease. Obstet Gynecol. 2010;115(1):41–8.
62. Groer MW, et al. Breastfeeding status and maternal cardiovascular variables across the postpartum. J Women's Health. 2013;22(5):453–9.
63. Park S, Choi NK. Breastfeeding and maternal hypertension. Am J Hypertens. 2018;25:4825441.
64. Lupton SJ, et al. Association between parity and breastfeeding with maternal high blood pressure. Am J Obstet Gynecol. 2013;208(6):7.
65. Peters SA, et al. Parity, breastfeeding and risk of coronary heart disease: a pan-European case-cohort study. Eur J Prev Cardiol. 2016;23(16):1755–65.
66. Peters SAE, et al. Breastfeeding and the risk of maternal cardiovascular disease: a prospective study of 300 000 Chinese women. J Am Heart Assoc. 2017;6(6):006081.
67. Natland Fagerhaug T, et al. A prospective population-based cohort study of lactation and cardiovascular disease mortality: the HUNT study. BMC Public Health. 2013;13(1070):1471–2458.

HRT and Cardiovascular Disease

11

Jenifer Sassarini and Mary Ann Lumsden

11.1 Introduction

Cardiovascular events are the main cause of death in women, particularly in those over the age of 70 years. However, one third of all non-fatal cardiovascular events before age 80 occur in women below age 60 (Writing Group [1]).

Until the late 1990s, oestrogen was thought to protect against coronary heart disease (CHD) [2]. Many cohort studies showed that menopausal hormone therapy HRT was associated with a 40–50% reduction in the incidence of CHD. However, an RCT, the Women's Health Initiative (WHI) found an early, transient increase in coronary events in the combined HRT (oestrogen plus progestogen), but not the oestrogen alone arm [3]. However, the average age of participants in WHI was 63 years old, 12 years older than the average age of menopause in the UK and Western Europe; therefore it is possible that the women in these studies had established subclinical atherosclerosis and the impact of HRT might be different in younger women. This 'window of opportunity concept has subsequently been supported by several publications [4–7].

In a meta-analysis of clinical outcomes, the 2015 Cochrane review of RCT data found that HRT initiated fewer than 10 years after menopause onset lowered CHD in postmenopausal women (RR, 0.52; 95% CI, 0.29–0.96) [8]. It also found a reduction in all-cause mortality (RR, 0.70; 95% CI, 0.52–0.95) and no increased risk of stroke but an increased risk of VTE (RR, 1.74; 95%CI, 1.11–2.73), similar to the findings of a prior meta-analysis of studies in women who initiated HRT within 10 years of menopause onset and/or in women aged younger than 60 years [9].

J. Sassarini
Glasgow Royal Infirmary, Glasgow, UK
e-mail: Jenifer.sassarini@ggc.scot.nhs.uk

M. A. Lumsden (✉)
University of Glasgow, Glasgow, UK
e-mail: Maryann.Lumsden@glasgow.ac.uk

© International Society of Gynecological Endocrinology 2019
R. D. Brinton et al. (eds.), *Sex Steroids' Effects on Brain, Heart and Vessels*,
ISGE Series, https://doi.org/10.1007/978-3-030-11355-1_11

These include the subgroup analysis of data, from the WHI trials, which examined HRT use stratified by age and time since menopause and demonstrated more favourable results for all-cause mortality and myocardial infarction in women aged 50–59 and those close to menopause [10] than 60 years [9].

The Danish Osteoporosis Prevention Study (DOPS) [11], an open-label RCT, showed that HRT was associated with a reduction in cardiovascular disease in women of the same age group.

For CEE alone, of the Women's Health Initiative study, CHD, total MI, and coronary artery bypass grafting or percutaneous coronary intervention showed a lowered HR in women aged younger than 60 years and fewer than 10 years since menopause onset, even in intention-to-treat analyses [10]. Age group analysis in the WHI CEE/MPA trial was an outlier. In the 50- to 59-year-old age group, the HR for CHD was elevated but not statistically significant at 1.34 (95% CI, 0.82–2.19) for CEE/MPA.

11.2   IMS Global Statement [12]

This Statement, endorsed by Menopause Societies from all around the world, states that randomized clinical trials and observational data as well as meta-analyses provide evidence that standard-dose oestrogen-alone HRT may decrease myocardial infarction and all-cause mortality in women younger than 60 years of age and within 10 years of menopause.

Data on oestrogen plus progestogen HRT in women younger than 60 years or within 10 years of menopause show a less compelling trend for mortality benefit, and evidence on cardioprotection is less robust with inconsistent results compared to the oestrogen alone group.

The *NICE Guideline on Menopause (NG23)* published in 2016 [13] provides guidance on the use of HRT and the risk of cardiovascular risk, and this is summarized below.

11.2.1 HRT and the Risk of Cardiovascular Disease in Women with No Previous CV Events

The baseline risk of coronary heart disease for women around menopausal age varies from one woman to another according to the presence of cardiovascular risk factors. Baseline risk estimated 26.3/1000 over 7.5 years.

- HRT does not increase the risk of cardiovascular disease when started in women aged under 60 years.
- HRT does not affect the risk of dying from cardiovascular disease.

11.2.2 Women with Pre-existing Cardiovascular Risk Factors

- Optimise cardiovascular risk factors.
- HRT is not contraindicated in this group.
- Use transdermal preparations in women who are obese.

11.3 North American Menopause Society [14]

11.3.1 Cardiovascular Disease and All-Cause Mortality

Newer observational data and reanalysis of older studies by age or time since menopause, including the WHI, suggest that for healthy, recently menopausal women, the benefits of HRT (oestrogen alone or with a progestogen) outweigh its risks, with fewer CVD events in younger versus older women.

11.3.2 Advice Must Be Given to Modify Their Risk Factors for CV Events

11.3.2.1 BMI and Obesity
Women should maintain or lose weight through an appropriate balance of physical activity, caloric intake, and formal behavioural programme to maintain/achieve a BMI of between 18.5 and 24.9 kb/m^2 and a waist circumference ≤35 in. Recommendations may vary between different ethnic groups, e.g. South Asians where increased risk occurs at lower BMI than in Europeans [15].

11.3.2.2 Smoking
Compared to non-smokers, female current smokers have a relative risk of myocardial infarction of 2.24 (range 1.85–2.71) [16]. Second-hand smoke also increases the risk of CHD. Smoking cessation, but not reduction, reduces the risk of myocardial infarction.

11.3.2.3 Exercise and Physical Activity
Lower fitness levels are associated with a 4.7-fold increased risk for CHD. It is now accepted that women should undertake 150 min/week of moderate to vigorous physical activity [17].

11.3.2.4 Hypertension
Treating hypertension reduces the risk of CHD. For every 1 mmHg decrease in systolic blood pressure, there is a decrease in risk of a cardiovascular event even in those whose blood pressure is at the higher end of the normal range [18].

11.3.3 Women with a Past History of Cardiovascular Events

- HRT should be discontinued after myocardial infarction (MI).
- The decision to initiate HRT after MI should be made after full discussion between the woman, the menopause specialist, and a cardiologist.

The current recommendation is to discontinue HRT after MI, despite there being no evidence that a cardiovascular event takes a more serious course in HRT users than in non-users. In fact, there is some data that HRT users have a lower mortality rate after MI than non-users [19–21]. The 30-day mortality after a cardiovascular event appears primarily determined by conventional risk factors and the degree of cardiac impairment.

Risk of cardiovascular events may then increase in stopping HRT [22].

11.4 Stroke

The baseline risk of stroke for women around menopausal age varies from one woman to another according to the presence of cardiovascular risk factors such as hypertension. Baseline risk estimated to be 11.3/1000, respectively, over 7.5 years.

The attributable risk of stroke in women under the age of 60 years or within 10 years of menopause was subject to meta-analysis of studies. No increased risk was demonstrated in women aged younger than 60 years or who were within 10 years of the menopause [8]. In a subgroup analysis, the attributable risk of stroke in the WHI for women who initiated MHT aged less than 60 years was rare (<1/1000 person years) and statistically nonsignificant for CEE/MPA, with an absolute risk of 5/10,000 person-years in women aged younger than 60 years or within 10 years of initiation [10], similar to other studies [10, 23].

For CEE alone the WHI, findings were inconsistent. For women aged 50 to 59 years at randomization, a decrease of 1/10,000 person-years was seen for stroke, whereas for women fewer than 10 years from menopause onset, an increase in 13 strokes/10,000 person-years was seen [4]. In observational studies, lower doses of either oral [24] or transdermal [25] oestrogen may have less risk of stroke. No head-to-head data comparing oral to transdermal are available although one study suggests transdermal oestrogen may pose less risk.

There is no increase in the risk of haemorrhagic stroke associated with HRT.

- *Taking oral (but not transdermal) oestrogen is associated with a small increase in the risk of stroke.*

11.4.1 Past History of Stroke

Oestrogen has a procoagulatory activity, and thromboembolism is the common pathomechanism of ischaemic strokes.

* Initiating HRT after stroke or TIA is contraindicated.

Women on oral low- and standard-dose oestrogen therapy, the risk of stroke was appreciably elevated (rate ratio 1.28, 95% CI 1.15–1.42); however, it should be noted that transdermal oestrogen up to a dosage of 50 µg/day—mostly combined with micronized progesterone—in women with a past history of stroke was not associated with an increased risk of stroke versus controls (rate ratio 0.81, 95% CI 0.62–1.05). However, this is a nested case-control study, not an RCT [26].

11.4.2 Venous Thromboembolism

In a meta-analysis of trials of women who began MHT treatment within 10 years of the menopause or who were aged under 60 years, strong evidence of increased risk of VTE was found in the MHT group compared with placebo (RR 1.74; 95% CI, 1.11–2.73) [8]. Lower doses of oral ET may confer less VTE risk than higher doses [25], but comparative RCT data are lacking. Micronized progesterone may be less thrombogenic than other progestins [19]. Limited observational data suggest less risk with transdermal HT than oral [27, 28]. No excess risk has been seen with vaginal oestrogen.

11.4.3 Premature Ovarian Insufficiency

Women with an untreated premature menopause are at increased risk of CHD [29]. Regulatory bodies recommend the use of HRT in premature ovarian failure up till the average age of the natural menopause.

11.4.4 Alternative Treatments for Vasomotor Symptoms

See RCOG Guidance (link) and below for further reading.

References

1. Writing Group Members. Heart disease and stroke statistics – 2017 update: a report from the American Heart Association. Circulation. 2017;135:e146–603.
2. Grodstein F, Mansori JE, Golditz FA, Willit WC, Speizer FD, Stampfer MJ. A prospective, observational study of postmenopausal hormone therapy and primary prevention of cardiovascular disease. Ann Intern Med. 2000;133:933–41.
3. Writing Group for the Women's Health Initiative Investigators. Risk and benefits of estrogen plus progestin in healthy postmenopausal women: principal results from the Women's Health Initiative randomized controlled trial. JAMA. 2002;288(3):321–33.
4. Manson JE, Chlebowski RT, Stefanick ML, et al. Menopausal hormone therapy and health outcomes during the intervention and extended poststopping phases of the Women's Health Initiative randomized trials. JAMA. 2013;310(13):1353–68. Pubmed Central PMCID: 3963523.
5. Salpeter SR, Walsh JM, Greybar E, Salpeter EE. Brief report: coronary heart disease events associated with hormone therapy in younger and older women. A meta-analysis. J Gen Intern Med. 2006;21:363–6.
6. Savolainen-Peltonen H, Tuomikoski P, Korhonen P, et al. Cardiac death risk in relation to the age at initiation or the progestin component of hormone therapies. J Clin Endocrinol Metab. 2016;101:2794–801.
7. Carrasquilla GD, Berglund A, Gigante B, et al. Does menopausal hormone therapy reduce myocardial infarction risk if initiated early after menopause? A population-based case-control study. Menopause. 2015;22:598–606.
8. Boardman HM, Hartley L, Eisinga A, et al. Hormone therapy for preventing cardiovascular disease in post-menopausal women. Cochrane Database Syst Rev. 2015;3:CD002229.
9. Salpeter SR, Cheng J, Thabane L, Buckley NS, Salpeter EE. Bayesian meta-analysis of hormone therapy and mortality in younger postmenopausal women. Am J Med. 2009;12:1016–22.
10. Rossouw JE, Prentice RL, Manson JE, et al. Postmenopausal hormone therapy and risk of cardiovascular disease by age and years since menopause. JAMA. 2007;297:1465–77.
11. Schierbeck LL, Rejnmark L, Tofteng CL, et al. Effect of hormone replacement therapy on cardiovascular events in recently postmenopausal women: randomized trial. BMJ. 2012;345:e6409.
12. de Villiers TJ, Hall JE, Pinkerton JV, Pérez SC, Rees M, Yang C, Pierroz DD. Revised global consensus statement on menopausal hormone therapy. Maturitas. 2016;91:153–5.
13. NICE. NICE guidance: ng23. Diagnosis and management of menopause. London: NICE. https://www.nice.org.uk/guidance/ng23/
14. The NAMS 2017 Hormone Therapy Position Statement Advisory Panel. The 2017 hormone therapy position statement of the North American Menopause Society. Menopause. 2017;24:728–53.
15. Kidy FF, Dhalwani N, Harrington DM, Gray LJ, Bodicoat DH, Webb D, Davies MJ, Khunti K. Associations between anthropometric measurements and cardiometabolic risk factors in White European and South Asian adults in the United Kingdom. Mayo Clin Proc. 2017;92(6):925–33.
16. Aune D, Schlesinger S, Norat T, Riboli E. Tobacco smoking and the risk of sudden cardiac death: a systematic review and meta-analysis of prospective studies. Eur J Epidemiol. 2018;33(6):509–21. https://doi.org/10.1007/s10654-017-0351-y.
17. Iliodromiti S, Ghouri N, Celis-Morales CA, Sattar N, Lumsden MA, Gill JM. Should physical activity recommendations for South Asian adults be ethnicity-specific? Evidence from a cross-sectional study of South Asian and White European men and women. PLoS One. 2016;11(8):e0160024.
18. Hong Z, Wu T, Zhou S, Huang B, Wang J, Jin D, Geng D. Effects of anti-hypertensive treatment on major cardiovascular events in populations within prehypertensive levels: a system-

atic review and meta-analysis. J Hum Hypertens. 2018;32(2):94–104. https://doi.org/10.1038/s41371-017-0026-x.

19. Windler E, Stute P, Ortmann O, Mueck AO. Is postmenopausal hormone replacement therapy suitable after a cardio- or cerebrovascular event? Arch Gynecol Obstet. 2015;291(1):213–7.

20. Shlipak MG, Angeja BG, Go AS, et al. Hormone therapy and in-hospital survival after myocardial infarction in postmenopausal women. Circulation. 2001;104(19):2300–4.

21. Tackett AH, Bailey AL, Foody JM, et al. Hormone replacement therapy among postmenopausal women presenting with acute myocardial infarction: insights from the GUSTO-III trial. Am Heart J. 2010;160(4):678–84.

22. Mikkola TS, Tuomikoski P, Lyytinen H, et al. Increased cardiovascular mortality risk in women discontinuing postmenopausal hormone therapy. J Clin Endocrinol Metab. 2015;100(12):4588–94.

23. LaCroix AZ, Chlebowski RT, Manson JE, et al. Health risks and benefits after stopping the Women's Health Initiative trial of conjugated equine estrogens in postmenopausal women with prior hysterectomy. JAMA. 2011;305(13):1305–14. https://doi.org/10.1001/jama.2011.382.

24. Canonico M, Carcaillon L, Plu-Bureau G, Oger E, et al. Postmenopausal hormone therapy and risk of stroke: impact of the route of estrogen administration and type of progestogen. Stroke. 2016;47:1734–41.

25. Speroff L. Transdermal hormone therapy and the risk of stroke and venous thrombosis. Climacteric. 2010;13:429–32.

26. Renoux C, Dell'aniello S, Garbe E, Suissa S. Transdermal and oral hormone replacement therapy and the risk of stroke: a nested case-control study. BMJ. 2010;340:c2519.

27. Canonico M, Oger E, Plu-Bureau G, et al., Estrogen and Thromboembolism Risk (ESTHER) Study Group. Hormone therapy and venous thromboembolism among postmenopausal women: impact of the route of estrogen administration and progestogens: the ESTHER study. Circulation. 2007;115:840–5.

28. Canonico M, Alhenc-Gelas M, Plu-Bureau G, Olie V, Scarabin PY. Activated protein C reseistance among postmenopausal women using transdermal estrogens: importance of progestogen. Menopause. 2010;17:1122–7.

29. Peters SA, Woodward M. Women's reproductive factors and incident cardiovascular disease in the UK Biobank. Heart. 2018;pii:heartjnl-2017-312289.

Further Reading

BMS consensus statements. www.thebms.org.uk

NICE. NICE guidance: ng23. Diagnosis and management of menopause. London: NICE. https://www.nice.org.uk/guidance/ng23/

RCOG. Alternatives to HRT for the management of symptoms of the menopause (SAC opinion paper 6). London: RCOG; 2010. http://www.rcog.org.uk/womens-health/clinical-guidance/alternatives-hrt-management-symptoms-menopause

Unique Vascular Benefits of Estetrol, a Native Fetal Estrogen with Specific Actions in Tissues (NEST)

J. M. Foidart, U. Gaspard, C. Pequeux, M. Jost, V. Gordenne,
E. Tskitishvili, A. Gallez, M. C. Valera, P. Gourdy, C. Fontaine,
D. Henrion, Andrea R. Genazzani, F. Lenfant, and J. F. Arnal

Abbreviations

Ang II	Angiotensin II
CEE	Combined equine estrogen
CHD	Coronary heart disease
COCs	Combined oral contraceptives
CVD	Cardiovascular disease
DRSP	Drospirenone
DVT	Deep venous thrombophlebitis

J. M. Foidart (✉) · U. Gaspard · C. Pequeux · E. Tskitishvili · A. Gallez
Laboratory of Tumor and Development Biology, GIGA-Cancer, University of Liège, Liege, Belgium
e-mail: jmfoidart@uliege.be; c.pequeux@uliege.be; ekaterine.tskitishvili@uliege.be;
anne.gallez@uliege.be

M. Jost · V. Gordenne
Mithra Pharmaceuticals, Liège, Belgium
e-mail: mjost@mithra.com; vgordenne@mithra.com

M. C. Valera · P. Gourdy · C. Fontaine · F. Lenfant · J. F. Arnal
I2MC, Institut National de la Santé et de la Recherche Médicale (INSERM) U 1048,
University of Toulouse 3, Toulouse, France
e-mail: pierre.gourdy@inserm.fr; coralie.fontaine@inserm.fr; francoise.lenfant@inserm.fr;
jean-francois.arnal@inserm.fr

D. Henrion
MITOVASC Institute, CARFI Facility, INSERM U1083, UMR CNRS, 6015, University
of Angers, Angers, France
e-mail: daniel.henrion@univ-angers.fr

A. R. Genazzani
Division of Obstetrics and Gynecology, Department of Clinical and Experimental Medicine,
University of Pisa, Pisa, Italy

International School for Gynecological and Reproductive Endocrinology, International
Society of Gynecological Endocrinology, Locarno, Switzerland

© International Society of Gynecological Endocrinology 2019
R. D. Brinton et al. (eds.), *Sex Steroids' Effects on Brain, Heart and Vessels*,
ISGE Series, https://doi.org/10.1007/978-3-030-11355-1_12

E   Estrogen
E2   Estradiol
E4   Estetrol
eNOS   Endothelial nitric oxide synthase
ERα   Estrogen receptor alpha
ERα$^{-/-}$ Estrogen receptor alpha KO
FMR   Flow-mediated arteriolar remodeling
HF   High flow
HT   Hormone therapy
LNG   Levonorgestrel
MPA   Medroxyprogesterone acetate
NEST   Native estrogen with selective actions in tissues
NF   Normal flow
NIH   National Institutes of Health
NO   Nitric oxide
PE   Pulmonary embolism
RR   Relative risk
VTE   Venous thromboembolism
WHI   Women's Health Initiative

12.1   Introduction

For several decades, the role of hormone replacement therapy (HRT) has been debated. Early observational data on HRT showed many benefits, including a reduction in coronary atherosclerosis, coronary heart disease (CHD), osteoporosis, CHD mortality, and all-cause mortality as well as the risk of Alzheimer's disease [1–3]. As CHD has the highest case fatality rate, the reduction in CHD with HRT was considered to have the greatest impact on mortality, with all-cause mortality cases being decreased by 20–40% in the observational studies [4, 5]. Meta-analyses of these and other data suggested that use of HRT would result in one to two additional years of life, which is large in epidemiological terms. More recently, randomized trials in women with established coronary disease (secondary prevention trials), as well as the Women's Health Initiative (WHI), which studied mostly women many years after the onset of menopause, showed no such benefit and an increased risk of CHD and breast cancer [6, 7]. In 2002, the NIH, who sponsored the WHI, emphatically stated that HRT caused more harm than good and that this pertained to women of all ages and occurred with all types of HRT.

In 2006, the first study from WHI emerged that carried out an age stratification for coronary disease outcomes. The use of conjugated equine estrogens (CEE) had a protective effect in women aged 50–59 years, but not in those women aged ≥60 years [8]. In 2007, another manuscript from the WHI showed that in women aged 50–59 years or those <10 years from menopause onset, total mortality decreased significantly by 30% [9]. This figure is in accordance with reports from the original observational studies and suggests that the protective effects of HRT are dependent on the "timing" of initiation, as was originally proposed by Clarkson.

Recent randomized (ELITE, KEEP) and observational data (COMPREHEND) and several meta-analyses, including a Cochrane analysis, now consistently show reductions in CHD and mortality when HRT is initiated soon after menopause [10–12].

Finally the WHI writing group published in September 2017 that among 27,347 postmenopausal women, HRT with CEE plus medroxyprogesterone acetate (MPA) for a median of 5.6 years or with CEE alone for a median of 7.2 years was not associated with risk of all-cause, cardiovascular, or cancer mortality during a cumulative follow-up of 18 years. Younger women (aged 50–59 years) tended to have lower HRs than older women did for mortality due to CVD, cancer, and other causes during the intervention phases of the two trials [13].

In summary, the WHI had a considerable negative impact; the originally reported adverse cardiovascular effects have been proven incorrect, when taking into account the time of initiation of HRT. The relationship of HRT to breast cancer is also complex, controversial, and confusing. In WHI, CEE alone showed a decrease in breast cancer, and only prior users of HRT before randomization into the WHI trial who used combination CEE and MPA showed some increase in breast cancer risk over time.

Objective analyses of the data allow concluding that observational studies and randomized trials are concordant in showing some increase in stroke (RR 1.3–1.4), modest increase in endometrial cancer with estrogen alone, a decrease in colon cancer, and an increase in venous thrombosis with oral HRT [14]. Ischemic stroke in younger (aged <60 years) women is rare and has been proposed to be due to a thrombotic mechanism [15, 16]. This suggests that a non-oral route of estrogen administration or an estrogen, which is devoid of thrombotic tendencies, may reduce stroke incidence. Transdermal estradiol, in standard doses, does not to increase the risk of stroke [17].

Finally, in 2017, the WHI writing group published its latest long-term follow-up of the hormone trials. They acknowledged that WHI only assessed one dose, one formulation, and one route of administration in each trial. The group conceded that the results are not necessarily generalizable to other hormone preparations, in contrast to their initial statement [13, 18]. The predominance of data has been generated with CEE. However, clinical data suggest that estradiol has similar efficacy. Since orally administered estradiol increases the risk of deep venous thrombophlebitis and pulmonary embolism and is contraindicated in obese women with high levels of plasma triglycerides, transdermal E2, which avoids the first liver pass effect, has the benefit of not increasing the risks of thrombosis and is well suited for more high-risk women [19]. The type of estrogen is of critical importance, and the development of a new, safe, oral estrogen which would maintain the benefits of estrogens in use today but which provides a safer profile is a worthwhile goal.

Combined oral contraception (COC) use is associated with a three- to sevenfold relative increased risk of DVT and pulmonary embolism (PE) [20]. This increased risk is the consequence of the changes that occur in the coagulation cascade brought on by E [21]. E causes an increase in plasma levels of thrombogenic clotting factors (factors I, II, VII, VIII, X) as well as a decrease in plasma levels of clotting inhibitors (antithrombin, protein S, protein C, tissue factor pathway inhibitor (TFPI), etc.) that shift the balance to favor clot formation. Several studies have shown that the type of progestogen used in a COC influences the magnitude of the E-induced changes in these hemostatic proteins [22–24]. The biological mechanism of this progestogen effect seems to be through modification of the E impact on the liver rather than a direct effect, because progestogen-only contraception with levonorgestrel (LNG) or drospirenone (DRSP) does not increase VTE risk [25, 26].

The high levels of E seen by the liver following oral dosing are supraphysiologic. While E2 is rapidly converted to less potent estriol and estrone following the first pass, synthetic ethinylestradiol (EE) is more stable and reactivates during prolonged period of time the liver cell synthesis of clotting factors during recirculation. The lower estrogenic imprinting of E2 versus EE explains why the E2-based COC is less thrombogenic than the third- and fourth-generation COCs that contain EE [27]. The risk of thromboembolism from using COCs with norethisterone, levonorgestrel, desogestrel, or gestodene decreases with decreasing E dose [20]. The same progestins and DRSP in the absence of EE do not increase the VTE risk ([20, 25] [26]). These data indicate that it is the E and not the progestin that causes the DVT risk.

The second-generation pills containing EE + LNG as a progestin cause a three-fold increased risk of DVT, while the third- and fourth-generation pills containing desogestrel, gestodene, or DRSP are associated with a six- to sevenfold increase and with considerably higher plasma levels of clotting factors [20]. The third- or fourth-generation progestin has a lower androgenic profile of activity, with less acne and seborrhea, weight gain, and oily hair in comparison to LNG. Their antiestrogenic activity decreased also significantly [28, 29]. Consequently, the liver impact of EE, the E predominantly used in COCs, is more important in users of third- and fourth-generation pills [30]. This causes a significantly higher increase in coagulation factors and a more profound decrease in coagulation inhibitors.

Due to the low absolute incidence of DVT (0.02–0.04%), prospective trials require 5–10 years to obtain reliable estimates for the DVT risk associated with the use of a particular COC. Surrogate hemostasis markers are therefore useful tools to estimate the thrombogenic risk of new COCs or E. Measurement of activated protein C (APC) resistance via thrombin generation is a validated test for determining the thrombogenicity of hormonal contraceptives [31, 32]. Sex hormone-binding globulin (SHBG) has also been suggested to be a marker for the risk of venous thrombosis [31, 33].

In summary, the E used in COCs are responsible for procoagulatory changes in hemostasis markers. The development of new safer E that would have a minimal impact on liver metabolism and on coagulation would provide great vascular advantage to women's healthcare.

In this review, we highlight recent data on the impact of estetrol (E4) on the vascular system in comparison to that of E2 and propose that it may provide a more attractive risk-benefit ratio compared to other oral estrogens in use today. We will also report on recent clinical data of the effects of E4 for the relief of the climacteric symptoms and for contraception.

12.2   Estetrol (E4)

Estetrol (E4) is an estrogen of fetal origin, which was the last estrogen discovered. E4 differs from all other natural estrogens because it is present only in pregnant primates (at 100-fold higher levels in human pregnant women compared to other primates). It is exclusively synthesized by the human fetal liver (which has the capacity to hydroxylate estradiol at the 15 and 16 carbon positions) and circulates at high levels (up to 20–30 ng/mL) in fetal blood. It is present in maternal blood and urine from the ninth week of gestation and reaches the maternal circulation through the placenta. Maternal plasma levels increase during pregnancy to high concentrations toward the end of gestation ($\geq$3–6 ng/mL) [34, 35]. E4 maternal plasma levels are about 12–20 times levels lower than in the fetal plasma at parturition.

12.3 Estetrol: The NEST Concept

E4 can be described as the first NEST [Native (natural and human) Estrogen with Specific action in Tissues]. The Nest property is the consequence of its unique mode of action, which is distinctly different from a selective estrogen receptor modulator (SERM). All estrogens bind to two subpopulations of estrogen receptor alpha: the nuclear ERα which induces gene transcription and the membrane ERα which initiates rapid signaling also called "membrane-initiated steroid signaling" (MISS) effects (for a review, see [36]). In a similar fashion to other estrogens, E4 activates the nuclear ERα and induces gene transcription. However, in contrast to the other estrogens, E4 antagonizes the activity of membrane ERα (Fig. 12.1) [37]. Evidence has accumulated over the last two decades that ERα is not only present in the cell nucleus but is associated with the plasma membrane and activates nonnuclear

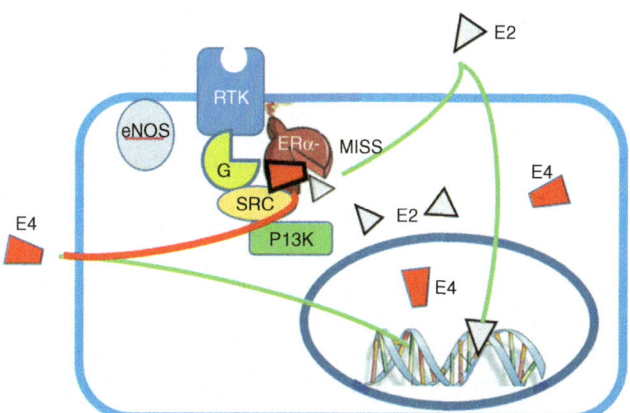

Fig. 12.1 ERα localization in the nucleus and at the cell surface. ERα is localized in the nucleus and at the cell surface. E_2 and classical E bind and activate both types of ERα (green arrows). The nuclear ERα activation upon E binding induces gene transcription, while the cell surface-associated ERα initiates a series of rapid membrane-initiated steroid signaling (MISS) that contribute to regulate cyclic AMP synthesis, Ca++ entry, and kinase activation (receptor tyrosine kinase-RTK, MAPKs, ERK1/2, and/or PI3K/Akt, SRC) that are essential for the modulation of transcription and nongenomic functions in many target cells. As an example, the MISS effect may enhance cell proliferation and endothelial NO synthase (eNOS) activity (for a review, see [36]). E4 binds and activates the nuclear ERα (green arrow), but its binding to the membrane ERα results in a blockade of the MISS signaling (red arrow) [37]. E4 displays thus mixed agonist and antagonist estrogenic activities

signaling from this site. These rapid/nongenomic/MISS actions have been characterized in a variety of cell lines and in particular in cancer cell lines and in endothelial cells. The development of selective pharmacological tools that specifically activate MISS and the generation of knock-out mice expressing either an ERα protein which is impeded for membrane action or for the nuclear action has allowed for the more precise delineation of the role of the nuclear and membrane forms of ERα [36, 38]. Thus the vascular profile of E4 activity can be compared with that of E2 17β. These actions of E4 (NEST activity) are distinctly different from SERMs which induce conformational changes in the ER and accordingly recruit coactivators or co-inhibitors in different tissues to allow for varied expression of agonistic or antagonistic activities.

12.4 Experimental Data

12.4.1 E4 Does Not Accelerate Endothelial Healing and Does Not Enhance Endothelial NO Production but Induces Endothelium-Dependent Vasodilation

E2 accelerates re-endothelialization after removal of the carotid artery endothelium by electric injury [39]. It also increases endothelial nitric oxide synthase (eNOS) phosphorylation and thereby endothelial NO production [40]. Stimulation of endothelial healing and eNOS activation is now recognized as two established actions of E2 dependent on membrane ERα activation [41, 42].

E4 (at doses of 0.3, 1, and 6 mg/kg/day) failed to accelerate endothelial cell proliferation/migration as well as to stimulate eNOS phosphorylation or endothelial NO production. E4 was not only devoid of ERa membrane-initiated steroid signaling (MISS) in the endothelium but was also able to antagonize the E2 effects, in line with its NEST activity profile that antagonizes the membrane ERα [37].

Does this mean that E4 is less effective than E2 on the vascular system?

Acceleration of endothelial healing and NO production are usually considered as features, which are protective for arteries. Would an absence of endothelial NO synthase stimulation by E4 result in a lack of E4-mediated vasodilation and in a poorer endothelium-mediated vascular protection in comparison to E2? The answer to this essential question is no. Several studies have confirmed that NO production, which is essential for proper vasodilation and endothelial function, is controlled by multiple factors besides estrogen. In addition, E4 causes vasodilation of animal arteries by a specific mechanism distinct from NO production.

Vascular tone by endothelium-derived nitric oxide is mediated by multiple controlling mechanisms, including physical factors, such as increases in shear stress and reduction in temperature, as well as a large number of neurohumoral mediators through the activation of specific endothelial cell membrane receptors and/or post-translational modifications (Fig. 12.2). The main physiological driver of NO production is not estrogen but shear stress [43–45], and estrogen is considered to play a limited role in regulating endothelial-derived NO production and vasodilation.

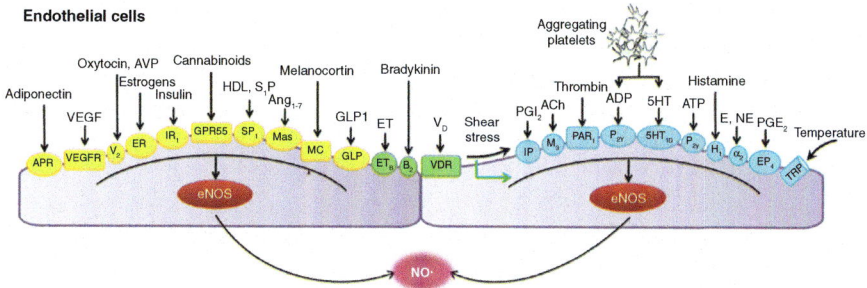

Fig. 12.2 Regulation of vascular tone by endothelium-derived nitric oxide (NO). Physical factors (increases in shear stress and temperature lowering) and neurohumoral mediators (through activation of specific endothelial cell membrane receptors) cause instantaneous increases in the release of endothelium-derived NO by endothelial nitric oxide synthase (eNOS). Color code: Signals leading to activation of eNOS dependent mainly on increases in Ca2+ concentration, mainly on posttranslational modifications, or on both are indicated by blue, yellow, and green, respectively. These factors include α2: alpha adrenergic mediators, E (epinephrine); NE (norepinephrine); Ach (acetylcholine); ADP (adenosine diphosphate); Ang1–7 (angiotensin1–7); adiponectin; AVP (arginine vasopressin); bradykinin; PGE2 (prostaglandin E2); estrogen; ET (endothelin-1); GLP1 (glucagon-like peptide 1); histamine; HDL (high-density lipoprotein); 5HT (serotonin, 5-hydroxytryptamine); insulin; PGI2 (prostacyclin); SP1 (sphingosine 1-phosphate); VEGF (vascular endothelial growth factor); VD (vitamin D); melanocortin; thrombin; ATP; cannabinoids; oxytocin; etc. (Reproduced from Vanhoutte PM, Zhao Y, Xu A, et al. Thirty years of saying NO: sources, fate, actions, and misfortunes of the endothelium-derived vasodilator mediator. Circ Res 2016; 119: 375–96, by permission of Wolters Kluwer)

In addition, pharmacological studies suggest that E4 induces vasodilation through a distinct mechanism. It has been shown that E4 induces vasodilation at very high concentrations (10 μM or more) in ewe uterine arteries [46] and relaxing responses in rat uterine, thoracic, aortic, carotid, mesenteric, pulmonary, renal, middle cerebral, and septal coronary arteries [47]. The vasodilation induced by E4 in rat arteries was ER dependent since it was abrogated by ICI 182780, an ERα antagonist. Blockade of eNOS by N(ω)-nitro-L-arginine methyl ester (L-NAME) blunted E2-mediated but not E4-mediated relaxing responses, demonstrating that E2 but not E4 induces vasodilation by stimulating eNOS activity. Only, the soluble guanylate cyclase (sGC) inhibitor, ODQ, blocked E4 relaxation. These studies concluded that E4 caused relaxation of precontracted rat uterine arteries via both an endothelium-dependent mechanism involving ER and a guanylate cyclase mechanism. Furthermore, E4 inhibited smooth muscle cell Ca++ entry and contraction. However, a discrepancy between the micromolar range estrogenic effects on ex vivo vasorelaxation and the nanomolar range of circulating estrogen levels in vivo is unclear. It may be the consequence of the experimental conditions of the in vitro perfusion model used. The observations made on the effects of estrogens using ex vivo vasorelaxation models are pharmacological in nature and require further validation in vivo and if possible in human.

As we will see below, E2-mediated acceleration of endothelial healing and NO production does not summarize the "physiological vascular benefit," and E4, as E2, can mediate numerous vasculoprotective actions that are independent on membrane ERα and fully dependent on nuclear ERα. In summary, we believe that the E2-mediated acceleration of endothelial healing and NO production should not convey a unique "physiological benefit" of E2 17β, and the impact of E4 on arterial and capillary vessels also should be as beneficial.

12.4.2 E4 Has an Atheroprotective Effect as Mediated Through Nuclear ERa

The scientific community believes that the increase in endothelium-derived NO plays an important role in the vascular protective actions of estrogen, by preventing or attenuating arterial atheroma formation [48, 49]. A validated model to study atheroprotection by estrogens [50, 51] was used to compare the effect of E2 (80 μg/kg/day) and E4 (0.6 and 6 mg/kg/day). Lipid deposition was evaluated at the aortic sinus from ERa+/+LDLr−/− or ERa−/−LDLr−/− (low-density lipoprotein receptor) mice fed with a high-cholesterol diet. E4 in a dose-dependent fashion prevented lipid deposition in ovariectomized ERa+/+LDLr−/− mice (Fig. 12.3), decreasing atheroma deposition by up to 80% [37], a level of protection similar to that obtained using a high dose of E2 [53, 54]. Deletion of ERα in ERa−/− LDLr−/− mice abolished this E4 protection, indicating that ERa is necessary to mediate the atheroprotective effect of E4 [37]. Taken together these studies indicate that E4 is able to prevent atherosclerosis, by activating the nuclear ERα, without enhancement of NO. The capacity of E4 to prevent atherosclerosis and the persistence of the atheroprotection by estrogen in transgenic mice lacking the membrane ERα indicate that this membrane receptor subpopulation does not contribute to atheroprotection [55]. Accordingly, we propose that the atheroprotective effects of E4 should be similar to the effects of E2 17β and are not likely to be less in spite of not activating the membrane receptor subpopulation and not enhancing NO production.

12.4.3 E4 Protects Against Neointimal Hyperplasia

Neointimal hyperplasia arises when vascular smooth muscle cells cross the internal elastic lamina to migrate and proliferate in the intima [56, 57]. In human pathology, this process frequently occurs after the treatment of symptomatic atherosclerosis, which involves mechanical endovascular ballooning (angioplasty) followed by stenting. Neointimal hyperplasia leads to a narrowing of the arterial lumen and restenosis [58]. E2 antagonizes this process [59].

We used an experimental model of femoral artery injury to trigger neointimal hyperplasia of vascular smooth muscle cells (VSMC) [60]. Using transgenic mice and selective deletion of ERα in VSMC or in endothelial cells, we demonstrated that, contrary to a common belief, E2 and E4 prevent neointimal hyperplasia by a direct inhibitory effect on SMC proliferation and migration but not by

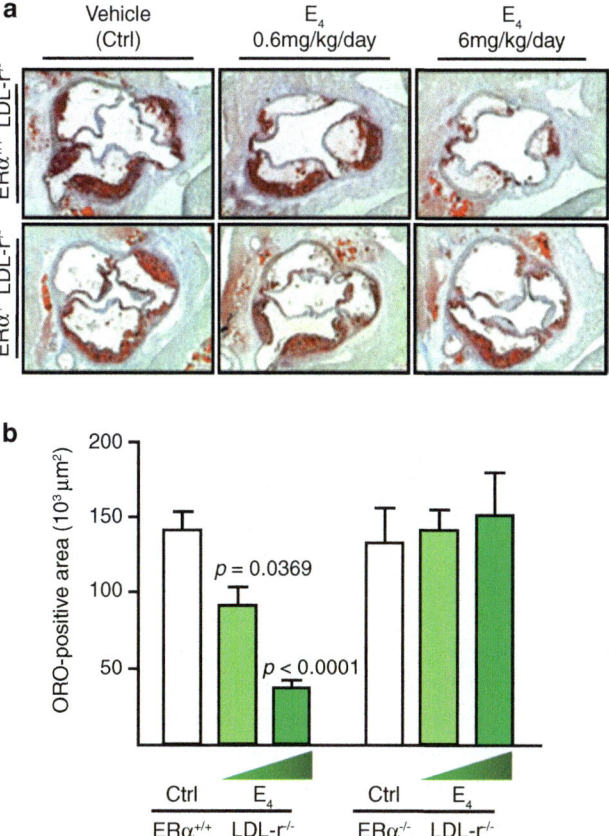

Fig. 12.3 E4 prevents aortic sinus lipid deposition in hypercholesterolemic mice. Four-week-old ovariectomized ERa$^{+/+}$LDL-r$^{-/-}$ (estrogen receptor α-positive/low-density lipoprotein receptor-negative) or ERa$^{-/-}$LDL-r$^{-/-}$ (estrogen receptor α-negative/low-density lipoprotein receptor-negative) mice were switched to atherogenic diet from the age of 6 to 18 weeks added with placebo (Ctrl) or E4 (0.6 or 6 mg/kg/day). (**a, b**) Representative micrographs of oil red-O (ORO) lipid-stained cryosections of the aortic sinus (**a**) and quantification of lipid deposition (**b**) are represented (from Abot et al. 2014 EMBO Mol Med. 2014, 10:1328–46 Fig. 5, p. 1338; reproduced with permission from Wiley online Library)

acting on endothelial cells. E4 prevented neointimal hyperplasia formation to the same extent as E2 (Fig. 12.4).

12.4.4 E4 Favors Flow-Mediated Arteriolar Remodeling (FMR)

Chronic increases in blood flow induce outward hypertrophic remodeling in resistance arteries and improvement of nitric oxide (NO)-dependent dilation [61–63]. Resistance arteries control local blood flow, and their capacity to remodel in

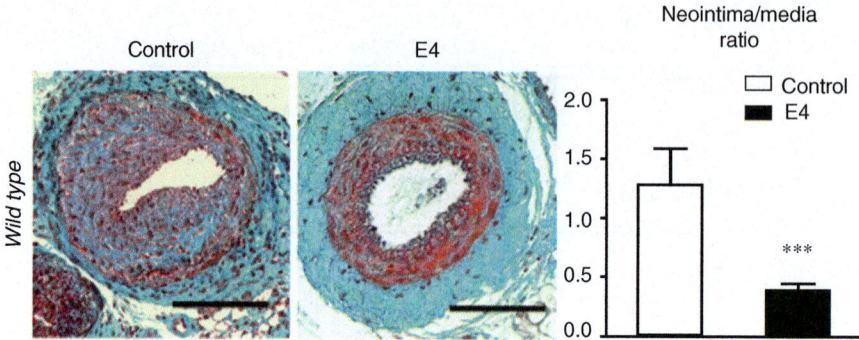

Fig. 12.4 E4 protects against neointimal hyperplasia. Four-week-old wild-type female mice were ovariectomized and subcutaneously implanted with control or E4 (6 mg/Kg/day) eluting osmotic minipumps. Two weeks later, animals were submitted to mechanical injury of the femoral artery. Arteries were harvested 28 days after the injury for morphometric analysis. Left, representative image of cross section of femoral arteries of mice stained with Masson trichrome. Bars, 100 μm. Right, quantitative analysis of neointima/media ratio of mice. Values are presented as mean ± SEM ($n = 7–12$ mice per group) and statistically compared with Mann–Whitney U test. ***$p < 0.001$ (from Smirnova NF et al. (Fig. 12.5b) Circ Res. 2015; 117:770–8 reproduced with permission of Wolters Kluwer)

response to chronic changes in the hemodynamic environment is necessary to maintain their full efficiency. Chronic increases in blood flow occur in physiological situations, such as growth, pregnancy, or exercise. In response to a chronic increase in blood flow, arterial diameters increase until the shear stress is normalized. In addition to angiogenesis, high-flow-mediated remodeling of resistance arteries plays a key role in revascularization of ischemic tissues after occlusion of a large artery [64]. Physiologically, chronic increases in blood flow in resistance arteries cause the diameter to expand with a compensatory increase in wall mass and an increased responsiveness of the endothelium to vasodilator stimuli. Besides pressure-associated medial hypertrophic remodeling that characterizes hypertension, outward remodeling at the level of arterioles occurs in response to increased blood flow and shear stress at the surface of endothelial cells.

Flow-mediated arteriolar remodeling (FMR) consists in vascular enlargement or outward remodeling induced by flow (shear stress) in small collateral arteries surrounding ischemic areas. This remodeling is essential in postischemic revascularization or collateral arteries growth since it contributes to the prevention of further tissue injury, in limb or myocardial ischemia [65]. FMR has been shown to be reduced by hypertension [66, 67], diabetes [68, 69], and aging [70, 71].

Two weeks after arterial ligation of some mesenteric arteries, the arterial diameter of the intact arteries was determined in vitro in response to stepwise increases in intraluminal pressure (Fig. 12.5a). As expected, passive arterial diameter was significantly higher in high-flow (HF) than in normal-flow (NF) arteries in WT mice. Ovariectomy caused a complete loss of FMR (Fig. 12.5b). A chronic treatment with E4 allowed flow arteriolar remodeling to occur in ovariectomized mice

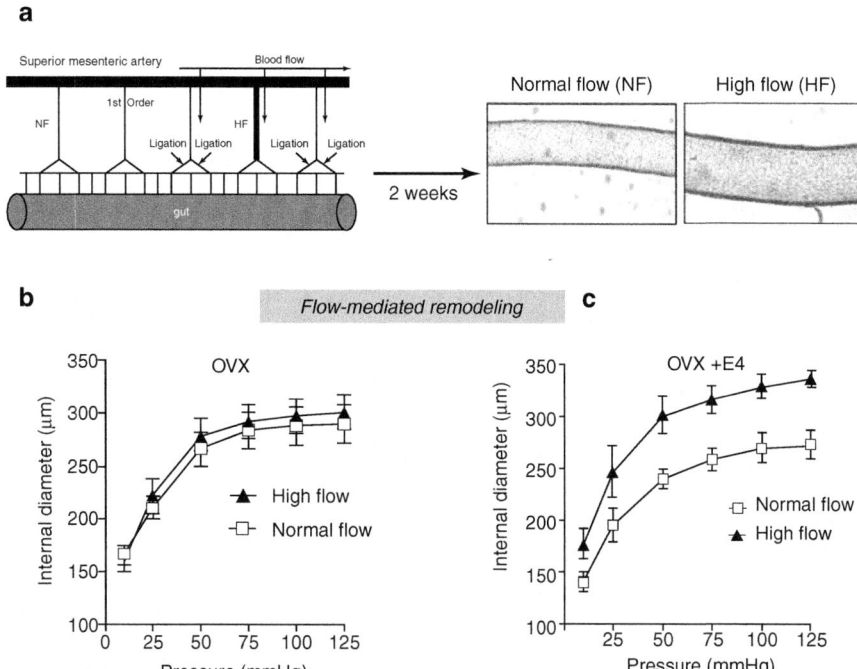

Fig. 12.5 Flow-mediated remodeling is promoted by E4. Experimental model: Blood flow was increased in the mesenteric artery of 4- to 5-month-old female mice using a model in which two mesenteric arteries are ligated, leading to a chronic increase in blood flow in the central artery without a change in the systemic hemodynamic environment [52]. Arterial diameter was then measured in vitro after cannulation in response to stepwise increases in pressure in the mesenteric arteries submitted chronically to high flow (HF) or to normal flow (NF). Briefly, three consecutive first-order mesenteric arteries were used and surgery consisted in ligatures of second-order branches. The artery located between the two ligated arteries was designated as the high-flow (HF) artery. Arteries located at distance of the ligated arteries were used as controls (normal flow, NF). Mice were sacrificed after 14 days and mesenteric arteries were collected. For the measurement of the pressure–diameter relationship in mesenteric arteries, in vitro arterial segments were cannulated at both ends and mounted in a video-monitored perfusion system (Living System, LSI, Burlington, VT). (**a**) FMR was evaluated in mesenteric arteries isolated from ovariectomized mice treated chronically with vehicle or E4 during 2 weeks ($n = 6$). Arterial diameter was measured in response to stepwise increases in pressure in mesenteric arteries submitted chronically to high flow (HF) or to normal flow (NF). After ovariectomy, no FMR is observed in HF mesenteric arteries. (**b**) Treatment with E4 for 2 weeks restored the capacity of HF mesenteric arteries to develop FMR

(Fig. 12.5c). Importantly, we assessed the short-term acute flow-mediated dilation in pressurized precontracted mesenteric arteries, i.e., in physiological ex vivo conditions (compared to vascular rings). E4 or vehicle caused quite similar vasodilating response to stepwise increase in intraluminal flow, demonstrating that E4 does not impair the vasodilatory response to the most important and physiological stimulus of NO production: endothelial shear stress [55].

Taken altogether these data indicate that E4 has a similar vasoprotective capacity compared to E2 and allows flow-mediated remodeling to occur, which is essential for proper arterial functioning in health and diseases.

12.4.5 E4 Protects Mice from Angiotensin II-Induced Hypertension

Hypertension affects one in four women worldwide, and its prevalence is particularly high among women over 60 years of age. The first decade after menopause is accompanied by an increase in blood pressure and has been associated with a higher risk of atherosclerosis, myocardial infarction, and stroke [72]. Up to the time of menopause, endogenous estrogen plays a protective role against high blood pressure. In line with these epidemiological data, clinical and preclinical studies show considerable evidence that estrogen modulates cardiovascular physiology and function and is cardioprotective [73].

We therefore tested the capacity of E4 to reduce the effects of angiotensin II (AngII) and to prevent hypertension in animals.

In the WT littermate control ovariectomized mice, 4 weeks of AngII infusion increased systolic blood pressure (SBP) [55]. The hypertensive effect of AngII was significantly more exacerbated in ovariectomized mice or in mice lacking ERα (ERα$^{-/-}$), showing that the beneficial effect of endogenous estrogen is ERα dependent. This finding is in agreement with previous work showing that hypertension induced by angiotensin II is lower in females than in males [74, 75]. Furthermore, the hypertensive effect of AngII was significantly more exacerbated in mice lacking nuclear ERα but not in mice lacking membrane ERα. Importantly and quite consistently, both E2 and E4 protected WT female mice from AngII-induced hypertension (Fig. 12.6).

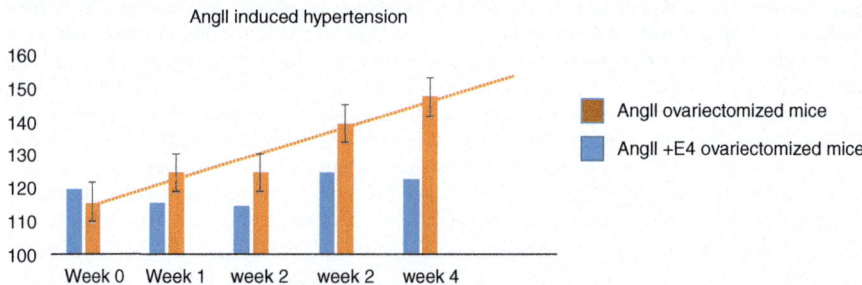

Fig. 12.6 E4 protects against AngII-induced hypertension. Effect of E4 on AngII treatment was evaluated in wild-type female mice ovariectomized 2 weeks before sham-surgery or simultaneous implantation with osmotic minipumps delivering angiotensin II (1 month) (AngII, solubilized in NaCl 0.9%, 0.5 mg/kg per day and E4 6 mg/kg per day, solubilized in 50% PBS + 50% DMSO) ($n = 7$). Mean of systolic blood pressure (SBP) measurements for 5 days was represented as weekly evolution of blood pressure pre- (week 0) and during AngII treatment (reproduced with permission modified from Guivarc'h et al. 2018)

12.4.6 E4 Protects from Arterial and Venous Thrombosis in Mice

12.4.6.1   E4 Like E2 Has a Minimal Impact on Coagulation Factors

In the mouse, estrogens do not alter circulating coagulation factors toward a procoagulant profile [76] as they do in women [20, 77, 78]. We verified that chronic E4 treatment (6 mg/Kg/day) did not modify the platelet counts, prothrombin time, and the level of plasma fibrinogen. A small decrease of the activated partial thromboplastin time and a modest increase in factors II and IX were observed. The conclusion of these studies suggests that E4 only has a moderate effect on coagulation factors in the mouse.

12.4.6.2   Estetrol Increases the Bleeding Time in Mice

Chronic administration of E4 for 3 weeks led to an increased tail-bleeding time in mice. The tail-bleeding time of untreated ovariectomized mice was 5.2 min (SD ± 2.4, $n = 12$), which is in the normal range [79]. Among 18 mice treated with E4, the bleeding time was so prolonged that there was no overlapping time with the vehicle-treated mice. The tail-bleeding time was prolonged above 30 min in 6 out of 18 mice [80].

12.4.6.3   E4 Protects Against Arterial Thrombus Formation

All ovariectomized control mice ($n = 12$) died from occlusive thromboembolism within 10 min after an injection in the jugular vein of 0.4 mg/kg collagen and 60 µg/kg epinephrine. Six E4-treated mice (E4) died, while four mice were protected from thromboembolism ($p = 0.028$). Histological analysis of mouse lungs harvested 10 min after the injection showed marked protection from occlusive thrombi in vessels of surviving E4-treated mice compared to E4-treated and control mice that died. The occlusive pulmonary thrombi in surviving E4-treated mice were mostly observed in small vessels and rarely in large vessels [80]. Using transthoracic echocardiography, we found that *left ventricular* geometry, assessed by the *sphericity index* (*SI*, an indicator of right ventricular pressure overload), was altered from the moment of injection in ovariectomized mice and in E4-treated mice that died. In contrast, E4-treated mice protected from collagen-/epinephrine-induced thromboembolism showed *normal* left ventricular function.

12.4.6.4   E4 Protects from Venous Thrombus Formation

We induced venous thrombosis by partial or total ligation of the inferior vena cava (IVC) [81]. In these models, blood flow decreased or arrested leading to endothelial cell activation and extensive thrombosis. Thrombus mass was quantified 24 h (for total ligation) or 48 h (partial ligation) after stasis or stenosis induction. As compared to ovariectomized control mice, E4-treated mice had significantly smaller thrombi in both models of IVC stenosis. In the total ligation model, the mean thrombus weight was 6.1 mg (SD ± 1.9, $n = 13$) in control ovariectomized mice and 2.3 mg (SD ± 0.5, $n = 7$) following E4 treatment. In the partial ligation model, the mean thrombus weight was again significantly reduced by E4 treatment (4.2 mg SD ± 1.3, $n = 8$ and 0.7 mg SD ± 0.5, $n = 7$, respectively).

12.4.6.5   E4 Decreases Thrombus Growth on Collagen Under Ex Vivo Arterial Flow Conditions

Platelet adhesion and thrombus formation were evaluated ex vivo under arterial flow conditions (60 dynes/cm^2, 1500 s^{-1}) using a flow-based adhesion assay where heparinized whole blood was perfused over a collagen matrix. While blood from untreated mice exhibited robust formation of densely packed platelet thrombi on collagen, platelets from E4-treated mice formed 33% smaller thrombi. To assess the stability of the thrombi formed, a low shear rate (20 dynes/cm^2, 500 s^{-1}) was first applied during 2 min followed by an acute increase of blood flow to reach a pathological shear rate (160 dynes/cm^2, 4000 s^{-1}) for 2 min. In all groups, the thrombi formed did not detach from the collagen matrix and even grew further but at a slower rate with blood from E4-treated mice compared to control untreated mice. These results indicate that while platelet aggregation in suspension was not significantly modified, platelet thrombus growth under arterial shear rate on collagen matrix was reduced following E4 treatment. Finally, we generated hematopoietic chimera with bone marrow cells deficient for nuclear ERα. Deletion of hematopoietic nuclear ERα significantly reduced E4-induced protection against thromboembolism, while this deletion did not affect the increased tail-bleeding time. Taken altogether, these data, combined with the human studies (see below), concur to define E4 as a unique, native estrogen. It could be a promising candidate for oral contraception as well as for HRT, as it has minimal impact on coagulation and is even protective in the animal models used. To what extent this observed antithrombotic effect in animal studies relates to women remains to be determined in clinical studies. Such preliminary clinical data are emerging and will be reviewed below.

12.4.7   Other Effects

E4 Antagonizes E2-Stimulated Tumoral Angiogenesis.

Most solid tumors need a blood supply and can grow only if they induce the development of new blood vessels from pre-existing ones, a process known as tumor angiogenesis. Tumor vascularization is a complex event that involves tumor cells and host endothelial cells, stromal cells, immune cells, and circulating bone marrow stem cells. Multiple endocrine factors, cytokines, and chemokines regulate tumoral angiogenesis [82]. The physiopathology of tumoral angiogenesis and the role of estrogens in this process are beyond the scope of this review. It is however noteworthy to mention that in experimental models of tumoral angiogenesis, E4 antagonizes the effect of E2 on blood vessels formation and tumor growth (Fig. 12.7). This observation is in line with the demonstration that E4 antagonizes the stimulation of endothelial cells proliferation and migration elicited by E2 [37].

E2 17β potentiates tumor growth even when cancer cells lack ERα and are therefore E insensitive [83]. E2 activates normal host stromal (endothelial) cells ERα to increase intratumoral vessel density. E2 improves vessels structure and functionality that deliver more oxygen to the tumor [83]. E4, which does not stimulate endothelial

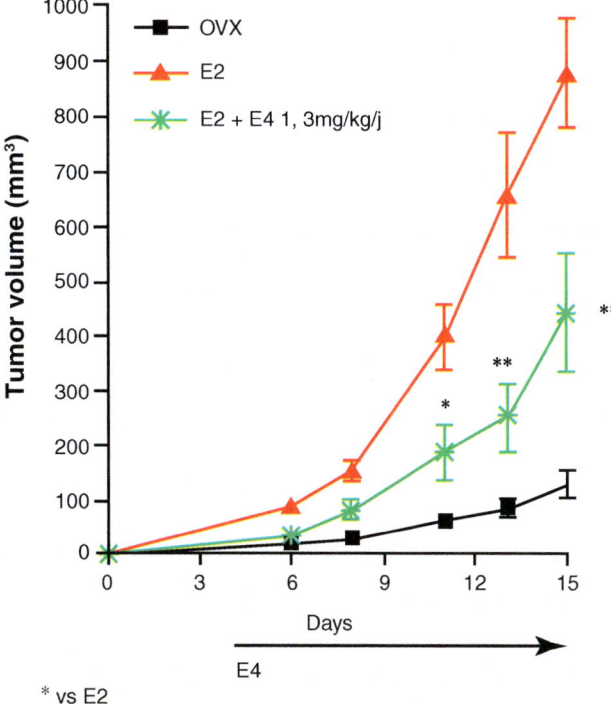

Fig. 12.7 Reduction by E4 of E2 stimulated B16 melanoma tumor growth. Four weeks old, ovariectomized C57 black/6 mice were inoculated with a pellet releasing E2 (80 µg/kg/day) as described in Pequeux et al. [83]. Two weeks later, mice were inoculated with 4×10^5 ERα-negative B16K2 melanoma cells. Some mice were injected with an E4 pellet (1.3 mg/kg/day) 4 days after tumor cell injection. Tumor growth was monitored for 15 days ($*p < 0.05$; $**p < 0.01$). While E2 stimulates the ERα-negative B16 melanoma tumor growth, E4 antagonizes this effect

cells proliferation and migration (see above), is able to partially antagonize the enhancement of tumoral angiogenesis and tumor growth elicited by E2 in ER-negative tumors (Fig. 12.7). These data confirm that E4 is an antagonist of the membrane ERα subpopulation and antagonizes the effect of E2 on tumoral angiogenesis.

12.5   Clinical Data

12.5.1   Five or Ten Milligram E4 Has a Minimal Impact on Hemostasis in Young Reproductive Age Women

Hepatic estrogenicity and hemostasis markers are in the list of the European Medicines Agency (EMA) advised to evaluate potential risk for thrombotic side effects of hormonal contraceptives [84]. Five or ten milligram E4 was therefore evaluated, in a phase 2 clinical trial, as an oral contraceptive in combination with 3 mg drospirenone (DRSP) [77] and compared to a classical combined oral contraceptive containing 20 µg EE combined with 3 mg DRSP (Yaz®). Healthy women 18–35 years of age with a body mass index (BMI) of 18–30 kg/m² were eligible for inclusion. Spontaneous ovulation between day 9 (±1) and day 24 (±1) was verified in the pretreatment cycle by a progesterone concentration ≥ 16 nM (5 ng/mL) and a luteal phase duration of ≥6 days. The study included three treatment groups: 20 µg EE combined with 3 mg DRSP (EE/DRSP), 5 mg E4 combined with 3 mg DRSP (5 mg E4/DRSP), and 10 mg E4 combined with 3 mg DRSP (10 mg E4/DRSP). All subjects were stratified according to the day of ovulation in the pretreatment cycle and then assigned to a treatment group. Oral treatment was started on the first day of menstruation following the pretreatment cycle and continued daily for 24 days followed by a 4-day break.

In the EE/DRSP group, both SHBG and angiotensinogen increased significantly in the third cycle (to 381% and 256% of baseline, respectively) (Fig. 12.8a, b). In contrast, SHBG and angiotensinogen were 100% (i.e., no change) and 125% of baseline in the 5 mg E4/DRSP group and 143% and 131% of baseline in the 10 mg E4/DRSP group. Thus, compared to 20 µg EE, both 5 mg E4 and 10 mg E4 had considerably lower effect on SHBG and minor impact on angiotensinogen.

At variance to EE + DRSP which induced dramatic changes in the hemostasis markers (Fig. 12.9), E4, at the daily dose of 5 or 10 mg, had little or no effect on coagulation factors (Fig. 12.9 and Table 12.1 [77]). The influence of EE and E4 was also evaluated on the three most relevant coagulation inhibitors (free TFPI, protein S, and antithrombin) and on the global coagulation inhibition test (ETP-based APCr). Five and 10 mg E4 had no effect on antithrombin, protein S activity, or APCr (Fig. 12.10) and had only a considerably smaller impact on free TFPI than EE which considerably decreased the plasma levels of these coagulation inhibitors, thereby promoting coagulation.

Five weeks after stopping treatment, previous exposure to, 20 µg EE + 3 mg DRSP still caused an elevation of SHBG, angiotensinogen, and ETP-APC resistance that remained 10–15% of the maximal values observed. Protein S activity and free TFPI were still decreased [77].

Finally, the global activation of coagulation was evaluated. EE + DRSP increased D-dimer and prothrombin fragments F1.2, corresponding to a global activation of coagulation. COCs containing 5 or 10 mg E4 did not increase either marker, but rather decreased them.

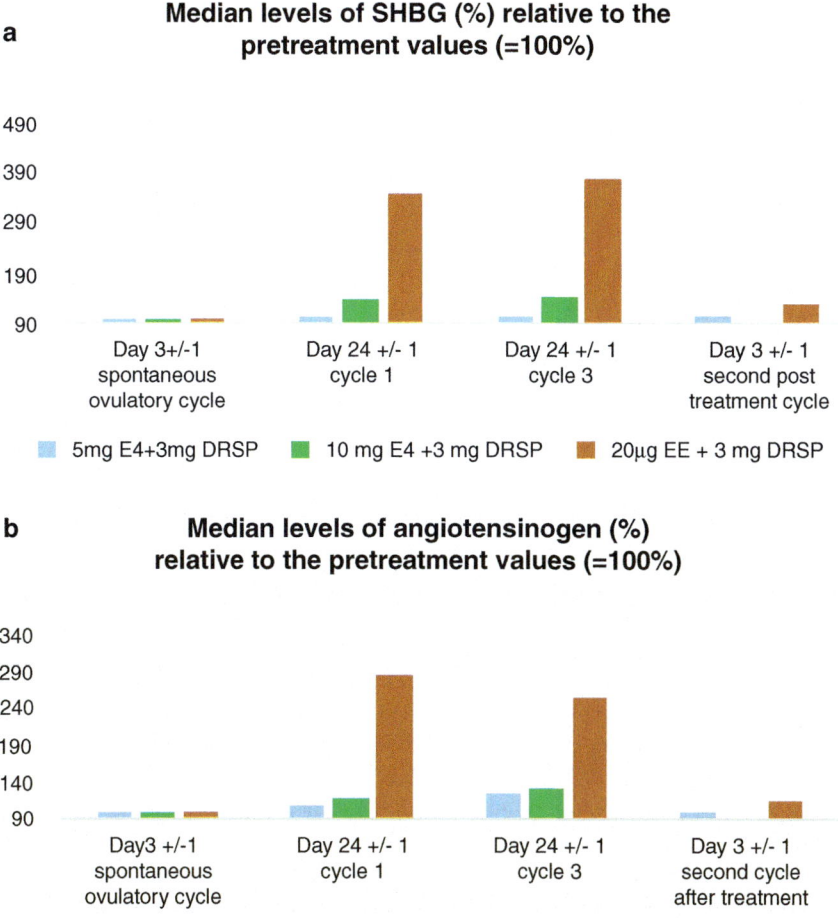

Fig. 12.8 Estrogenicity markers on liver. Changes in median plasma levels of SHBG (**a**) and angiotensinogen (**b**), relative to the pretreatment value (=100%), in women receiving for 3 cycles either 5 or 10 mg E4 combined with 3 mg DRSP. A classical COC containing 20 μg EE + the same dose of DRSP was used as a comparator. Paired statistics: Wilcoxon signed rank test see Table 12.1. In the EE/DRSP group, both SHBG and angiotensinogen increased significantly in the third cycle (to 381% and 256% of baseline, respectively) (**a**, **b**). In contrast, SHBG and angiotensinogen were 100% (i.e., no change) and 125% of baseline in the 5 mg E4/DRSP group and 143% and 131% of baseline in the 10 mg E4/DRSP group. Thus, compared to 20 μg EE, both 5 mg E4 and 10 mg E4 had nearly no effect on SHBG and minor on angiotensinogen (modified from Kluft et al. 2017 reproduced with permission from Elsevier)

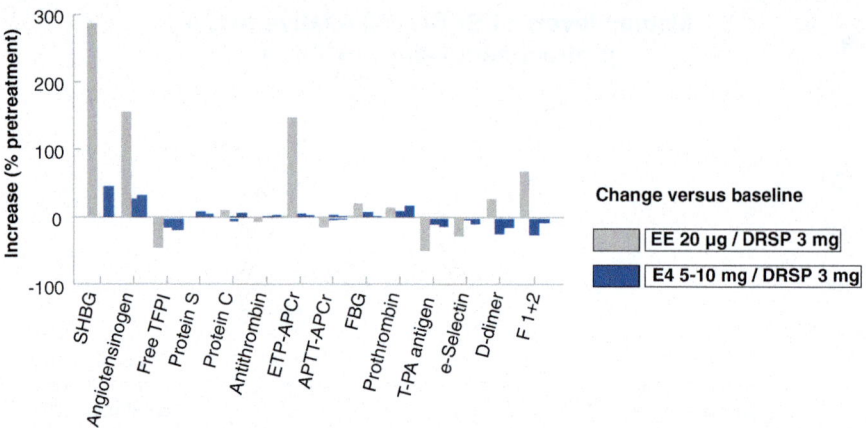

Fig. 12.9 Changes in hemostasis versus baseline in women receiving either a classical combined oral contraceptive (COC) containing 20 µg EE + 3 mg DRSP or 5 or 10 mg E4 + 3 mg DRSP. The markers of estrogenicity in liver (SHBG, angiotensinogen) of coagulation (prothrombin, prothrombin fragment 1.2, ETP-based APCr, APTT APCr, D-dimers, protein C, fibrinogen), of coagulation inhibitors (free TFPI, protein S, antithrombin), and of fibrinolysis (tissue plasminogen activator (TPA)) show considerably lower changes versus baseline (spontaneous ovulatory cycle) in the groups treated with 5 or 10 mg E4 + DRSP than in the group treated with EE 20 µg + DRSP. Ideally a COC would not modify any surrogate marker of hemostasis

The considerably lower impact of E4/DRSP compared to EE/DRSP on a number of hemostatic parameters confirms the importance of the E selected for COC use and indicates how neutral DRSP is in terms of coagulation.

Recently the influence of three COCs on hemostasis parameters was compared in three groups of about 30 women exposed for six cycles to either 20 µg EE + 3 mg DRSP or 30 µg EE + 150 µg LNG or 15 mg E4 + 3 mg DRSP. Changes of hemostasis parameters during EE/LNG and EE/DRSP were similar to those reported in literature. The effects of E4/DRSP and EE/LNG on hemostasis parameters were less important than those of EE/DRSP. Several coagulation parameters were lower in the E4/DRSP group than in the EE + LNG group (Mithra data on file).

Altogether these studies indicate that the lower impact of E4/DRSP compared to EE/DRSP on a number of hemostatic parameters confirms the importance of the estrogen selected for COC use. Larger studies on DRSP alone and on E4/DRSP combination are not yet available and will be required in order to document the putative reduced incidence of VTE among women using COCs containing E4 and DRSP.

Table 12.1 Plasma levels of estrogenic and hemostasis markers at the end of treatment cycle 3 expressed as percentage of the individual pretreatment values (=100%): median and (Q1–Q3 range)

	YAZ®	5 mg E4-DRSP	10 mg E4-DRSP
Number[a]	$n = 17$	$n = 15$	$n = 15$
Estrogenicity markers			
SHBG antigen	381 (313–462)	100 (90–125)	143 (129–176)
	$p \leq 0.001$	$p > 0.05$	$p \leq 0.001$
Angiotensinogen	256 (229–344)	125 (92–146)	131 (113–145)
	$p < 0.001$	$p \leq 0.05$	$p \leq 0.01$
Global assays, markers			
APTT-based	92 (83–97)	103 (90–106)	100 (90–105)
APC global	$p \leq 0.001$	$p > 0.05$	$p > 0.05$
ETP-based APCr	275 (196–348)	105 (93–129)	99 (87–154)
	$p \leq 0.001$	$p > 0.05$	$p > 0.05$
D-dimer antigen (FbDP)	127 (101–154)	74 (48–92)	74 (57–94)
	$p \leq 0.05$	$p \leq 0.01$	$p \leq 0.05$
F 1 + 2 antigen	163 (131–193)	77 (68–83)	97 (76–114)
	$p \leq 0.001$	$p \leq 0.001$	$p > 0.05$
Levels			
Fibrinogen activity	119 (113–126)	107 (97–116)	99 (93–107)
	$p \leq 0.001$	$p > 0.05$	$p > 0.05$
Prothrombin antigen	113 (96–134)	110 (88–123)	118 (108–141)
	$p \leq 0.05$	$p > 0.05$	$p \leq 0.01$
Protein C activity	111 (107–125)	99 (88–102)	99 (91–106)
	$p \leq 0.001$	$p > 0.05$	$p > 0.05$
Protein S activity	73 (67–80)	107 (101–116)	103 (96–117)
	$p \leq 0.001$	$p > 0.05$	$p > 0.05$
Free TFPI antigen	55 (46–58)	85 (77–101)	83 (80–92)
	$p \leq 0.001$	$p \leq 0.01$	$p \leq 0.001$
Antithrombin activity	95 (90–99)	99 (94–110)	102 (95–107)
	$p \leq 0.01$	$p > 0.05$	$p > 0.05$
t-PA antigen	52 (43–68)	92 (75–104)	90 (60–104)
	$p \leq 0.001$	$p > 0.05$	$p > 0.05$
$E-Selectin antigen	80 (74–88)	101 (96–114)	92 (82–105)
	$p \leq 0.001$	$p > 0.05$	$p > 0.05$

Paired statistics: Wilcoxon signed rank test
From Kluft et al. reproduced with permission from Elsevier
[a]Evaluated number of individuals with data from all sampling points

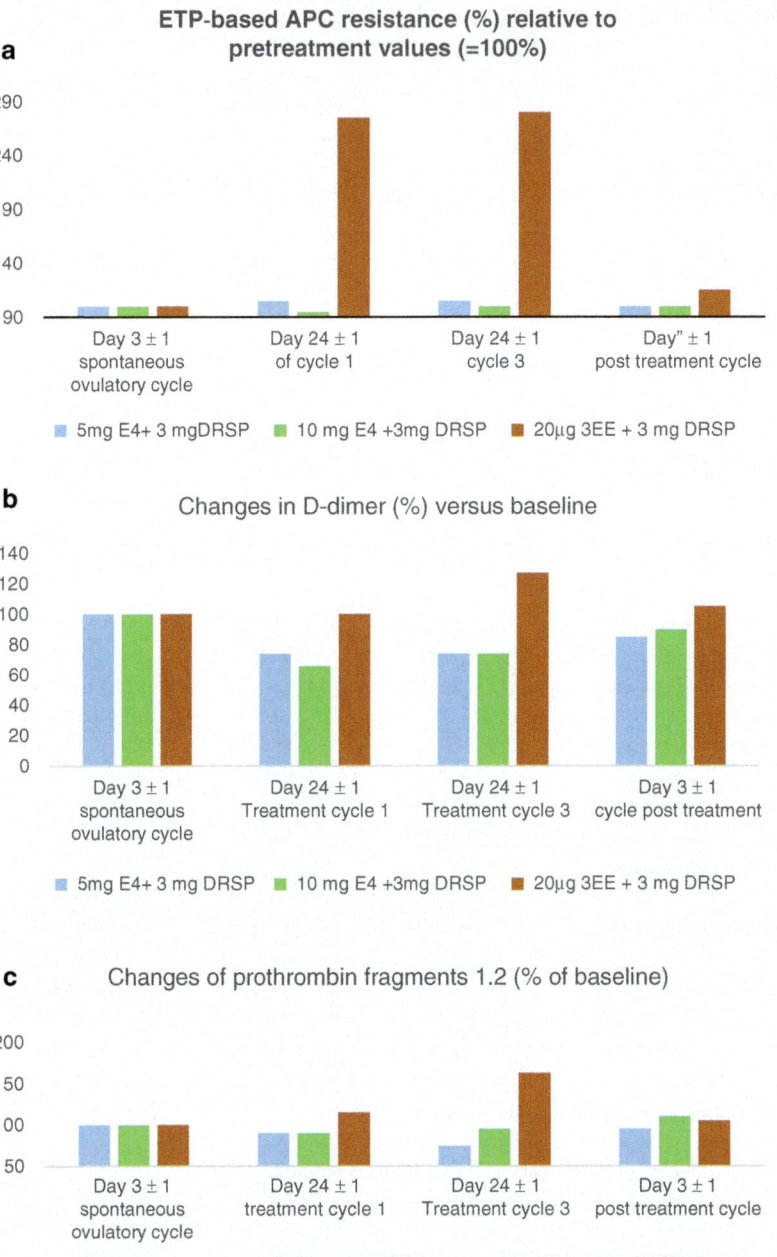

Fig. 12.10 Changes in ETP-based APC resistance (**a**), D-Dimer (**b**), and prothrombin fragment 1.2 (**c**), in the presence of 5 or 10 mg E4 + 3 mg DRSP versus 20 μg EE + 3 mg DRSP. The global marker of coagulation inhibition test (ETP-based APC resistance) and of coagulation activation (D-Dimers and prothrombin fragment 1.2) demonstrates considerable differences of EE versus E4 in association with the same dose of DRSP. EE causes major procoagulatory changes, while E4 does not. (Modified from Kluft et al. 2017 with permission from Elsevier)

12.5.2   Fifteen Milligram E4 Has No Impact on Hemostasis in Postmenopausal Women

E4 relief is a prospective, multicenter, randomized, placebo-controlled, double-blinded, dose-finding study in both hysterectomized and non-hysterectomized postmenopausal women. The primary objective was to select the optimal effective oral dose of E4 for the treatment of VMS in postmenopausal women. Secondary efficacy objectives included the evaluation of safety, the effects of different doses of E4 on vulvar and vaginal atrophy (VVA scoring system; maturation index), bone biomarkers, and health-related quality of life. No significant changes in any markers of coagulation or angiotensinogen were documented in the 250 women receiving for 12 weeks 2.5, 5, 10, or 15 mg E4 (Mithra data on file).

Taken altogether these phase 2 clinical data indicate that E4 is a unique molecule, which does not appear to increase the risk of thrombosis in that it does not affect coagulation factors when compared to effects elicited by orally administered classical and synthetic estrogens.

12.6   Conclusion

Experimental and clinical observational and prospective randomized trials indicate that estrogens convey multiple benefits. Their use is also associated with unwanted side effects. For example, women using COCs or oral HRT have an increased incidence of DVT and PE. There is also an increased incidence of stroke among postmenopausal women treated with oral HRT. The identification of safer estrogenic compounds for HRT and for combined oral contraceptives (COCs) that would selectively preserve the beneficial effects of estrogens on symptoms of menopause, the bone, and urogenital system while reducing their unwanted side effects is largely needed. In particular, the precise delineation of the activity/safety profile of E4 requires both preclinical and clinical studies. This estrogen is human (primate) specific and synthesized in large amounts (3–5 mg/day) by the human fetus. Selected by natural evolution, this fetal estrogen acts selectively in tissues, with mixed agonist and antagonist activities. This NEST (Native Estrogen that has Selective action in Tissues) property is the consequence of the selective activation by E4 of the nuclear ERα and of the blockade of the membrane ERα as demonstrated by combined genetic and pharmacological approaches [37, 85].

This review has summarized the preclinical (and limited clinical) information about the impact of E4 on the vascular system. The impact of E4 on the vascular system may be summarized in one integrated concept (Fig. 12.11). The membrane ERα is neither necessary nor sufficient for eliciting beneficial effect of estrogens on arteries (i.e., protection against neointimal hyperplasia, atheroma, hypertension, and induction of FMR). E4 by selectively activating the nuclear ERα is able to convey, at least in animal models, all the beneficial vascular effects of E2. In contrast to E2, E4 does not enhance endothelial NO production but does not alter the flow-induced vasodilation, the most potent physiological stimulus of NO production. This neutrality could confer an advantage in a tumoral context, as E4

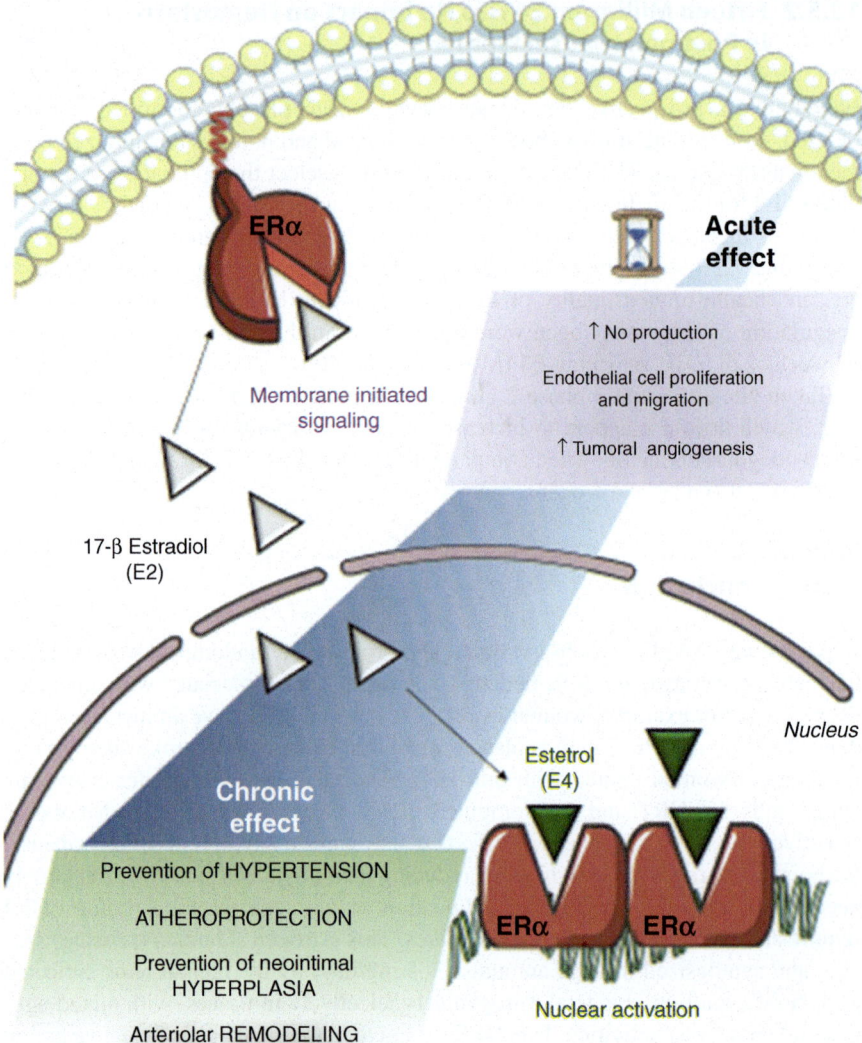

Fig. 12.11 The key role of nuclear ERα activation in controlling the E4 vascular effects. The beneficial actions of ERα activation by E4 on atheroma, hypertension, neointimal hyperplasia and arterial remodeling all rely on nuclear ERα. ERα membrane-initiated signaling is not stimulated by E4 which does not enhance tumoral angiogenesis (reproduced with permission modified from Guivarc'h et al. 2018)

does not enhance tumoral angiogenesis in contrast to E2 and may even antagonize this unwanted effect elicited by E2. Finally, E4 may induce an arterial vasodilation by a guanylate cyclase dependent mechanism. In clinical studies, E4 in contrast to EE and E2 has a minimal impact on the synthesis of hemostasis parameters and of liver proteins induced by estrogens, including SHBG and angiotensinogen.

E4, a fetal estrogen, which is devoid of thrombogenic activity but carries the vascular beneficial effects of E2 17β, may prove to be an efficacious and safer estrogen for clinical use. Phase 3 clinical studies in progress should contribute to further confirm these encouraging data.

Acknowledgments The authors warmfully thank Professor Rogerio A. Lobo, Columbia University College of Physicians and Surgeons, and Professor Mitchell Creinin, Division of Family Planning, Department of Obstetrics and Gynecology, University of California, Davis, Sacramento, California, for helpful discussions and comments in the preparation and reviewing process of this manuscript.

References

1. Grodstein F, Stampfer MJ, Colditz GA. Postmenopausal hormone therapy and mortality. N Engl J Med. 1997;336:1769–75.
2. Stampfer MJ, Colditz GA. Estrogen replacement therapy and coronary heart disease: a quantitative assessment of the epidemiologic evidence. Prev Med. 1991;20:47–63.
3. Yaffe K, Sawaya G, Lieberburg I, Grady D. Estrogen therapy in postmenopausal women: effects on cognitive function and dementia. JAMA. 1998;279:688–95.
4. Grady D, et al. Hormone therapy to prevent disease and prolong life in postmenopausal women. Ann Intern Med. 1992;117:1016–37.
5. Henderson BE, Paganini-Hill A, Ross RK. Decreased mortality in users of estrogen replacement therapy. Arch Intern Med. 1991;151:75–8.
6. Hulley S, Grady D, Bush T, Furberg C, Herrington D, Riggs B, Vittinghoff E. Randomized trial of estrogen plus progestin for secondary prevention of coronary heart disease in postmenopausal women. Heart and Estrogen/progestin Replacement Study (HERS) Research Group. JAMA. 1998;280:605–13.
7. Rossouw JE, Anderson GL, Prentice RL, LaCroix AZ, Kooperberg C, Stefanick ML, Jackson RD, Beresford SA, Howard BV, Johnson KC, Kotchen JM, Ockene J, Writing Group for the Women's Health Initiative Investigators. Risks and benefits of estrogen plus progestin in healthy postmenopausal women: principal results from the Women's Health Initiative randomized controlled trial. JAMA. 2002;288:321–33.
8. Hsia J, et al. Conjugated equine estrogens and coronary heart disease: the Women's Health Initiative. Arch Intern Med. 2006;166:357–65.
9. Rossouw JE, et al. Postmenopausal hormone therapy and cardiovascular disease by age and years since menopause. JAMA. 2007;297:1465–77.
10. Carrasquilla GD, et al. The association between menopausal hormone therapy and coronary heart disease depends on timing of initiation in relation to menopause onset: results based on pooled individual participant data from the Combined Cohorts of Menopausal Women — Studies of Register Based Health Outcomes in Relation to Hormonal Drugs (COMPREHEND) study [abstract S17]. Menopause. 2015;22:1373.
11. Hodis HN, Mack WJ, Henderson VW. Effects of early versus late postmenopausal treatment with estradiol. N Engl J Med. 2016;374:1221–31.
12. Lobo Pickar JH, Stevenson JC, Mack WJ, Hodis HN. Back to the future: Hormone replacement therapy as part of a prevention strategy for women at the onset of menopause. Atherosclerosis. 2016;254:282–90.
13. Manson JE, Aragaki AK, Rossouw JE, Anderson GL, Prentice RL, LaCroix AZ, Chlebowski RT, Howard BV, Thomson CA, Margolis KL, Lewis CE, Stefanick ML, Jackson RD, Johnson KC, Martin LW, Shumaker SA, Espeland MA, Wactawski-Wende J, Investigators WHI. Menopausal hormone therapy and long-term all-cause and cause-specific mortality: the women's health initiative randomized trials. JAMA. 2017;318:927–38.

14. Lobo RA. Hormone-replacement therapy: current thinking. Nat Rev Endocrinol. 2017;13: 220–31.
15. Grodstein F, Manson JE, Stampfer MJ, Rexrode K. Postmenopausal hormone therapy and stroke: role of time since menopause and age at initiation of hormone therapy. Arch Intern Med. 2008;168:861–6.
16. Lobo RA, Clarkson TB. Different mechanisms for benefit and risk of coronary heart disease and stroke in early postmenopausal women: a hypothetical explanation. Menopause. 2011;18:237–40.
17. Sare GM, Gray LJ, Bath PM. Association between hormone replacement therapy and subsequent arterial and venous vascular events: a meta-analysis. Eur Heart J. 2008;29:2031–41.
18. NHLBI. NHLBI stops trial of estrogen plus progestin due to increased breast cancer risk and lack of overall benefit. South Med J. 2002;95:795–7.
19. Mohammed K, Abu Dabrh AM, Benkhadra K, Al Nofal A, Carranza Leon BG, Prokop LJ, Montori VM, Faubion SS, Murad MH. Oral vs transdermal estrogen therapy and vascular events: a systematic review and meta-analysis. J Clin Endocrinol Metab. 2015;100:4012–20.
20. Lidegaard Ø, Nielsen LH, Skovlund CW, Skjeldestad FE, Løkkegaard E. Risk of venous thromboembolism from use of oral contraceptives containing different progestogens and oestrogen doses: Danish cohort study, 2001–9. BMJ. 2011;25:343.
21. Han L, Jensen JT. Does the progestogen used in combined hormonal contraception affect venous thrombosis risk? Obstet Gynecol Clin N Am. 2015;42:683–98.
22. Kemmeren JM, Algra A, Meijers JC, Tans G, Bouma BN, Curvers J, Rosing J, Grobbee DE. Effect of second- and third-generation oral contraceptives on the protein C system in the absence or presence of the factor VLeiden mutation: a randomized trial. Blood. 2004;103:927–33.
23. Oral Contraceptive and Hemostasis Study Group. The effects of seven monophasic oral contraceptive regimens on hemostatic variables: conclusions from a large randomized multicenter study. Contraception. 2003;67:173–85.
24. Vandenbroucke JP, Koster T, Briët E, Reitsma PH, Bertina RM, Rosendaal FR. Increased risk of venous thrombosis in oral-contraceptive users who are carriers of factor V Leiden mutation. Lancet. 1994;344(8935):1453–7.
25. Mantha S, Karp R, Raghavan V, Terrin N, Bauer KA, Zwicker JI. Assessing the risk of venous thromboembolic events in women taking progestin-only contraception: a meta-analysis. BMJ. 2012;345:e4944.
26. Regidor PA, Colli E, Schindler AE. Drospirenone as estrogen-free pill and hemostasis: coagulatory study results comparing a novel 4 mg formulation in a 24 + 4 cycle with desogestrel 75 μg per day. Gynecol Endocrinol. 2016;32:749–51.
27. Dinger J, Do Minh T, Heinemann K. Impact of estrogen type on cardiovascular safety of combined oral contraceptives. Contraception. 2016;94:328–39.
28. Sitruk-Ware R. New progestagens for contraceptive use. Hum Reprod Update. 2006;12:169–78.
29. Wiegratz I, Lee JH, Kutschera E, Winkler UH, Kuhl H. Effect of four oral contraceptives on hemostatic parameters. Contraception. 2004;70:97–106.
30. van Vliet HA, Frolich M, Christella M, Thomassen LG, Doggen CJ, Rosendaal FR, Rosing J, Helmerhorst FM. Association between sex hormone-binding globulin levels and activated protein C resistance in explaining the risk of thrombosis in users of oral contraceptives containing different progestogens. Hum Reprod. 2005;20:563–8.
31. Raps M, Helmerhorst F, Fleischer K, Thomassen S, Rosendaal F, Rosing J, Ballieux B, VAN Vliet H. Sex hormone-binding globulin as a marker for the thrombotic risk of hormonal contraceptives. J Thromb Haemost. 2012;10:992–7.
32. Rosing J, Middeldorp S, Curvers J, Christella M, Thomassen LG, Nicolaes GA, Meijers JC, Bouma BN, Büller HR, Prins MH, Tans G. Low-dose oral contraceptives and acquired resistance to activated protein C: a randomised cross-over study. Lancet. 1999;354:2036–40.
33. Odlind V, Milsom I, Persson I, Victor A. Can changes in sex hormone binding globulin predict the risk of venous thromboembolism with combined oral contraceptive pills? Acta Obstet Gynecol Scand. 2002;81:482–90.

34. Hickey M, Hart R, Keelan JA. The relationship between umbilical cord estrogens and perinatal characteristics. Cancer Epidemiol Biomark Prev. 2014;23:946–5.
35. Kundu N, Wachs M, Iverson GB, Petersen LP. Comparison of serum unconjugated estriol and estetrol in normal and complicated pregnancies. Obstet Gynecol. 1981;58(3):276–81.
36. Arnal JF, Lenfant F, Metivier R, Flouriot G, Henrion D, Adlanmerini M, Fontaine C, Gourdy P, Chambon P, Katzenellenbogen B, Katzenellenbogen J. Membrane and nuclear estrogen receptor alpha actions: from tissue specificity to medical implications. Physiol Rev. 2017;3: 1045–87.
37. Abot A, Fontaine C, Buscato M, Solinhac R, Flouriot G, Fabre A, Drougard A, Rajan S, Laine M, Milon A, Muller I, Henrion D, Adlanmerini M, Valéra MC, Gompel A, Gerard C, Péqueux C, Mestdagt M, Raymond-Letron I, Knauf C, Ferriere F, Valet P, Gourdy P, Katzenellenbogen BS, Katzenellenbogen JA, Lenfant F, Greene GL, Foidart JM, Arnal JF. The uterine and vascular actions of estetrol delineate a distinctive profile of estrogen receptor α modulation, uncoupling nuclear and membrane activation. EMBO Mol Med. 2014;10:1328–46.
38. Gourdy P, Guillaume M, Fontaine C, Adlanmerini M, Montagner A, Laurell H, Lenfant F, Arnal JF. Estrogen receptor subcellular localization and cardiometabolism. Mol Metab. 2018;15:56–69.
39. Brouchet L, Krust A, Dupont S, Chambon P, Bayard F, Arnal JF. Estradiol accelerates reendothelialization in mouse carotid artery through estrogen receptor-alpha but not estrogen receptor-beta. Circulation. 2001;103:423–8.
40. Wu Q, Chambliss K, Umetani M, Mineo C, Shaul PW. Non-nuclear estrogen receptor signaling in the endothelium. J Biol Chem. 2011;286:14737–43.
41. Adlanmerini M, Solinhac R, Abot A, Fabre A, Raymond-Letron I, Guihot AL, Boudou F, Sautier L, Vessieres E, Kim SH, et al. Mutation of the palmitoylation site of estrogen receptor alpha in vivo reveals tissue-specific roles for membrane versus nuclear actions. Proc Natl Acad Sci U S A. 2014;111:E283–90.
42. Chambliss KL, Wu Q, Oltmann S, Konaniah ES, Umetani M, Korach KS, Thomas GD, Mineo C, Yuhanna IS, Kim SH, et al. Non-nuclear estrogen receptor alpha signaling promotes cardiovascular protection but not uterine or breast cancer growth in mice. J Clin Invest. 2010;120:2319–30.
43. Vanhoutte PM. Nitric oxide: from good to bad. Ann Vasc Dis. 2018;11:41–51.
44. Vanhoutte PM, Zhao Y, Xu A, Leung SW. Thirty years of saying no: sources, fate, actions, and misfortunes of the endothelium-derived vasodilator mediator. Circ Res. 2016;119:375–96.
45. Yamazaki Y, Kondo Y, Kamiyama Y. Estimation of shear-stress-induced endothelial nitric oxide production from flow-mediated dilation. Conf Proc IEEE Eng Med Biol Soc. 2013;2013:4521–4.
46. Levine MG, Miodovnik M, Clark KE. Uterine vascular effects of estetrol in nonpregnant ewes. Am J Obstet Gynecol. 1984;148(6):735–8.
47. Hilgers RH, Oparil S, Wouters W, Coelingh Bennink HJ. Vasorelaxing effects of estetrol in rat arteries. Endocrinology. 2012;215:97–106.
48. Arnal JF, Fontaine C, Billon-Gales A, Favre J, Laurell H, Lenfant F, Gourdy P. Estrogen receptors and endothelium. Arterioscler Thromb Vasc Biol. 2010;30:1506–12.
49. Chambliss KL, Shaul PW. Estrogen modulation of endothelial nitric oxide synthase. Endocr Rev. 2002;23:665–86.
50. Mallat Z, Tedgui A. Cytokines as regulators of atherosclerosis in murine models. Curr Drug Targets. 2007;8:1264–72.
51. Weber C, Zernecke A, Libby P. The multifaceted contributions of leukocyte subsets to atherosclerosis: lessons from mouse models. Nat Rev Immunol. 2008;8:802–15.
52. Tarhouni K, Guihot AL, Freidja ML, Toutain B, Henrion B, Baufreton C, Pinaud F, Procaccio V, Grimaud L, Ayer A, Loufrani L, Lenfant F, Arnal JF, Henrion D. Key role of estrogens and endothelial estrogen receptor alpha in blood flow-mediated remodeling of resistance arteries. Arterioscler Thromb Vasc Biol. 2013;33:605–11.
53. Billon-Gales A, Fontaine C, Douin-Echinard V, Delpy L, Berges H, Calippe B, Lenfant F, Laurell H, Guery JC, Gourdy P, Arnal JF. Endothelial estrogen receptor-alpha plays a cru-

cial role in the atheroprotective action of 17beta-estradiol in low-density lipoprotein receptor-deficient mice. Circulation. 2009;120:2567–76.

54. Billon-Gales A, Krust A, Fontaine C, Abot A, Flouriot G, Toutain C, Berges H, Gadeau AP, Lenfant F, Gourdy P, et al. Activation function 2 (AF2) of estrogen receptor-{alpha} is required for the atheroprotective action of estradiol but not to accelerate endothelial healing. Proc Natl Acad Sci U S A. 2011;108:13311–6.

55. Guivarc'h E, Buscato M, Guihot A.L, Favre J, Vessières E, Grimaud L, Wakim J, Melhem NJ, Zahreddine R, Adlanmerini M., Loufrani M, Knauf C, Katzenellenbogen JA, Katzenellenbogen BS, Foidart JM, Gourdy P, Lenfant F, Arnal JF, Henrion D, Fontaine C Predominant role of nuclear *versus* membrane estrogen receptor (ER)α in arterial protection: implications for ERα modulation in cardiovascular prevention/safety. J Am Heart Assoc. 2018. https://doi.org/10.1161/JAHA.118.008950.

56. Hui DY. Intimal hyperplasia in murine models. Curr Drug Targets. 2008;9:251–60.

57. Smirnova NF, Gayral S, Pedros C, Loirand G, Vaillant N, Malet N, Kassem S, Calise D, Goudounèche D, Wymann MP, Hirsch E, Gadeau AP, Martinez LO, Saoudi A, Laffargue M. Targeting PI3Kγ activity decreases vascular trauma-induced intimal hyperplasia through modulation of the Th1 response. J Exp Med. 2014;211:1779–92.

58. Costa MA, Simon DI. Molecular basis of restenosis and drug eluting stents. Circulation. 2005;111:2257–73.

59. Chandrasekar B, Sirois MG, Geoffroy P, Lauzier D, Nattel S, Tanguay JF. Local delivery of 17beta-estradiol improves reendothelialization and decreases inflammation after coronary stenting in a porcine model. Thromb Haemost. 2005;94:1042–7.

60. Smirnova NF, Fontaine C, Buscato M, Lupieri A, Vinel A, Valera MC, Guillaume M, Malet N, Foidart JM, Raymond-Letron I, Lenfant F, Gourdy P, Katzenellenbogen BS, Katzenellenbogen JA, Laffargue M, Arnal JF. The activation function-1 of estrogen receptor alpha prevents arterial neointima development through a direct effect on smooth muscle cells. Circ Res. 2015;117:770–8.

61. Bouvet C, Belin de Chantemèle E, Guihot AL, Vessieres E, Bocquet A, Dumont O, Jardel A, Loufrani L, Moreau P, Henrion D. Flow-induced remodeling in resistance arteries from obese Zucker rats is associated with endothelial dysfunction. Hypertension. 2007;50:248–54.

62. Dumont O, Loufrani L, Henrion D. Key role of the NO-pathway and matrix metalloprotease-9 in high blood flow-induced remodeling of rat resistance arteries. Arterioscler Thromb Vasc Biol. 2007;27:317–24.

63. Pourageaud F, De Mey JG. Vasomotor responses in chronically hyperperfused and hypoperfused rat mesenteric arteries. Am J Phys. 1998;274:H1301–7.

64. Carmeliet P. Angiogenesis in life, disease and medicine. Nature. 2005;438:932–6.

65. Silvestre JS, Smadja DM, Levy BI. Postischemic revascularization: from cellular and molecular mechanisms to clinical applications. Physiol Rev. 2013;93:1743–802.

66. Dumont O, Kauffenstein G, Guihot AL, Guerineau NC, Abraham P, Loufrani L, Henrion D. Time-related alteration in flow- (shear stress-) mediated remodeling in resistance arteries from spontaneously hypertensive rats. Int J Hypertens. 2014;2014:859793.

67. Tuttle JL, Sanders BM, Burkhart HM, Fath SW, Kerr KA, Watson WC, Herring BP, Dalsing MC, Unthank JL. Impaired collateral artery development in spontaneously hypertensive rats. Microcirculation. 2002;9:343–51.

68. Belin de Chantemele EJ, Vessieres E, Guihot AL, Toutain B, Maquignau M, Loufrani L, Henrion D. Type 2 diabetes severely impairs structural and functional adaptation of rat resistance arteries to chronic changes in blood flow. Cardiovasc Res. 2009;81:788–96.

69. Freidja ML, Tarhouni K, Toutain B, Fassot C, Loufrani L, Henrion D. The age-breaker alt-711 restores high blood flow-dependent remodeling in mesenteric resistance arteries in a rat model of type 2 diabetes. Diabetes. 2012;61:1562–72.

70. Dumont O, Pinaud F, Guihot AL, Baufreton C, Loufrani L, Henrion D. Alteration in flow (shear stress)-induced remodelling in rat resistance arteries with aging: Improvement by a treatment with hydralazine. Cardiovasc Res. 2008;77:600–8.

71. Tarhouni K, Guihot AL, Vessieres E, Toutain B, Procaccio V, Grimaud L, Loufrani L, Lenfant F, Arnal JF, Henrion D. Determinants of flow-mediated outward remodeling in female rodents: respective roles of age, estrogens, and timing. Arterioscler Thromb Vasc Biol. 2014;34:1281–9.
72. Barton M, Meyer MR. Postmenopausal hypertension: mechanisms and therapy. Hypertension. 2009;54:11–8.
73. Regitz-Zagrosek V, Kararigas G. Mechanistic pathways of sex differences in cardiovascular disease. Physiol Rev. 2017;97:1–37.
74. Barsha G, Denton KM, Mirabito Colafella KM. Sex- and age-related differences in arterial pressure and albuminuria in mice. Biol Sex Differ. 2016;7:57.
75. Sampson AK, Moritz KM, Jones ES, Flower RL, Widdop RE, Denton KM. Enhanced angiotensin II type 2 receptor mechanisms mediate decreases in arterial pressure attributable to chronic low-dose angiotensin II in female rats. Hypertension. 2008;52:666–71.
76. Valera MC, Gratacap MP, Gourdy P, Lenfant F, Cabou C, Toutain CE, Marcellin M, Saint Laurent N, Sie P, Sixou M, Arnal JF, Payrastre B. Chronic estradiol treatment reduces platelet responses and protects mice from thromboembolism through the hematopoietic estrogen receptor alpha. Blood. 2012;120:1703–12.
77. Kluft C, Zimmerman Y, Mawet M, Klipping C, Duijkers IJ, Neuteboom J, Foidart JM, Bennink HC. Reduced hemostatic effects with drospirenone-based oral contraceptives containing estetrol vs. ethinyl estradiol. Contraception. 2017;95:140–7.
78. Shapiro S. Oral contraceptives, hormone therapy and cardiovascular risk. Climacteric. 2008;11:355–63.
79. Jirouskova M, Shet AS, Johnson GJ. A guide to murine platelet structure, function, assays, and genetic alterations. J Thromb Haemost. 2007;5:661–9.
80. Valéra MC, Noirrit-Esclassan E, Dupuis M, Fontaine C, Lenfant F, Briaux A, Cabou C, Garcia C, Lairez O, Foidart JM, Payrastre B, Arnal JF. Effect of estetrol, a selective nuclear estrogen receptor modulator, in mouse models of arterial and venous thrombosis. Mol Cell Endocrinol. 2018;477:132–9. S0303-7207(18) 30196-5
81. Geddings J, Aleman MM, Wolberg A, von Bruhl ML, Massberg S, Mackman N. Strengths and weaknesses of a new mouse model of thrombosis induced by inferior vena cava stenosis: communication from the SSC of the ISTH. J Thromb Haemost. 2014;12:571–3.
82. Donnem T, Reynolds AR, Kuczynski EA, Gatter K, Vermeulen PB, Kerbel RS, Harris AL, Pezzella F. Non-angiogenic tumours and their influence on cancer biology. Nat Rev Cancer. 2018;18:323–36.
83. Péqueux C, Raymond-Letron I, Blacher S, Boudou F, Adlanmerini M, Fouque MJ, Rochaix P, Noël A, Foidart JM, Krust A, Chambon P, Brouchet L, Arnal JF, Lenfant F. Stromal estrogen receptor-α promotes tumor growth by normalizing an increased angiogenesis. Cancer Res. 2012;72:3010–9.
84. EMA. European Medicines Agency, Committee for Medicinal Products for Human Use. Guideline on clinical investigation of steroid contraceptives in women. London: EMA; 2005. EMEA/CPMP/EWP/519/98 rev 1
85. Benoit T, Valera MC, Fontaine C, Buscato M, Lenfant F, Raymond-Letron I, Tremollieres F, Soulie M, Foidart JM, Game X, Arnal JF. Estetrol, a fetal selective estrogen receptor modulator, acts on the vagina of mice through nuclear estrogen receptor α activation. Am J Pathol. 2017;187:2499–507.

Vascular Effects of Progestogens

13

Xiangyan Ruan and Alfred O. Mueck

13.1 Clinical Endpoint Studies

About 30 observational studies suggest that estrogen(E)-only and, with a more limited evidence, combined HRT are associated with a significant reduction in cardiovascular mortality and morbidity. Most studies have been performed before the Women's Health Initiative (WHI) [1, 2], but also newer studies suggest cardiovascular prevention if HRT is early started. For example, a recent Danish randomized case-control study including only patients between 45 and 58 years did found after 10 years a significantly reduced risk of mortality, heart failure, or myocardial infarction, without any apparent increase in risk of cancer, venous thromboembolism, or stroke [3].

This evidence, however, has not been supported by randomized placebo-controlled studies summarized in Table 13.1 with clinical endpoints or with coronary arteriography or intima-media thickness measurements at the carotid artery (CIMT) as primary indirect clinical endpoints, resp.

The most important trial, the *Women's Health Initiative (WHI)*, which allows the assessment of a progestogen effect based on clinical endpoints by comparison of estrogen(E)-only with a combined HRT, has used medroxyprogesterone acetate (MPA) added to conjugated equine estrogens (CEE) [1]. In the CEE-only arm, a trend to reduction of coronary heart disease (CHD) was found in the age group of 50–59 years missing scarcely a significance [2]. Although the most recent follow-up of 18 years in both groups did not demonstrate an increased mortality [4], neither total nor specific (cardiovascular, cancer) mortality, this difference of risk between the cohorts during the interventional phase of WHI points at a crucial role of

X. Ruan · A. O. Mueck (✉)
Beijing Obstetrics and Gynecology Hospital, Capital Medical University, Beijing, China

Department of Women's Health, University Hospitals of Tuebingen, Tuebingen, Germany
e-mail: Alfred.Mueck@med.uni-tuebingen.de

© International Society of Gynecological Endocrinology 2019
R. D. Brinton et al. (eds.), *Sex Steroids' Effects on Brain, Heart and Vessels*,
ISGE Series, https://doi.org/10.1007/978-3-030-11355-1_13

Table 13.1 Randomized placebo-controlled interventional studies investigating the risk of arterial cardiovascular diseases during HRT

		n (ITT) (incl. Placebo)	HRT (dosage/day)	Remarks
1. Studies with clinical endpoints (myocardial infarction, stroke)				
WHI	Women's *H*ealth *I*nitiative study			
	Combined arm	16.608	CEE 0.625 mg/ MPA 2.5 mg	
	Estrogen-only arm	10.739	CEE 0.625 mg	
WISDOM	Women's *I*nternational *S*tudy of long *D*uration *O*estrogen after *M*enopause	5.700		(1)
HERS I	*H*eart and *E*strogen/progestin *R*eplacement Study (Teil I)	2.763	CEE 0.625 mg/ MPA 2.5 mg	
ESPRIT	*ES*trogen for *P*revention of *ReI*nfarct *T*rial	1.017		
PHASE	*P*apworth *HRT A*thero*S*clerosis *E*strogen study	255	Estradiol 80 µg/ NETA 120 g	(2)
WHISP	Womens' *H*ormone *I*ntervention *S*econdary *P*revention study	100	Estradiol 1 mg/ NETA 0.5 mg	
WEST	Women's *E*strogen for *S*troke *T*rial	664	Estradiol 1 mg	
2. Studies with indirect endpoints				(3)
2.1 Coronary angiography (primary endpoint)				
ERA	*E*strogen/progestin *R*eplacement and *A*therosclerosis trial	309	CEE 0.625 mg/ MPA 2.5 mg	
WAVE	Women's *A*ngiographic *V*itamin and *E*strogen/ progestin trial	423	CEE 0.625 mg/ MPA 2.5 mg	(4)
WELLHART	Women's *E*strogen/progestin *L*ipid-*L*owering *H*ormone *A*therosclerosis *R*egression *T*rial	226	Estradiol 1 mg// MPA 5 mg seq.	
2.2 Carotid Intima Media Thickness (primary endpoint)				
PHOREA	*P*ostmenopausal *HO*rmone *RE*placement against *A*therosclerosis	321	Estradiol 1 mg/ gestodene 0.025 mg	(5)
HERS B	*H*eart and *E*strogen/progestin *R*eplacement *S*tudy using *B* Mode	362	CEE 0.625 mg/ MPA 2.5 mg	
OPAL	*O*steoporosis *P*revention and *A*rterial effects on *L*ivial	866	Tibolone 2.5 mg; CEE 0.625 mg/ MPA 2.5 mg	
EPAT	*E*strogen in *P*revention of *A*therosclerosis *T*rial	222	Estradiol 1 mg	

Table 13.1 (continued)

		n (ITT) (incl. Placebo)	HRT (dosage/day)	Remarks
KEEPS	Kronos Early Estrogen Prevention Study	727	Estradiol 0.025 mg; CEE 0.3 mg	(6)
			Progesterone 100–200 mg seq.	
ELITE	Early versus Late Intervention Trial with Estradiol/ progesterone	643	Estradiol 1 mg/ progesterone 100 mg	(6)

ITT Intent to Treat Analysis

CEE conjugated equine estrogens, *NETA* norethisterone acetate, *MPA* medroxyprogesterone acetate

Remarks:

(1) WISDOM: in plan n = 32.000 patients, different HRT regimens, but was stopped in Oct 2002 due to recruitment problems caused by WHI results

(2) PHASE: transdermal HRT: 2 weeks E2 patch releasing 80 µg/day, sequential combi patch, releasing additionally 120 µg NETA/day

(3) Various studies with lipids and/or markers of glucose metabolism as indirect study endpoints, e.g., PEPI (Postmenopausal Estrogen/Progestin Intervention Trial) (n = 596): CEE-only (0.625 mg/day) vs. CEE + seq. MPA (10 mg/day; 12 days) vs. CEE + cont. MPA (2.5 mg/day) vs. CEE + seq. Progesteron (200 mg/day; 12 days) vs. Placebo

(4) WAVE: additional study-arm vitamine E (400 E/day) plus vitamine C (500 mg/day)

(5) PHOREA: use of gestodene monthly or 3-monthly (long-cycle); study indeed only single-blind design

(6) KEEPS, ELITE: must recent studies as described within the text

progestogen addition, which can antagonize the beneficial cardiovascular protective effect regarding the risk of CHD.

Most other studies do not allow to conclude about the progestogen effect because they do not compare with E-only medication. From the studies listed in Table 13.1, the two most recent studies, the KEEPS (Kronos Early Estrogen Prevention Study) [5] and the ELITE (Early versus Late Intervention Trial with Estradiol) studies [6], are remarkable because they demonstrate not only the possibilities but also the limitations of clinical cardiovascular research.

13.2   KEEPS and ELITE Studies

In *KEEPS* [5] 727 healthy menopausal women within 3 years since last menstrual period (mean age 52.7 years) were recruited and followed during 4 years with either low-dose CEE (0.45 mg/day) or patch estradiol (E2) (50 µg/day) with oral progesterone (200 mg for 12 days per month) or placebo. HRT had no significant effect on CIMT progression or on the CAC (coronary artery calcification) score.

In *ELITE* [6] 643 healthy postmenopausal women were stratified less than 6 years or 10 or more years past menopause receiving oral E2 (1 mg daily) or placebo. Women with uterus also received progesterone (45 mg) as a 4% vaginal gel (10 days per month) in the E2 group, in the placebo group placebo gel. The CIMT was measured every 6 months during a median 5-year follow-up period. Among women less than 6 years past menopause, the mean CIMT increase was significantly lower, and also the absolute CIMT values were lower compared to the women 10 years or more past menopause. CT values of coronary-artery calcium, total stenosis, and plaque (secondary endpoints) did not differ significantly between the placebo and the E2 group in either postmenopause stratum.

In summary the results of ELITE suggest a small effect of primary cardiovascular prevention if HRT is early started which has been suggested in about 30 observational studies and in experimental research ("Window of opportunity"), whereas in KEEPS no effect could be demonstrated, perhaps because the women have been too healthy for any preventive estrogen effect. Important seems that in both studies obviously progesterone did not antagonize the cardiovascular preventive effect of estradiol, which, however, needs "historical" conclusion comparing with other studies using E-only.

From several observational studies, a lower risk using E-only compared to combined HRT can be suggested, e.g., from the analysis of *Danish registry (n = 698.098)*, the highest risk for myocardial infarction was concluded for combined HRT regimens, whereas lower or no increased risk was found with cyclic combined or unopposed estrogen regimens [7].

Mechanisms of the potential negative progestogen action cannot be concluded from clinical studies although there is evidence that they may be very important: The 1.5–3-fold increased risk of cardiac and stroke death in the first year after stop of HRT, shown in a *huge cohort of Finnish women (n = 432.775)* [8] treated with HRT between 1994 and 2013 and compared with the age-matched female background population, can be explained by reactive vasoconstrictory effects and/or destabilization of arterial plaques, both mainly dependent on the progestogen component as suggested from experimental studies (see below).

13.3 Importance of Direct Vascular Effects

In contrast to clinical endpoint studies, the differential effect of the various progestogens in terms of vascular effects has been demonstrated in numerous studies, e.g., the well-known negative effect of androgenic progestogens on HDL-cholesterol or different actions in the glucose metabolism. Here only should be mentioned that many studies on metabolic effects using HRT have been performed showing in summary a more neutral metabolic action if progesterone or its isomer dydrogesterone have been used.

Progestogens can be characterized according to their partial effects on the androgen, glucocorticoid, and mineralocorticoid receptor. Vascular systems can be influenced positively or negatively based on these "partial" progestagenic effects. For an advanced differentiated assessment in vascular systems, the research currently is strongly focused on so-called vascular active biochemical markers, since

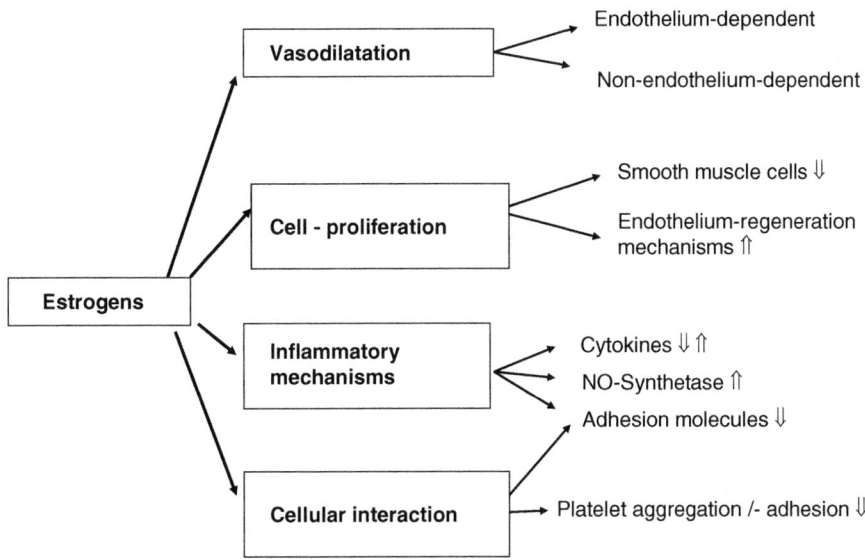

Fig. 13.1 Direct vascular effects of estrogens. Note: All effects can be influenced by addition of progestogens, mostly antagonizing the estrogen effect dependent on type and dosage of the progestogen (see text)

it is expected that risk assessment and monitoring during therapy is possible by means of simple and cost-saving measurement of blood concentrations of these biological mediators, comparable to the measurements in the lipid and carbohydrate system for prediction of a cardiovascular risk. The main mechanism of the cardioprotection of estrogens appears to be a direct effect on the vasculature via those vascular active biomarkers resulting in an improvement of endothelial function and inhibition of atherogenesis, summarized in Fig. 13.1. The beneficial E-effects mostly are antagonized by addition of synthetic progestogens, whereas progesterone and its isomer dydrogesterone mostly react "neutral," like in the metabolic systems [9–11].

Since the net effect on all those vasoactive markers, responsible for the clinical action, is complex and difficult to predict, these more "neutral" progestogens should be preferred in cardiovascular-risk patients. Recent research especially has focused on the neutral or even beneficial effects of progesterone [12–18]. This may be explained that it is more and more used in HRT based on clinical observational studies suggesting that combining natural progestogen with E2 may also reduce the risk of venous thromboembolism and especially of breast cancer, according also to official guidelines, for example, of the International Menopause Society [19].

In the following the action of those vasoactive markers and some typical examples of different progestagenic effects, based on own investigations and selected from the literature of more than 100 experimental studies on this issue, are described. Action of estrogens and progestogens on all of the following various markers has been described, and mostly a beneficial (i.e., suggesting cardiovascular preventive) effect of estrogen was seen antagonized by synthetic progestogens, with the exception of inflammatory markers where results have been controversial.

13.3.1 Effects of the Most Important Vascular Biomarkers

13.3.1.1 Markers with Effect on Vasotonus

Nitric oxide (NO) is known to be the strongest vasodilatator. It also acts antiaggregatory, antiproliferative, antiinflammatoric, and antioxidative [20]. Since the half-lifetime is very short, direct measurement is very complex. Therefore indirect measurements of the oxidation products, i.e., nitrite and nitrate, or of the second messenger cGMP are performed which can reflect NO production. *Prostacyclin*, like NO synthesized in the endothelium, also has strong vasodilative and antiaggregatoric effects [21]. Its counterpart, *thromboxane*, is produced mainly in thrombocytes. The ratio of prostacyclin to thromboxane can reflect the overall positive or negative effect on vasotonus. *Endothelin* is one of the most as yet known vasoconstrictory compounds. It is mainly synthesized in the vascular endothelial cells and has direct effects on the vascular smooth muscle cells [22].

13.3.1.2 Pro-inflammatory Markers

The inflammatory marker *C-reactive protein* (CRP) has gained attention as independent marker of upcoming coronary events and may be also a mediator in atherogenesis, because it elicits numerous negative direct effects on the vasculature [23].

The cytokine *interleukin-6* (IL-6) is a potent inducer of the hepatic acute phase response and hence a regulator of CRP and may have a key role in the etiology of coronary heart disease [24]. *Adhesion molecules* play a crucial role in the early stages of atherogenesis [25]. These molecules mediate the adhesion, rolling and tethering of leucocytes on endothelial cells. Chemokines, such as the *monocyte-attracting protein-1* (MCP-1), are synthesized by vascular cells in the follow-up of inflammatory processes in order to recruit monocytes using their chemotacting properties [26]. Thus, the activity of this molecule is decisive in the early stages of atherosclerosis.

13.3.1.3 Markers for Plaque Stabilization

Plaque stabilization has been shown to be important in preventing acute coronary syndromes such as myocardial infarct or stroke. Several factors contribute to plaque stabilization; these include collagenases such as *matrix metalloproteinase-1* (MMP-1) which can be synthesized by macrophages and endothelial cells [27].

Increased serum concentrations of *plasminogen activator inhibitor-1* (PAI-1) shift the fibrinolytic/coagulatory balance toward an increased risk for arterial thrombosis and may accelerate arterial thrombosis following plaque rupturing. It may be an independent risk factor for cardiovascular diseases [28].

13.4   Examples of Progestogen Effects on Vascular Biomarkers

Simoncini et al. investigated the effects of progesterone (P), MPA, dydrogesterone (DYD), and its dihydro-metabolite (DHD) on endothelial synthesis of NO and characterized the signaling events [29]. DYD alone or in combination with E2 resulted in neutral effects. DHD and P enhanced eNOS through the regulation of the ERK 1/2 mitogen-activated protein kinase cascade and potentiated also eNOS induction by E2. On the contrary, MPA did not trigger eNOS enzymatic activation and decreased the extent of eNOS induction by E2.

These findings clearly support the concept that the more natural progestogens that act "neutral" or even beneficial and synthetic progestogens can antagonize vascular positive E-effects and/or can induce vasoconstrictory mechanism. In contrast the vasodilative genomic and non-genomic effects of progesterone, increasing endothelial NO production and enhancing E2-induced vasodilatation, have been seen in a variety also of other recent studies whereby obviously membrane-bound steroid receptors and secondary reduction of calcium entry in smooth muscle cells seem to play a decisive role [12–18]. This clearly must lead to the recommendation to use the natural progestogen in cardiovascular-risk patients!

Regarding other biomarkers of endothelial function and atherosclerotic plaque characteristics, we compared the effects of MPA vs. NET on E2-induced changes in human female coronary endothelial cell cultures [30]. E2 induced a significant increase of endothelial *prostacyclin* (suggesting vasodilative effects) and enhanced the production of the MMP-1, which is crucial for atherosclerotic plaque stability, and was able to significantly decrease the synthesis of *endothelin, PAI-1, E-selectin*, and intercellular *adhesion molecule-1*. Neither MPA nor NET addition negatively interfered with these E2-induced benefits. However, MPA, but not NET, antagonized the E2-induced significant reduction of TNF-alpha-stimulated *MCP-1* synthesis, so contrary effects of synthetic progestogens can exist regarding early stages of atherosclerosis. However, in the PEPI study, CEE combined with progesterone significantly lowered serum MCP-1 levels, suggesting a neutral effect of natural progesterone also regarding this marker [31]. Different effects of synthetic progestogens on arterial plaques and markers for plaque stabilization, respectively, have been seen also in other experimental studies [32, 33].

We also tested the effect of tibolone compared with E2-only and E2 combined with progestogens on the production of the following markers in endothelial cells from human female coronary arteries [34]: eNOS, prostacyclin, endothelin, PAI-1, E-selectin, intercellular adhesion molecule-1 (ICAM-1), MCP-1, and pro-MMP-1. Tibolone, its 3-hydroxy metabolites, E2/NET, E2/MPA, and E2 alone had similar significant but mostly smaller effects on markers tested like E2/NET and E2/MPA suggesting that also tibolone can exert cardiovascular preventive effects.

Interestingly we could demonstrate that addition of a statin can additively increase the beneficial effects of E2-induced production of prostacyclin and NO and E2-induced reduction of endothelin production in human female coronary artery

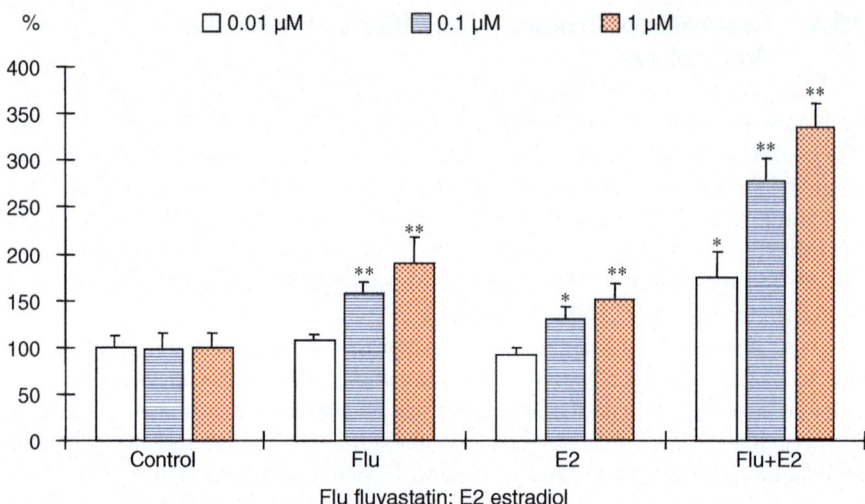

Fig. 13.2 Stimulation of prostacyclin in human vascular endothelial coronary cells comparing statin, E2-only, and the combination. Note: Modified according Mueck AO et al. [35]. Using the combination of statin+E2, resulting in an enlarged positive additive effect, will increase the chance that the possible negative impact of added progestogen will not neglect the beneficial cardioprotective estrogenic action

cells [35] (Fig. 13.2). These enlarged positive effects will increase the chance that antagonizing effects of added progestogen will not neglect the beneficial estrogen action. The combination of estrogen with statin for therapy of postmenopausal women is of interest because both substance classes exert beneficial effects not only on the lipid profile but also on the vasculature, and combined therapy may decrease additively the cardiovascular risk. This has been suggested in HERS [36] and in a large observational study (n = 40.958 statin users) of the Karolinska Institute in Sweden [37].

However, the results in clinical studies are controversial. Negative effects of MPA [38] or NETA [39] regarding the E2-induced increase of nitrate/nitrite levels have been observed in postmenopausal women. But a Finnish study [40] did not see any effect of NETA added to oral or transdermal E2, whereas our own study [41] showed antagonizing effect of oral NETA but not of transdermal NETA (using combi-patches) added to oral or transdermal E2, resp. In another own study comparing E2valerat-only and E2valerat combined with dienogest prospectively, we did not find any significant difference of cGMP (NO) production suggesting a vascular neutral effect of dienogest added to estrogen regarding protective vasodilating mechanisms [42].

We think we can explain some of those controversial data. In terms of beneficial effects, it always has to be considered *that the preconditions are intact vascular cells and results may vary not only due to the type and dosages of the hormones but also due to the different atherosclerotic stages of the vessels.* To investigate the endothelial potency of vasodilatation (perhaps the most important mechanism for cardiovascular protection during HRT), we compared healthy postmenopausal women ($n = 22$) vs. postmenopausal patients with coronary artery disease (CAD) ($n = 26$), diagnosed by coronary arteriography, within two paralyzed, randomized, double-blind, placebo-controlled crossover studies [43]. Application of 4 mg sublingual estradiol (E2) increased the cGMP production in both crossover studies significantly higher compared to placebo during bicycle ergometry, which reflects a standardized vasoconstrictory stress situation like adding vasoconstrictory-acting progestogens. But the most important result was that the absolute amount of increase of NO production was threefold higher in the healthy group. *Thus the results in clinical studies, likewise also regarding other vascular biomarkers, may be strongly dependent from the preconditions of vascular function using estradiol (e.g., regarding vasodilatation) and progestogens (e.g., regarding vasoconstriction).*

13.5 Summary and Practical Recommendations

Although evidence strongly supports some of these markers as predictors of acute events, it remains to be established that modifying circulating levels of these markers will influence outcomes. Therefore, routinely measurement presently cannot be recommended, and it has to be stressed that vasoactive biochemical markers only "surrogate" on clinical effects and never can replace clinical studies.

Despite of these limitations, in the future also vascular markers may become a tool to predict risk and could be most useful to monitor therapy, especially as soon as the measurement will be able to be performed quickly and cost-sparingly like metabolic markers such as lipids. Although also lipids are "only" "surrogate markers," their measurement in most guidelines is recommended as first-line to predict risk. In analogy vascular markers may follow for the recommendation in the clinical routine! Our above described ergometry experiment with assessment of those markers during stress situation could be a standardized test for the endothelial function in risk patients.

References

1. Writing Group for the Women's Health Initiative Investigators. Risks and benefits of estrogen plus progestin in healthy postmenopausal women. JAMA. 2002;288:321–33.
2. Women's Health Initiative Steering Committee. Effects of conjugated equine estrogen in postmenopausal women with hysterectomy. JAMA. 2004;291:1701–12.
3. Schierbeck L. Primary prevention of cardiovascular disease with hormone replacement therapy. Climacteric. 2015;18:1–6.
4. Manson JE, Aragaki AK, Rossouw JE, et al. (WHI Investigators). Menopausal hormone therapy and long-term all-cause and cause-specific mortality: the women's health initiative randomized trials. JAMA. 2017;318:927–38.
5. Harman SM, Black DM, Naftolin F, et al. Arterial imaging outcomes and cardiovascular risk factors in recently menopausal women: a randomized trial. Ann Intern Med. 2014;161:249–60.
6. Hodis HN, Mack WJ, Henderson VW, et al. Vascular effects of early versus late postmenopausal treatment with estradiol. N Engl J Med. 2016;374:1221–31.

7. Lokkegaard E, Andreasen AH, Jacobsen RK, Lars Hougaard Nielsen LH, Carsten Agger C, Lidegaard O. Hormone therapy and risk of myocardial infarction: a national register study. Eur Heart J. 2008;29:2660–8.

8. Venetkoski MM, Savolainen-Peltonen HM, Rahkola-Soisalo PK, Hoti F, Vattulainen P, Gissler MVJ, Ylikorkala O, Mikkola TS. Increased cardiac and stroke death risk in the first year after discontinuation of postmenopausal hormone therapy. Menopause. 2017;25(4):375. https://doi.org/10.1097/GME.0000000000001023.

9. Mendelsohn ME, Karas RH. The protective effects of estrogen on the cardiovascular system. N Engl J Med. 1999;340:1801–11.

10. Cid MC, Schnaper HW, Kleinman HK. Estrogens and the vascular endothelium. Ann N Y Acad Sci. 2002;966:143–57.

11. Mueck AO, Seeger H. Estrogens acting as cardiovascular agents: direct vascular actions. Curr Med Chem Cardiovasc Hematol Agents. 2004;2:35–42.

12. Pang Y, Dong J, Thomas P. Progesterone increases nitric oxide synthesis in human vascular endothelial cells through activation of membrane progesterone receptor-α. Am J Physiol Endocrinol Metab. 2015;308:E899–911.

13. Pang Y, Thomas P. Additive effects of low concentrations of estradiol-17β and progesterone on nitric oxide production by human vascular endothelial cells through shared signaling pathways. J Steroid Biochem Mol Biol. 2017;165:258–67.

14. Yuan XH, Fan YY, Yang CR, Gao XR, Zhang LL, Hu Y, Wang YQ, Jun H. Progesterone amplifies oxidative stress signal and promotes NO production via H2O2 in mouse kidney arterial endothelial cells. J Steroid Biochem Mol Biol. 2016;155:104–11.

15. Thomas P, Pang Y. Protective actions of progesterone in the cardiovascular system: potential role of membrane progesterone receptors (mPRs) in mediating rapid effects. Steroids. 2013;78:583–8.

16. He Y, Gao Q, Han B, Zhu X, Zhu D, Tao J, Chen J, Xu Z. Progesterone suppressed vasoconstriction in human umbilical vein via reducing calcium entry. Steroids. 2016;108:118–25.

17. Miller NR, Dolinsky BM, Napolitano PG. Micronized progesterone reduces vasoconstriction in the placenta. J Matern Fetal Neonatal Med. 2015;28:1581–4.

18. Ramírez-Rosas MB, Cobos-Puc LE, Sánchez-López A, Gutiérrez-Lara EJ, Centurión D. Pharmacological characterization of the mechanisms involved in the vasorelaxation induced by progesterone and 17β-estradiol on isolated canine basilar and internal carotid arteries. Steroids. 2014;89:33–40.

19. Baber RJ, Panay N, Fenton A. (on behalf of the IMS Writing Group). 2016 IMS Recommendations on women's midlife health and menopause hormone therapy. Climacteric. 2016;19:109–50.

20. Anggard E. Nitric oxide: mediator, murderer, and medicine. Lancet. 1994;343:1199–206.

21. Vane JR, Botting RM. Pharmacodynamic profile of prostacyclin. Am J Cardiol. 1995;75:3A–10A.

22. Levin EL. Endothelins. New Engl J Med. 1995;333:356–63.

23. Rifai N, Ridker PM. High-sensitivity C-reactive protein: a novel and promising marker of coronary heart disease. Clin Chem. 2001;47:403–11.

24. Yudkin JS, Kumari M, Humphries SE, Mohamed-Ali V. Inflammation, obesity, stress and coronary heart disease: is interleukin-6 the link? Atherosclerosis. 2000;148:209–14.

25. Chia MC. The role of adhesion molecules in atherosclerosis. Crit Rev Clin Lab Sci. 1998;35:573–602.

26. Reape TJ, Groot TH. Chemokines and atherosclerosis. Atherosclerosis. 1999;147:213–25.

27. Galis ZS, Khatri JJ. Matrix metalloproteinases in vascular remodelling and atherogenesis. Circ Res. 2002;90:251–62.

28. Kohler HP, Grant PJ. Plasminogen-activator inhibitor type 1 and coronary artery disease. N Engl J Med. 2000;342:1792–801.

29. Simoncini T, Caruso A, Girett MS, Scorticati C, Fu X-D, Garibaldi S, Baldacci C, Mannella P, Fornari L, Genazzani A. Effects of dydrogesterone and of its stable metabolite

20-alpha-dihydrodydrogesterone, on nitric oxide synthesis in human endothelial cells. Fertil Steril. 2006;86(Suppl 3):1235–42.

30. Mueck AO, Seeger H, Wallwiener D. Medroxyprogesterone acetate versus norethisterone: effect on estradiol-induced changes of markers for endothelial function and atherosclerotic plaque characteristics in human female coronary endothelial cell cultures. Menopause. 2002;9:273–81.

31. Cushman M, Legault C, Barrett-Connor E, Stefanick ML, Kessler C, Judd HL, Sakkinen PA, Tracy RP. Effect of postmenopausal hormones on inflammation-sensitive proteins: the Postmenopausal Estrogen/Progestin Interventions (PEPI) Study. Circulation. 1999;100:717–22.

32. Freudenberger T, Deenen R, Kretschmer I, Zimmermann A, Seiler LF, Mayer P, Heim HK, Köhrer K, Fischer JW. Synthetic gestagens exert differential effects on arterial thrombosis and aortic gene expression in ovariectomized apolipoprotein E-deficient mice. Br J Pharmacol. 2014;171:5032–48.

33. Ito F, Mori T, Takaoka O, Tanaka Y, Koshiba A, Tatsumi H, Iwasa K, Kitawaki J. Effects of drospirenone on adhesion molecule expression and monocyte adherence in human endothelial cells. Eur J Obstet Gynecol Reprod Biol. 2016;201:113–7.

34. Seeger H, Kloosterboer HJ, Studen M, Wallwiener D, Mueck AO. In vitro effects of tibolone and its metabolites on human vascular coronary cells. Maturitas. 2007;58:42–9.

35. Mueck AO, Seeger H, Deuringer FU, Wallwiener D. Effect of estrogen/statin combination on biochemical markers of endothelial function in human coronary cell cultures. Menopause. 2001;8:216–21.

36. HERS Study Group. Statin therapy, cardiovascular events, and total mortality in the Heart and Estrogen/progestin Replacement Study. Circulation. 2002;105:2962–7.

37. Berglind IA, Andersen M, Citarella A, Linder M, Sundstrom A, Kieler H. Hormone therapy and risk of cardiovascular outcomes and mortality in women treated with statins. Menopause. 2014;22:369–76.

38. Imthurn B, Rosselli M, Jaeger AW, Keller PJ, Dubey RK. Differential effects of hormone-replacement therapy on endogenous nitric oxide (nitrite/nitrate) levels in postmenopausal women substituted with 17 beta-estradiol valerate and cyproterone acetate or medroxyprogesterone acetate. J Clin Endocrinol Metab. 1997;82:388–94.

39. Rosselli M, Imthurn B, Keller PJ, Jackson EK, Dubey RK. Circulating nitric oxide (nitrite/nitrate) levels in postmenopausal women substituted with 17beta-estradiol and norethisterone acetate. A two-year follow-up study. Hypertension. 1995;25:848–53.

40. Ylikorkala O, Cacciatore B, Paakkari I, Tikkanen MJ, Viinika L, Toivonen J. The long-term effects of oral and transdermal postmenopausal hormone replacement therapy on nitric oxide, endothelin-1, prostacyclin, and thromboxane. Fertil Steril. 1998;69:883–8.

41. Seeger H, Mueck AO, Teichmann AT, Lippert TH. Effect of sequential estrogen/progestin treatment on biochemical markers in postmenopausal women comparing oral and transdermal application. Clin Exp Obstet Gynecol. 2000;27:17–20.

42. Mueck AO, Seeger H, Lüdtke R, Gräser T, Wallwiener D. Effect on biochemical vasoactive markers during postmenopausal HRT: estradiol vs. estradiol/dienogest. Maturitas. 2001;38:305–13.

43. Mueck AO, Ruan X, Seeger H, Hanke H. Vasodilative potency induced with Estradiol in women with and without CAD during standardized stress:- two paralyzed, randomized, double-blind, placebo-controlled cross-over studies. 18th World Congress of Gynecological Endocrinology, Florence (Italy), March 7th-10th 2018, Abstract ID 6616.

Sex Differences, Progesterone, and Ischemic Stroke

14

Michael Schumacher and Rachida Guennoun

14.1 Introduction

The incidence, prevalence, and outcomes of ischemic stroke differ between women and men, whereas hemorrhagic stroke seems not to vary according to sex [1, 2]. Women have a higher lifetime risk of ischemic stroke, and male patients are on average younger than female patients when they get their first stroke [3, 4]. Women are indeed considered as being protected during their fertile years by their ovarian hormones [5–7]. However, women have in general worse stroke outcomes than men, and they may also respond differently to stroke therapies [5, 8]. It is interesting to note that the incidence of ischemic stroke has decreased between the years 1993 and 2010 but that this trend seems to be primarily driven by a decrease in ischemic stroke in men [2].

When discussing sex differences in ischemic stroke, the focus is largely on the estrogens. For example, in the case of menopausal hormone treatment (HT), synthetic progestins or progesterone are only considered for protecting the uterus against estrogen-induced hyperplasia, but their potential additional health benefits and protective effects on the brain are only rarely taken into consideration. There is however an extensive preclinical literature documenting the neuroprotective efficacy of progesterone [9–11].

Considering sex differences in stroke only in the context of ovarian hormones seems far too limited. As discussed in this review, different sources of steroid hormones, including adrenal steroids and neurosteroids synthesized within the brain, are likely to influence the incidence and outcome of ischemic stroke. Recently, we uncovered the importance of endogenous brain progesterone in the resistance of the

M. Schumacher (✉) · R. Guennoun
U1195 Inserm, University Paris-Sud, University Paris-Saclay, Kremlin-Bicêtre, France
e-mail: michael.schumacher@inserm.fr; rachida.guennoun@inserm.fr

© International Society of Gynecological Endocrinology 2019
R. D. Brinton et al. (eds.), *Sex Steroids' Effects on Brain, Heart and Vessels*,
ISGE Series, https://doi.org/10.1007/978-3-030-11355-1_14

brain to ischemic injury. We also showed that progesterone, a major female reproductive hormone, is an important cerebroprotective neurosteroid in males [12]. A
consequence of the local synthesis of progesterone by neural cells is that its circulating levels not necessarily reflect its brain levels. In fact, very little is known concerning changes in neurosteroids [13].

As shown by results of the "Framingham Heart Study," stroke risk raises with
age, but it is important to note that the increase is gradual until the age of 50 in both
women and men. It is only around age 75 that the incidence of stroke becomes comparable between both sexes, that is, long after the beginning of menopause. Stroke
risk only becomes higher in women than in men by the age of 80 [14]. It is important to remind here that testicular androgens also have an impact on cardiovascular
events in men, although their precise role remains controversial.

In addition to hormonal aging, other factors appear to be involved in the age-
dependent increase in stroke. In menopausal women, ischemic stroke risk has been
linked to abdominal adiposity, elevated levels of triglycerides and cholesterol,
enhanced insulin resistance, and increased blood pressure [15]. Besides stroke, obesity is related to several other disorders including diabetes, sleep disorders, hypertension, and atherosclerosis [16–18]. These comorbidities present a challenge for
the rehabilitation of stroke patients [19]. Interestingly, the deposition and distribution of adipose tissues differ between men and women [20]. When compared with
women, men show more visceral adipose deposits, which are associated with cardiovascular risk. In contrast, women before menopause have more subcutaneous
adipose deposits, a feature associated with lower cardiovascular risk. However, after
menopause, the decrease in estrogens leads to a shift in favor of the visceral fat,
comparable to that seen in men, and in a concomitant increase in cardiovascular
risks [21]. It is of note that the way for metabolic dysfunctions, cardiovascular problems, and generalized inflammation is paved by decreased ovarian functions [22].
Another risk factor is the elevated blood pressure in women after menopause.
Whereas blood pressure is in general lower in premenopausal women than in men,
the prevalence of hypertension increases in women after menopause [23]. In addition to these systemic health factors, age-dependent changes in brain structure and
function add to the increased vulnerability to ischemic stroke. Alterations include
degenerative processes, structural changes in white matter, small-vessel diseases,
reduced brain weight, and the intraneuronal accumulation of proteins such as tau
and α-synuclein [24].

14.2 Ischemic Stroke Incidence and Cardiovascular Events in Women and the Role of Steroids

A systemic review of observational studies examining the risk of ischemic
stroke in women with premature menopause or bilateral oophorectomy concluded that the lack of endogenous ovarian hormones is associated with an
increased risk of ischemic stroke. Importantly, age at menopause appeared to be
a more important risk factor than its cause, either early ovarian insufficiency or

surgical intervention [25]. In the "MAYO Clinic Cohort Study of Oophorectomy and Aging," the increased risk of stroke after bilateral oophorectomy before the age of 45 years could be reduced by estrogen therapy, pointing to a role of estrogen deprivation [26].

These observations are consistent with a protective role of estrogens in stroke, at least in women younger than age 50 years. Conversely, for postmenopausal women, the Women's Health Initiative (WHI) clinical trials reported deleterious effects on ischemic stroke for HT with estrogen alone or in combination with a progestin [27, 28]. More than 26,000 postmenopausal women were enrolled in this prospective and randomized trial, which comprised two arms: women receiving oral conjugated equine estrogens (CEE, 0.625 mg/day) together with the synthetic progestin medroxyprogesterone acetate (MPA, 2.5 mg/day) to protect the uterus against hyperplasia and women with prior hysterectomy receiving CEE alone. It is interesting to note that one of the inclusion criteria for the WHI was the absence of climacteric symptoms.

A subgroup of about 8300 women aged 65 or older from the two arms of the WHI were included in the Women's Health Initiative Memory Study (WHIMS) over a 2-year period to evaluate the effects of CEE + MPA or CEE alone on the incidence of mild cognitive impairment (MCI) or dementia. Neither HT prevented age-related cognitive decline when compared with placebo, but instead slightly increased the risk for both endpoints [29–31]. Of the WHIMS participants, about 1400 were examined by MRI for subclinical cerebrovascular disease as a possible cause of cognitive decline. Total ischemic lesion volume was a primary outcome. Hormone therapy was not associated with a significant increase in ischemic brain lesion volume relative to placebo [32]. However, brain MRI scans revealed slightly greater brain atrophy in women receiving CEE with or without MPA [33].

Questions raised by this large trial, its limitations, and the resulting confusion have been extensively discussed [34, 35]. One major concern was the late initiation of the HT, for the majority of women one to two decades after the onset of their menopause. Stratification of the WHI results by years since menopause indeed showed that starting HT earlier than 10 years from the last menstrual period was associated with less risk of coronary heart disease. Consistently, preclinical studies in nonhuman primates had provided evidence that estrogen treatment was effective in slowing the progression of coronary artery atherosclerosis only when administered soon after surgical menopause. These observations led to the emergence of the "timing hypothesis," suggesting that HT initiated during early menopause may slow the progression of atherosclerosis but that the cardiovascular benefits of HT may be lost several years later [36]. In contrast, the slight increase in stroke risk by HT appeared to be independent of years since menopause: the stroke hazard ratio was 1.23 for women receiving HT within less than 10 years since menopause and younger than 60 years, corresponding to 8 more strokes per 10,000 person years [37].

Other serious issues with the WHI trials were the elevated dose of orally administered conjugated equine estrogens (CEE, 0.625 mg/day) and the associated synthetic progestin, medroxyprogesterone acetate (MPA, 2.5 mg/day), known for its deleterious effects on the vascular and nervous systems. In addition to its binding to the progesterone receptors (PR), MPA has agonistic activity on both androgen and glucocorticoid receptors and inhibits the beneficial actions of estradiol [13, 38–42]. Thus, MPA has properties very distinct from natural progesterone.

Both the type of hormones used and their modes of administration are important to be considered. Thus, different types of progestins show different risks of venous thromboembolism (VTE), whereas natural micronized progesterone and pregnane derivatives appear safe [43]. A similar situation has been reported for ischemic stroke. In a case-control study, the use of natural progesterone, in contrast to a series of progestins, was not associated with increased stroke risk in postmenopausal women [44]. Another multicenter case-control study has documented the importance of the mode of administration of estrogens for the risk of VTE in postmenopausal women. Thus, transdermal estrogen was found to be safer with respect to thrombotic risk than oral estrogen [45]. As an explanation, orally administered steroids enter the enterohepatic circulation, and during their first-pass through the liver, they stimulate the production of inflammatory and procoagulant proteins, associated with increased risk of venous and arterial thrombosis [46, 47].

Observations related to the timing, formulation, dose, and route of delivery of HT provided the context for the recent "Kronos Early Estrogen Prevention Study" (KEEPS) and the "Early Versus Late Intervention Trial" (ELITE) [48]. The KEEPS trial tested the hypothesis that initiation of HT within 3 years of menopause would reduce the progression of atherosclerosis as determined by changes in carotid intima-media thickness (CIMT) and coronary artery calcification. For this trial, a lower dose of oral CEE was used than in the WHI trial (0.45 mg/day versus 0.625 mg/day), and instead of MPA, micronized natural progesterone was used to protect the uterus against hyperplasia (200 mg/day per os, 12 days per month). An additional group of women received transdermal natural estradiol instead of CEE (50 μg/day) together with progesterone. Importantly, in contrast to the WHI, the 727 women enrolled in the KEEP trial had low cardiovascular risk profiles. After 4 years of treatment, no adverse cardiovascular events were observed: progression of CIMT did not differ among the treated and placebo groups, and coronary arterial calcification tended to be reduced in the hormone-treated groups. Moreover, the HT had no longer-term effects on vascular function [49, 50]. It should be noted that after oral CEE and transdermal estradiol, serum levels of estradiol and estrone remained in the low picomolar range, and the doses may not have been sufficient for efficient vasoprotection [48]. However, climacteric symptoms, in particular hot flashes, night sweats, and sleep problems, were improved by both oral CEE and transdermal estradiol combined with natural progesterone [51, 52].

The ELITE trial was specifically designed to test the "timing hypothesis." It was a randomized, double-blind, placebo-controlled trial enrolling women who were 6 or 10 years past menopause. Oral estradiol (1 mg/day) with intermittent vaginal progesterone was administered for 5 years. Again, main outcomes were changes in CIMT and coronary arterial calcification. The mean age of women enrolled in the early group was 55 years and in the late group 65 years [53]. The rate of progression of CIMT was significantly lower in women in the early group who were treated during 5 years with estradiol compared with placebo. However, the increase in CIMT did not differ in the late group between women treated with estradiol or placebo. Coronary arterial calcification was similar among groups and was not affected by HT [54].

14.3   Ischemic Stroke Incidence in Men

In men, like in women, stroke rates markedly increase from the age of 50 onward [14]. However, in contrasts to the ovaries, there is no abrupt decline in testicular activity, but levels of testosterone instead gradually decrease in men from about 40 years onward [55, 56]. It is however important to be aware that the age-dependent decline in circulating testosterone shows very large interindividual differences. Already by the age of 60, the incidence of hypogonadal testosterone in men is around 20% [56].

The influence of testosterone on the incidence of stroke remains controversial. Because young men have a higher incidence of stroke than women, elevated levels of testosterone have been suspected to represent a risk factor. However, there is little evidence for this assumption, and the established link between anabolic steroid abuse and cardiovascular pathologies does not provide information on the role of endogenous natural testosterone [57]. Conversely, the age-dependent increase in the incidence and severity of stroke in men indicates protective effects of androgens. Nevertheless, in spite of reported benefits of the therapeutic normalization of low testosterone levels [58], concerns have been raised about the cardiovascular safety of testosterone therapy in aging men [59].

14.4   Differences Between Women and Men in Stroke Outcomes

The previous sections dealt with stroke prevalence and incidence. What about ischemic stroke outcomes, which reflect vulnerability to infarction, capacity of recovery, and responses to therapeutic intervention? In fact, it is well-known that sex and gonadal hormones have a considerable impact on stroke outcomes [60]. In general, women are doing worse than men. Moreover, women and men respond differently to stroke therapeutics [5, 8].

Thrombolytic treatment with tissue plasminogen activator (tPA) has been shown to have greater efficacy in women, but this difference only resulted from the fact that placebo-treated women fared worse than men and that sex differences were no longer observed after tPA treatment [61, 62]. Likewise, in another trial testing pro-urokinase as a thrombolytic agent, women showed a larger treatment effect, annulling the worse outcome for untreated women when compared with men [63]. In addition to lysis of the thrombus, endovascular thrombectomy has become a standard of care for large vessel ischemic stroke since 2015 [64]. A recent meta-analysis revealed that thrombectomy with a retriever stent benefits patients with acute ischemic stroke irrespective of their sex [64].

A small clinical trial showed that oral administration of the antibiotic minocycline was efficient in male but not in female stroke patients [65]. Remarkably, in a previous preclinical study using a mouse model of middle cerebral artery occlusion (MCAO), minocycline reduced infarct volume in males, but was ineffective in females [66]. Another preclinical example of sex-dependent responses to protective treatments was the observation that an antagomir to the microRNA Let7f, which targets IGF-1 signaling, was effective in intact female rats but not in males or ovariectomized females after ischemic stroke. This finding suggests that ovarian hormones affect miRNA actions [67]. These examples highlight the importance of considering sex differences in translational stroke research [68]. Particularly intriguing are sex differences in glial and neuroinflammatory responses after experimental ischemic stroke [69, 70]. It is conceivable that the omission of sex as an experimental or clinical variable may have contributed to the failure of translating stroke therapies into clinical practice [71].

14.5 Progesterone Is Cerebroprotective After Ischemic Stroke in Experimental Animal Models

Twenty-five years ago, Donald Stein showed that progesterone protects the brain of both female and male rats against traumatic injury [72, 73]. Particularly promising was the finding that the administration of progesterone reduced edema and brain damage in rats when its administration was delayed until 24 h after injury [74]. Later, it has been speculated that elevated levels of endogenous brain progesterone may contribute to the early resistance of the brain to traumatic damage and to the extended window of opportunity [75].

Cerebroprotective effects of progesterone were also demonstrated after occlusion of the middle cerebral artery (MCAO) in male rats and mice, an experimental model of ischemic cerebral stroke [76–78]. In this model, blood flow through the medial cerebral artery is interrupted by an occluding filament, either transiently followed by reperfusion or permanently. The translational significance of transient MCAO has been discussed because of abrupt reperfusion after removal of the obstructing filament, which contrasts with the more gradual reperfusion after thrombolytic treatment of ischemic stroke patients. However, since the recent advent of endovascular thrombectomy as a therapeutic intervention of choice, transient MCAO may be considered as a model of choice for testing the preclinical neuroprotective efficacy of molecules [79, 80].

Although rapid recanalization by removing the clot from the obstructed brain vessel is critical for clinical outcomes, complementary cerebroprotective strategies remain an important unmet medical need. Indeed, increasing the resistance of neural cells to oxygen and glucose deprivation and reducing neuroinflammatory responses may allow to prolong the narrow therapeutic window of just a few hours for restoring the blood flow [81, 82]. Protective therapies are also needed to reduce brain damage and vasogenic edema caused by reperfusion. In particular the endovascular methods expose patients to ischemic reperfusion injury [83, 84]. It is interesting to note here that so far no pharmacological agent has yet reached the clinics for improving the viability of neurons and glial cells, whatever the neurological condition.

A meta-analysis of experimental stroke studies, limited to rats and mice, has assessed the outcomes of progesterone treatments according to sex, age, and species [85]. This extensive review revealed that administration of exogenous progesterone significantly reduced infarct volume in male rats and mice. Most studies (11/19) involved young male animals, and none of them have used gonadally intact young females. Interestingly, data suggested that progesterone may lack efficacy in ovariectomized females. This indicates that additional ovarian factors may influence stroke outcomes in response to progesterone [85]. The results of one study suggested that progesterone may exert different protective effects whether it is administered to young ovariectomized female mice or to aged females with intact ovaries [86].

The studies conducted in male rats have provided important informations. Treatment with progesterone improved neurological outcomes and inflammatory responses following cerebral ischemia not only in young but also in middle-aged and very old (24 months) animals [87–91]. Time-window studies showed that progesterone still exhibits substantial cerebroprotection when administered as late as 6 h after MCAO, but not after 24 h [89, 92]. As for TBI, it has been proposed that endogenous brain progesterone may contribute to the wide therapeutic window [78].

14.6   Progesterone Is an Endogenous Hormone and Neurosteroid in Both Females and Males

The ovaries are the main source of circulating progesterone. In women, levels of progesterone are low during the follicular phase of the menstrual cycle (about 1–3 nM) and are markedly increased during the luteal phase (about 20–40 nM) [93, 94]. In female mice and rats, the reproductive cycle of 4–5 days is named the "estrus cycle" and is subdivided into proestrus, estrus, diestrus-1, and diestrus-2 (the latter two are also named metestrus and diestrus, respectively) [95]. Reference values for changes in steroid levels during the mouse and rat estrus cycle were recently obtained by sensitive and specific gas chromatography–tandem mass spectrometry (GC–MS/MS) method [96]. Highest levels of progesterone, produced by the placenta, are reached during pregnancy [97]. In both humans and rodents, progesterone levels reach 200–400 nM by the end of gestation [98–100].

Not only the ovaries and placenta but also the adrenal cortex produces significant amounts of circulating progesterone in humans and rodents. Like corticosterone in rodents and cortisol in humans, both synthesis and secretion of progesterone by the adrenal glands are stimulated by adrenocorticotropic hormone (ACTH) and thus respond to stress [101]. In men, circulating levels of progesterone are in the low nanomolar range, but they may play an important role in health. Regrettably, the role of progesterone in men has so far not attracted much attention, and for this reason, it has been qualified as the "forgotten hormone in men" [102]. Importantly, progesterone secretion by the adrenal glands is markedly increased in men in response to a variety of stressors [103, 104]. After TBI, circulating progesterone even transiently reached concentrations comparable to luteal levels in women, but returned to low basal nanomolar levels several hours later [105].

In addition to the steroidogenic endocrine glands, progesterone is also by neurons and glial cells in the nervous system. To refer to their site of synthesis, steroids synthesized in the brain have been named "neurosteroids" [106, 107]. In addition to their de novo synthesis from cholesterol, progesterone and its metabolites can be synthesized within the nervous system from circulating precursors: progesterone can be formed from circulating pregnenolone, 5α-dihydroprogesterone (5α-DHP) can be derived from circulating progesterone, and allopregnanolone can be derived from circulating progesterone or 5α-DHP [108].

It is important to realize that variations in progesterone levels within the brain may reflect changes either in local synthesis or in circulating levels. Steroid hormones produced by the gonads and adrenal glands indeed easily cross the blood–brain barrier by transmembrane diffusion [109, 110]. They also rapidly diffuse throughout the nervous tissues because of their low molecular weight and lipid solubility. So far, no conditional knockouts of neurosteroid biosynthetic pathways have been generated, and compelling evidence for the synthesis of progesterone and its metabolites within the nervous system mainly comes from the following findings: (1) expression and activity of enzymes involved in their biosynthesis; (2) the presence of progesterone and its metabolites in nervous tissues after removal of the peripheral steroidogenic glands; (3) changes in neurosteroid levels independent of changes in circulating hormone levels; and (4) the uncovering of endogenous neurosteroid tones affecting neuronal excitability [10, 106, 108, 111–113].

14.7   Brain Metabolism of Progesterone and Cerebroprotective Effects of Allopregnanolone

Progesterone is converted in the brain to 5α-dihydroprogesterone (5α-DHP) by two steroid 5α-reductase isoenzymes. These enzymes have multiple steroid substrates characterized by a 3-keto group and a Δ4,5 double bond, including progesterone, deoxycorticosterone, and testosterone. The type I isoenzyme is the major form in the brain [114]. It is widely expressed in the rat brain at all stages of development, whereas the type II enzyme shows a more restricted distribution [115, 116]. Both neurons and glial cells convert progesterone to its 5α-reduced metabolites [117].

Progesterone and 5α-DHP are ligands of the intracellular progesterone receptors (PR) and regulators of gene transcription in neural cells [118] (Fig. 14.1). Specific functions of 5α-DHP in the brain seem likely as its endogenous levels are elevated and selectively and strongly upregulated in response to trauma and ischemic injury

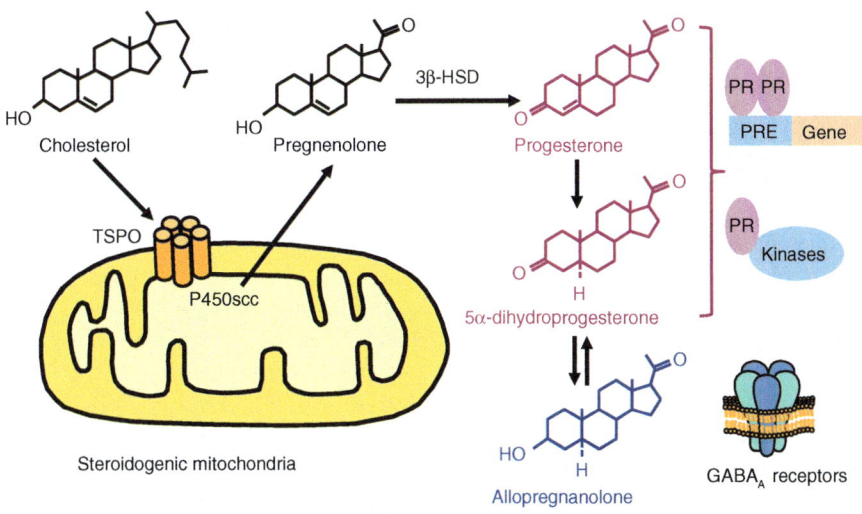

Fig. 14.1 Synthesis and metabolism of progesterone. The translocase (TSPO), the former peripheral benzodiazepine receptor, is involved in the transport of cholesterol from the cytoplasm to the inner mitochondrial membrane. At the level of the inner mitochondrial membrane, cholesterol is converted to pregnenolone by cytochrome P450scc, which cuts its carbon side chain. Pregnenolone is then metabolized to progesterone by the 3β-hydroxysteroid dehydrogenases (3β-HSD). Progesterone is irreversibly converted to 5α-dihydroprogesterone (5α-DHP) by the 5α-reductases. In neural cells, both progesterone and 5α-DHP bind to the intracellular progesterone receptors (PR), which regulate gene expression after binding to progesterone response element (PRE). The PR can also directly interact with membrane-associated kinases in the extranuclear compartment. 5α-DHP is metabolized by a 3α-hydroxysteroid dehydrogenase (3α-HSD) to allopregnanolone, a potent positive modulator of GABA$_A$ receptors

[12, 78]. Older studies suggested specific regulatory functions of 5α-DHP for neuroendocrine mechanisms [119, 120].

The metabolite 5α-DHP is further converted in the brain to allopregnanolone by NADPH-dependent cytosolic aldo–keto reductases (AKR) (Fig. 14.1). In rats, 5α-DHP is converted to allopregnanolone by a single AKR isoform, named the 3α-hydroxysteroid dehydrogenase (3α-HSD), whereas in humans and mice, there are multiple and less selective AKR isoforms [121]. Whereas the 5α-reduction of progesterone is an irreversible reaction, allopregnanolone can be converted back to 5α-DHP by NAD$^+$-dependent membrane-associated short-chain dehydrogenases/reductases, acting in vivo as 3α-hydroxysteroid oxidases [122, 123]. This is important, as the conversion back to 5α-DHP is a mechanism by which allopregnanolone could activate PR-dependent gene transcription [118].

In the brain, the 3α-HSD has been proposed to be restricted to glial cells [124]. However, a study of the distribution of 5α-reductase type I and 3α-HSD mRNA expression in the mouse brain has shown that both enzymes colocalize in principal glutamatergic neurons of the cerebral cortex, hippocampus, and olfactory bulbs and in glutamatergic output neurons of the thalamus and amygdala. Both enzymes are also present in GABAergic output neurons of the striatum and thalamus as well as in cerebellar Purkinje neurons, consistent with an autocrine/paracrine modulation of GABA$_A$ receptor signaling by locally produced allopregnanolone. Surprisingly, in this study, none of the enzymes were detected in astrocytes, previously considered to be a major source of 5α-reduced progesterone metabolites [125]. Another immunohistological study reported the presence of the two 5α-reductase isoenzymes and the 3α-HSD in neurons, astrocytes, and oligodendrocytes of the male rat spinal cord [126]. It is important to stress that there exists no specific 3α-HSD inhibitor, the frequently used indomethacin, or MPA being nonspecific. The only way to inhibit the formation of allopregnanolone is to inhibit the upstream 5α-reductase with drugs such as finasteride. It is thus not easy to distinguish between the effects of 5α-DHP and allopregnanolone, both metabolites being moreover interconvertible.

Whereas progesterone and 5α-DHP are ligands of PR in neural cells, allopregnanolone does not bind to the receptors but is instead a positive modulator of GABA$_A$ receptors [127] (Fig. 14.1). In the brain, the majority of fast inhibitory neurotransmission is mediated by GABA$_A$ receptors, which harbor a surprisingly large number of allosteric drug-binding sites for small molecules, including benzodiazepines, barbiturates, anesthetics, and steroids [128]. In 1986, it was shown that allopregnanolone (3α,5α-tetrahydroprogesterone) is part of the positive modulators of GABA$_A$ receptors [129]. This discovery provided a mechanistic explanation for some of the rapid effects of progesterone, in particular its anxiolytic, antidepressant, aesthetic, anticonvulsant, and analgesic effects. However, the interaction of allopregnanolone with GABA$_A$ receptors remained enigmatic until 2006, when finally two steroid-binding sites, located within the transmembrane domains of the α- and β-receptor subunits and distinct from the benzodiazepine binding site, were identified [130, 131].

Over the past years, much progress has been achieved in understanding how the potentiation of GABA$_A$ receptors by allopregnanolone affects neuronal excitability. Thus, allopregnanolone modulates both synaptic and extrasynaptic GABA$_A$ receptors, and variations in brain levels of allopregnanolone result in important changes in neuronal activity [132]. While synaptic GABA$_A$ receptors mediate rapid phasic inhibition of postsynaptic currents, the extrasynaptic receptors mediate a particular type of persistent inhibition of neuronal excitability, termed "tonic inhibition" [133, 134]. The extrasynaptic GABA$_A$ receptors differ from their synaptic counterparts by their subunit composition and pharmacological and functional properties [132]. For example, extrasynaptic GABA$_A$ receptors containing the δ subunit are insensitive to a variety of benzodiazepines, but are sensitive targets for allopregnanolone. Accordingly, δ subunit knockout mice show reduced sensitivity to neuroactive steroids [135, 136].

It has been proposed that allopregnanolone may mediate the cerebroprotective effects of progesterone after MCAO. This assertion was supported by the finding that administration of allopregnanolone was more potent than progesterone in attenuating cerebral damage after MCAO at single dose tested [137]. Both progesterone and allopregnanolone were also efficient in attenuating dysfunctions of the blood–brain barrier and in reducing neuroinflammatory responses [138]. The conversion to allopregnanolone has thus been considered as a key step in the cerebroprotective actions of progesterone. However, potential mechanisms relaying the protective effects of allopregnanolone remain elusive. Decreased neuronal excitability by allopregnanolone-activated $GABA_A$ receptors could be involved. In support of the hypothesis are the observations that benzodiazepines are neuroprotective after ischemic injury in rodents and that extracellular levels of GABA are increased in response to cerebral ischemia [139–141].

14.8   Multiple Target Proteins of Progesterone and Their Potential Role in Cerebroprotection

In addition to its effects mediated via allopregnanolone, progesterone itself acts at multiple targets in the brain. The best characterized are the intracellular progesterone receptors (PR). There exist two isoforms, named PR-A and PR-B, which are transcribed from two distinct promoters of a single gene [142, 143]. In the rat and mouse brain, both isoforms are widely expressed, but surprisingly, their specific functions have never been studied. This could however be done, as PR isoform-specific knockout mice are available since many years [144]. As already mentioned, both progesterone and 5α-DHP activate gene transcription in neuronal cells via PR [118]. Importantly, PR are expressed in the brain of both sexes [145, 146].

PR are well-known as hormone-dependent nuclear transcription factors. However, they can also interact with membrane-associated kinases and directly activate extranuclear signaling pathways [147] (Fig. 14.1). The regulation of signaling kinases by PR may play a particularly important role in the brain. In fact, outside the hypothalamus, neuronal PR are mainly located in axons and dendrites and at the level of synapses, thus far away from the nucleus [148]. Membrane translocation of PR, as for the other steroid receptors, involves palmitoylation of a highly conserved amino acid domain within the ligand-binding domain [149].

In addition to the intracellular PR, progesterone binds to many other target proteins within the cytoplasm and at the level of the cellular membrane. These include progesterone receptor membrane component 1 (PGRMC1) and the seven transmembrane domain receptors (mPRs) coupled to G proteins [150–152]. PGRMC1 has been shown to play an important role in the protective effects of progesterone in the brain, in particular via the stimulation brain-derived neurotrophic factor (BDNF) release [153]. More recently, it has been shown that the miRNA let-7i negatively regulates expression of PGRMC1 and BDNF and that treatment with a let-7i antagomir increases the cerebroprotective efficacy of progesterone after MCAO in ovariectomized female mice [154]. These results suggest a role of PGRMC1 in progesterone stroke protection.

Attention should also be paid to the mPRs, which comprise five isoforms encoded by distinct genes [155]. This is because of their wide distribution in the central nervous system and the neural cell-specific regulation of their expression. For example, in the normal mouse or rat brain, mPRα is mainly located in neurons. However, in response to traumatic brain injury, its expression is induced in oligodendrocytes, astrocytes, and reactive microglia, suggesting a role in neural responses to injury [156]. Importantly, mPRs only show low affinity for selective and potent progestin ligands of the classical intracellular PR [155, 157].

14.9   A Key Role of the Intracellular Progesterone Receptors in Cerebroprotection

Progesterone thus acts in the brain via multiple signaling mechanisms. According to the general consensus, allopregnanolone plays a key role in the cerebroprotective effects of progesterone. However, studies using male knockout mice have recently placed the intracellular PR in front of the stage. In homozygous total PR knockout mice (PR$^{-/-}$ mice), the vulnerability of the brain to ischemic damage was indeed markedly increased. Importantly, invalidation of a single allele of the PR gene (PR$^{+/-}$ mice) was sufficient to significantly increase the infarct volume [78]. This observation suggested that PR expression levels may even be a limiting factor for the cerebroprotective efficacy of progesterone. The greater resistance of wild-type mice to ischemic lesions in comparison to PR knockout mice was observed up to 24 h after MCAO and most likely involved endogenous brain progesterone signaling via PR. Prolonged cerebroprotection required the administration of exogenous progesterone. The effective dose (8 mg/kg) resulted in plasma levels reaching those of pregnancy. Again, progesterone therapy failed to be protective in PR knockout mice, consistent with a central role of the receptors [78].

Two important questions needed to be addressed after these experiments: (1) Does endogenous brain progesterone play a role in the resistance to damage shortly after the ischemic insult? In both sexes, neural cells of the adult brain are indeed exposed to significant levels of progesterone, either derived from the ovaries in females or in both females and males from the adrenal glands and from local synthesis (the neurosteroid concept). (2) Do brain PR play a key role in the cerebroprotective effects of progesterone? To answer these questions, we selectively invalidated PR in the brain of male and female mice using Cre–loxP recombination (PR^{NesCre} mice). Brain and plasma steroid levels were analyzed at different times after MCAO using sensitive and selective gas chromatography–tandem mass spectrometry (GC–MS/MS) [12].

In the male brain, levels of PR-active progesterone and 5α-DHP were rapidly and transiently upregulated between 1 and 24 h after MCAO, together reaching late pregnancy-like levels of about 200 nM (Fig. 14.2). 5α-DHP showed the greatest upregulation but only in the brain, not in plasma. This observation strongly suggested an increase in the local synthesis of 5α-DHP by neural cells in response to ischemia. Elevation of progesterone and 5α-DHP contributed to the resistance of neural cells to ischemic damage as the brain-specific invalidation of PR resulted in increased infarct volume and functional deficits already at 6 h after MCAO [12] (Fig. 14.3).

Unexpectedly, in contrast to males, progesterone and 5α-DHP were not significantly upregulated after MCAO in the female brain. However, invalidation of brain PR also resulted in increased brain infarct size in females, although to a lesser extent than in males, demonstrating a role of brain PR in the resistance to ischemic damage for both sexes. Somehow, the low brain levels of progesterone and 5α-DHP in

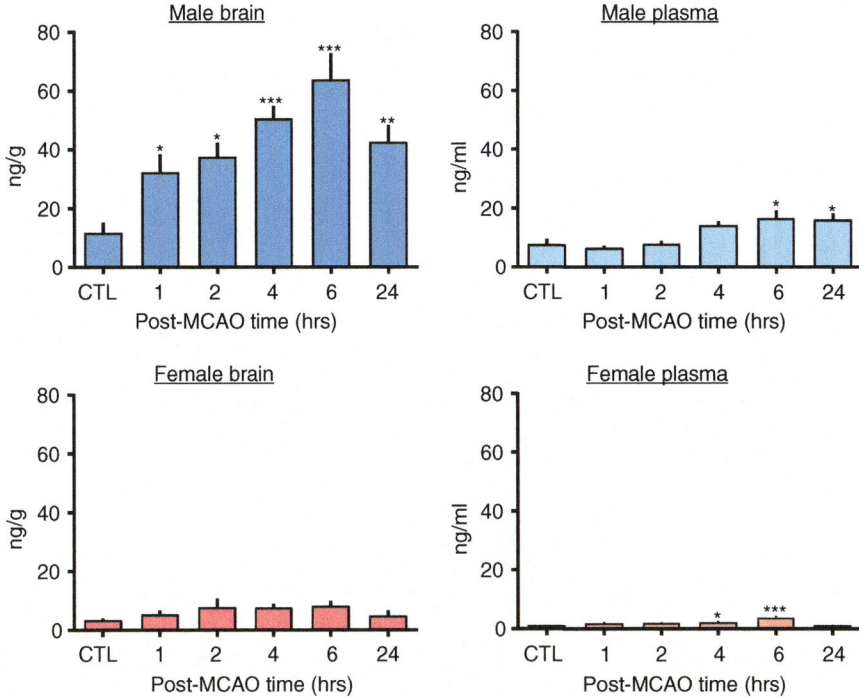

Fig. 14.2 Summed levels of progesterone and 5α-DHP, both agonist ligands of intracellular progesterone receptors (PR) in neural cells, at different times after transient middle cerebral artery occlusion (MCAO). Steroid levels were analyzed by gas chromatography–tandem mass spectrometry (GC–MS/MS) in the ischemic hemisphere and in plasma of young adult male and female mice ($***p \leq 0.001$, $**p \leq 0.01$, $*p \leq 0.05$ when compared to controls, CTL). Data from [12]

females were sufficient for providing protection, pointing to additional cerebroprotective mechanisms in females. An auxiliary endogenous cerebroprotective agent may be estradiol, despite the fact that similar low brain levels of the hormone were measured in both sexes and that they were not increased in response to MCAO. Females may indeed be more sensitive to the cerebroprotective effects of estradiol than males because estrogen receptor α (ERα) is rapidly upregulated in the ischemic brain of females but not males [158, 159]. In addition, estrogens may potentiate the cerebroprotective effects of progesterone in females.

As reviewed above, age is the most important risk factor for stroke and also a prognostic marker for poor outcomes [160]. Concordantly, preclinical studies report worse stroke outcomes in aged animals [161]. Our study confirmed that infarct volumes are larger and neurological deficits more severe in aging (12–14 months old) than in young (3 months old) mice. Notably, the brain-specific invalidation of PR also increased infarct size and aggravated neurological impairment in aging males and females [12] (Fig. 14.3). Thus, endogenous PR-dependent cerebroprotective mechanisms remain operational during aging. Previous studies had already shown that treatment with exogenous progesterone remains protective in aging rodents of both sexes [86, 87, 91].

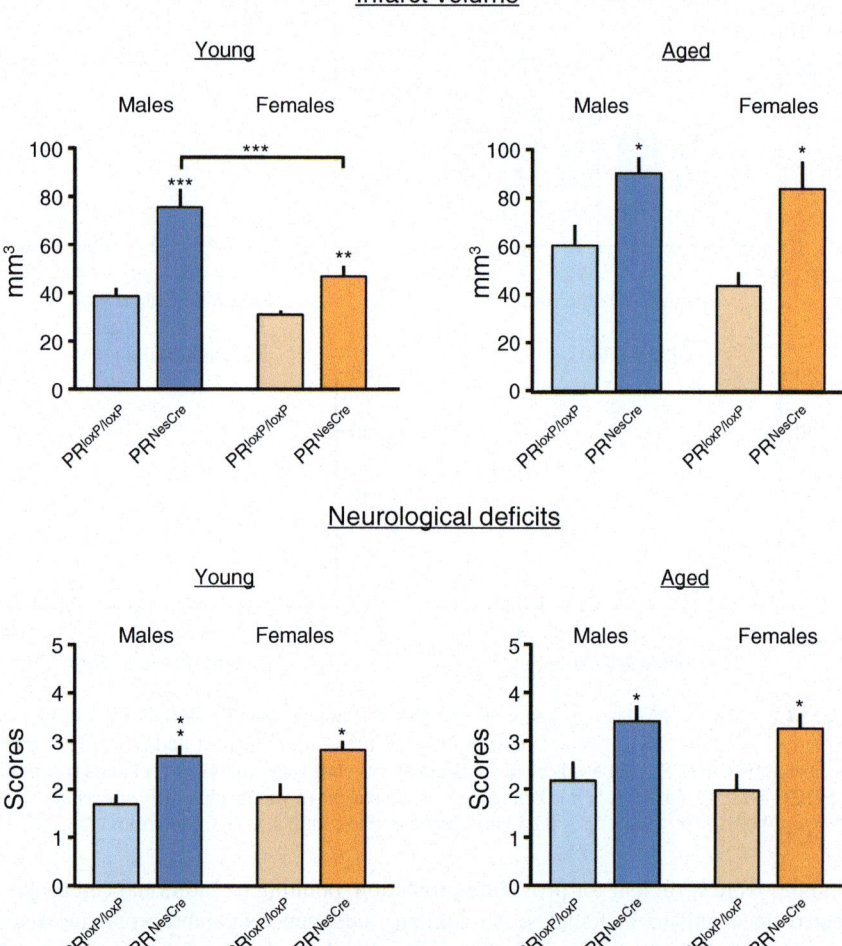

Fig. 14.3 Specific invalidation of the intracellular progesterone receptors (PR) in the central nervous system (PR^NesCre mice) resulted in increased brain infarct size and neurological deficits at 6 h post-MCAO. Male and female mice were either young (3 months old) or aged (12–14 months old). PR^loxP/loxP mice were used as controls. In these mice, exon 2 of the PR gene was flanked by loxP sites, which did not interfere with PR expression. Data from [12]. (***$p \leq 0.001$, **$p \leq 0.01$, *$p \leq 0.05$ when compared to control PR^loxP/loxP mice or as indicated)

14.10 The Role of Brain Progesterone Receptors in Cerebroprotection: Implications for Contraceptive Progestins

The identification of intracellular PR as major targets for the cerebroprotective effects of progesterone after ischemic brain injury has paved the way for the use of synthetic progestins in neuroprotective strategies. Indeed, synthetic progestins used for hormonal contraception or for the treatment of endocrine disorders have been designed to target PR. Moreover, most progestins are almost certainly not converted to GABA$_A$ receptor active metabolites with allopregnanolone-like properties. Thus, if the cerebroprotective actions of progesterone were to be mediated exclusively by allopregnanolone and the modulation of GABA$_A$ receptors, then synthetic progestins would not be expected to be useful for promoting the viability of neural cells.

Additional cerebroprotective health benefits have been demonstrated for the PR-selective and potent 19-norpregnane derivative Nestorone, developed for hormonal contraception in women and men [162, 163]. Nestorone is only poorly metabolized in the brain, as demonstrated by GC-MS, and its 3α,5α-metabolite tetrahydronestorone exhibited only limited activity on GABA$_A$ receptor-evoked responses [164]. However, at a 100-times lower dose than progesterone, the administration of Nestorone significantly decreased infarct volume and deficits in motor coordination assessed by the rotarod test [78], thus confirming a key role of PR.

References

1. van Asch CJ, Luitse MJ, Rinkel GJ, van der Tweel I, Algra A, Klijn CJ. Incidence, case fatality, and functional outcome of intracerebral haemorrhage over time, according to age, sex, and ethnic origin: a systematic review and meta-analysis. Lancet Neurol. 2010;9(2):167–76.
2. Madsen TE, Khoury J, Alwell K, Moomaw CJ, Rademacher E, Flaherty ML, Woo D, Mackey J, De Los Rios La Rosa F, Martini S, Ferioli S, Adeoye O, Khatri P, Broderick JP, Kissela BM, Kleindorfer D. Sex-specific stroke incidence over time in the Greater Cincinnati/Northern Kentucky Stroke Study. Neurology. 2017;89(10):990–6.
3. Appelros P, Stegmayr B, Terent A. Sex differences in stroke epidemiology: a systematic review. Stroke. 2009;40:1082–90.
4. Bushnell C, Howard VJ, Lisabeth L, Caso V, Gall S, Kleindorfer D, Chaturvedi S, Madsen TE, Demel SL, Lee SJ, Reeves M. Sex differences in the evaluation and treatment of acute ischaemic stroke. Lancet Neurol. 2018;17(7):641–50.
5. Reeves MJ, Bushnell CD, Howard G, Gargano JW, Duncan PW, Lynch G, Khatiwoda A, Lisabeth L. Sex differences in stroke: epidemiology, clinical presentation, medical care, and outcomes. Lancet Neurol. 2008;7(10):915–26.
6. Haast RA, Gustafson DR, Kiliaan AJ. Sex differences in stroke. J Cereb Blood Flow Metab. 2012;32(12):2100–7.
7. Gibson CL. Cerebral ischemic stroke: is gender important? J Cereb Blood Flow Metab. 2013;33(9):1355–61.
8. Sohrabji F, Park MJ, Mahnke AH. Sex differences in stroke therapies. J Neurosci Res. 2017;95(1-2):681–91.
9. De Nicola AF, Labombarda F, Deniselle MC, Gonzalez SL, Garay L, Meyer M, Gargiulo G, Guennoun R, Schumacher M. Progesterone neuroprotection in traumatic CNS injury and motoneuron degeneration. Front Neuroendocrinol. 2009;30:173–87.
10. Schumacher M, Mattern C, Ghoumari A, Oudinet JP, Liere P, Labombarda F, Sitruk-Ware R, De Nicola AF, Guennoun R. Revisiting the roles of progesterone and allopregnanolone in the nervous system: resurgence of the progesterone receptors. Prog Neurobiol. 2014;113:6–39.
11. Guennoun R, Frechou M, Gaignard P, Liere P, Slama A, Schumacher M, Denier C, Mattern C. Intranasal administration of progesterone: a potential efficient route of delivery for cerebroprotection after acute brain injuries. Neuropharmacology. 2019;145:283.

12. Zhu X, Frechou M, Liere P, Zhang S, Pianos A, Fernandez N, Denier C, Mattern C, Schumacher M, Guennoun R. A role of endogenous progesterone in stroke cerebroprotection revealed by the neural-specific deletion of its intracellular receptors. J Neurosci. 2017;37(45):10998–1020.
13. Schumacher M, Guennoun R, Ghoumari A, Massaad C, Robert F, el-Etr M, Akwa Y, Rajkowski K, Baulieu EE. Novel perspectives for progesterone in hormone replacement therapy, with special reference to the nervous system. Endocr Rev. 2007;28:387–439.
14. Petrea RE, Beiser AS, Seshadri S, Kelly-Hayes M, Kase CS, Wolf PA. Gender differences in stroke incidence and poststroke disability in the Framingham heart study. Stroke. 2009;40(4):1032–7.
15. Lisabeth L, Bushnell C. Stroke risk in women: the role of menopause and hormone therapy. Lancet Neurol. 2012;11(1):82–91.
16. Ford ES, Maynard LM, Li C. Trends in mean waist circumference and abdominal obesity among US adults, 1999-2012. JAMA. 2014;312(11):1151–3.
17. Ogden CL, Carroll MD, Fryar CD, Flegal KM. Prevalence of obesity among adults and youth: United States, 2011-2014. NCHS Data Brief. 2015;219:1–8.
18. Sharma N, Lee J, Youssef I, Salifu MO, McFarlane SI. Obesity, cardiovascular disease and sleep disorders: insights into the rising epidemic. J Sleep Disord Ther. 2017;6(1):260.
19. Nelson MLA, McKellar KA, Yi J, Kelloway L, Munce S, Cott C, Hall R, Fortin M, Teasell R, Lyons R. Stroke rehabilitation evidence and comorbidity: a systematic scoping review of randomized controlled trials. Top Stroke Rehabil. 2017;24(5):374–80.
20. White UA, Tchoukalova YD. Sex dimorphism and depot differences in adipose tissue function. Biochim Biophys Acta. 2014;1842(3):377–92.
21. Palmer BF, Clegg DJ. The sexual dimorphism of obesity. Mol Cell Endocrinol. 2015;402:113–9.
22. Della Torre S, Benedusi V, Fontana R, Maggi A. Energy metabolism and fertility-a balance preserved for female health. Nat Rev Endocrinol. 2014;10(1):13–23.
23. Lima R, Wofford M, Reckelhoff JF. Hypertension in postmenopausal women. Curr Hypertens Rep. 2012;14(3):254–60.
24. Chen RL, Balami JS, Esiri MM, Chen LK, Buchan AM. Ischemic stroke in the elderly: an overview of evidence. Nat Rev Neurol. 2010;6(5):256–65.
25. Rocca WA, Grossardt BR, Miller VM, Shuster LT, Brown RD Jr. Premature menopause or early menopause and risk of ischemic stroke. Menopause. 2012;19(3):272–7.
26. Rivera CM, Grossardt BR, Rhodes DJ, Brown RD Jr, Roger VL, Melton LJ 3rd, Rocca WA. Increased cardiovascular mortality after early bilateral oophorectomy. Menopause. 2009;16(1):15–23.
27. Wassertheil-Smoller S, Hendrix SL, Limacher M, Heiss G, Kooperberg C, Baird A, Kotchen T, Curb JD, Black H, Rossouw JE, Aragaki A, Safford M, Stein E, Laowattana S, Mysiw WJ. Effect of estrogen plus progestin on stroke in postmenopausal women: the Women's Health Initiative: a randomized trial. JAMA. 2003;289(20):2673–84.
28. Hendrix SL, Wassertheil-Smoller S, Johnson KC, Howard BV, Kooperberg C, Rossouw JE, Trevisan M, Aragaki A, Baird AE, Bray PF, Buring JE, Criqui MH, Herrington D, Lynch JK, Rapp SR, Torner J. Effects of conjugated equine estrogen on stroke in the Women's Health Initiative. Circulation. 2006;113(20):2425–34.
29. Rapp SR, Espeland MA, Shumaker SA, Henderson VW, Brunner RL, Manson JE, Gass ML, Stefanick ML, Lane DS, Hays J, Johnson KC, Coker LH, Dailey M, Bowen D. Effect of estrogen plus progestin on global cognitive function in postmenopausal women: the Women's Health Initiative Memory Study: a randomized controlled trial. JAMA. 2003;289(20):2663–72.
30. Espeland MA, Rapp SR, Shumaker SA, Brunner R, Manson JE, Sherwin BB, Hsia J, Margolis KL, Hogan PE, Wallace R, Dailey M, Freeman R, Hays J. Conjugated equine estrogens and global cognitive function in postmenopausal women: women's health initiative memory study. JAMA. 2004;291(24):2959–68.
31. Shumaker SA, Legault C, Kuller L, Rapp SR, Thal L, Lane DS, Fillit H, Stefanick ML, Hendrix SL, Lewis CE, Masaki K, Coker LH. Conjugated equine estrogens and incidence of probable dementia and mild cognitive impairment in postmenopausal women: women's health initiative memory study. JAMA. 2004;291(24):2947–58.

32. Coker LH, Hogan PE, Bryan NR, Kuller LH, Margolis KL, Bettermann K, Wallace RB, Lao Z, Freeman R, Stefanick ML, Shumaker SA. Postmenopausal hormone therapy and subclinical cerebrovascular disease: the WHIMS-MRI Study. Neurology. 2009;72(2):125–34.
33. Resnick SM, Espeland MA, Jaramillo SA, Hirsch C, Stefanick ML, Murray AM, Ockene J, Davatzikos C. Postmenopausal hormone therapy and regional brain volumes: the WHIMS-MRI Study. Neurology. 2009;72(2):135–42.
34. Gurney EP, Nachtigall MJ, Nachtigall LE, Naftolin F. The Women's Health Initiative trial and related studies: 10 years later: a clinician's view. J Steroid Biochem Mol Biol. 2014;142:4–11.
35. Valera MC, Gourdy P, Tremollieres F, Arnal JF. From the Women's Health Initiative to the combination of estrogen and selective estrogen receptor modulators to avoid progestin addition. Maturitas. 2015;82(3):274–7.
36. Clarkson TB, Melendez GC, Appt SE. Timing hypothesis for postmenopausal hormone therapy: its origin, current status, and future. Menopause. 2013;20(3):342–53.
37. Rossouw JE, Prentice RL, Manson JE, Wu L, Barad D, Barnabei VM, Ko M, LaCroix AZ, Margolis KL, Stefanick ML. Postmenopausal hormone therapy and risk of cardiovascular disease by age and years since menopause. JAMA. 2007;297(13):1465–77.
38. Adams MR, Register TC, Golden DL, Wagner JD, Williams JK. Medroxyprogesterone acetate antagonizes inhibitory effects of conjugated equine estrogens on coronary artery atherosclerosis. Arterioscler Thromb Vasc Biol. 1997;17(1):217–21.
39. Nilsen J, Brinton RD. Impact of progestins on estrogen-induced neuroprotection: synergy by progesterone and 19-norprogesterone and antagonism by medroxyprogesterone acetate. Endocrinology. 2002;143:205–12.
40. Nilsen J, Brinton RD. Divergent impact of progesterone and medroxyprogesterone acetate (Provera) on nuclear mitogen-activated protein kinase signaling. Proc Natl Acad Sci U S A. 2003;100:10506–11.
41. Littleton-Kearney MT, Klaus JA, Hurn PD. Effects of combined oral conjugated estrogens and medroxyprogesterone acetate on brain infarction size after experimental stroke in rat. J Cereb Blood Flow Metab. 2005;25:421–6.
42. Moore NL, Hickey TE, Butler LM, Tilley WD. Multiple nuclear receptor signaling pathways mediate the actions of synthetic progestins in target cells. Mol Cell Endocrinol. 2012;357:60–70.
43. Canonico M, Oger E, Plu-Bureau G, Conard J, Meyer G, Levesque H, Trillot N, Barrellier MT, Wahl D, Emmerich J, Scarabin PY. Hormone therapy and venous thromboembolism among postmenopausal women: impact of the route of estrogen administration and progestogens: the ESTHER study. Circulation. 2007;115(7):840–5.
44. Canonico M, Carcaillon L, Plu-Bureau G, Oger E, Singh-Manoux A, Tubert-Bitter P, Elbaz A, Scarabin PY. Postmenopausal hormone therapy and risk of stroke: impact of the route of estrogen administration and type of progestogen. Stroke. 2016;47(7):1734–41.
45. Canonico M, Plu-Bureau G, Lowe GD, Scarabin PY. Hormone replacement therapy and risk of venous thromboembolism in postmenopausal women: systematic review and meta-analysis. BMJ. 2008;336(7655):1227–31.
46. Scarabin PY, Alhenc-Gelas M, Plu-Bureau G, Taisne P, Agher R, Aiach M. Effects of oral and transdermal estrogen/progesterone regimens on blood coagulation and fibrinolysis in postmenopausal women. A randomized controlled trial. Arterioscler Thromb Vasc Biol. 1997;17(11):3071–8.
47. Lacut K, Oger E, Le Gal G, Blouch MT, Abgrall JF, Kerlan V, Scarabin PY, Mottier D. Differential effects of oral and transdermal postmenopausal estrogen replacement therapies on C-reactive protein. Thromb Haemost. 2003;90(1):124–31.
48. Miller VM, Harman SM. An update on hormone therapy in postmenopausal women: minireview for the basic scientist. Am J Physiol Heart Circ Physiol. 2017;313(5):H1013–h1021.
49. Harman SM, Black DM, Naftolin F, Brinton EA, Budoff MJ, Cedars MI, Hopkins PN, Lobo RA, Manson JE, Merriam GR, Miller VM, Neal-Perry G, Santoro N, Taylor HS, Vittinghoff E, Yan M, Hodis HN. Arterial imaging outcomes and cardiovascular risk factors in recently menopausal women: a randomized trial. Ann Intern Med. 2014;161(4):249–60.

50. Miller VM, Hodis HN, Lahr BD, Bailey KR, Jayachandran M. Changes in carotid artery intima-media thickness 3 years after cessation of menopausal hormone therapy: follow-up from the Kronos Early Estrogen Prevention Study. Menopause. 2019;26:24.
51. Santoro N, Allshouse A, Neal-Perry G, Pal L, Lobo RA, Naftolin F, Black DM, Brinton EA, Budoff MJ, Cedars MI, Dowling NM, Dunn M, Gleason CE, Hodis HN, Isaac B, Magnani M, Manson JE, Miller VM, Taylor HS, Wharton W, Wolff E, Zepeda V, Harman SM. Longitudinal changes in menopausal symptoms comparing women randomized to low-dose oral conjugated estrogens or transdermal estradiol plus micronized progesterone versus placebo: the Kronos Early Estrogen Prevention Study. Menopause. 2017;24(3):238–46.
52. Cintron D, Lahr BD, Bailey KR, Santoro N, Lloyd R, Manson JE, Neal-Perry G, Pal L, Taylor HS, Wharton W, Naftolin F, Harman SM, Miller VM. Effects of oral versus transdermal menopausal hormone treatments on self-reported sleep domains and their association with vasomotor symptoms in recently menopausal women enrolled in the Kronos Early Estrogen Prevention Study (KEEPS). Menopause. 2018;25(2):145–53.
53. Hodis HN, Mack WJ, Shoupe D, Azen SP, Stanczyk FZ, Hwang-Levine J, Budoff MJ, Henderson VW. Methods and baseline cardiovascular data from the Early versus Late Intervention Trial with Estradiol testing the menopausal hormone timing hypothesis. Menopause. 2015;22(4):391–401.
54. Hodis HN, Mack WJ, Henderson VW, Shoupe D, Budoff MJ, Hwang-Levine J, Li Y, Feng M, Dustin L, Kono N, Stanczyk FZ, Selzer RH, Azen SP. Vascular effects of early versus late postmenopausal treatment with estradiol. N Engl J Med. 2016;374(13):1221–31.
55. Andersson AM, Jensen TK, Juul A, Petersen JH, Jorgensen T, Skakkebaek NE. Secular decline in male testosterone and sex hormone binding globulin serum levels in Danish population surveys. J Clin Endocrinol Metab. 2007;92(12):4696–705.
56. Harman SM, Metter EJ, Tobin JD, Pearson J, Blackman MR. Longitudinal effects of aging on serum total and free testosterone levels in healthy men. Baltimore Longitudinal Study of Aging. J Clin Endocrinol Metab. 2001;86(2):724–31.
57. Quillinan N, Deng G, Grewal H, Herson PS. Androgens and stroke: good, bad or indifferent? Exp Neurol. 2014;259:10–5.
58. Sharma R, Oni OA, Gupta K, Chen G, Sharma M, Dawn B, Sharma R, Parashara D, Savin VJ, Ambrose JA, Barua RS. Normalization of testosterone level is associated with reduced incidence of myocardial infarction and mortality in men. Eur Heart J. 2015;36(40):2706–15.
59. Vigen R, O'Donnell CI, Baron AE, Grunwald GK, Maddox TM, Bradley SM, Barqawi A, Woning G, Wierman ME, Plomondon ME, Rumsfeld JS, Ho PM. Association of testosterone therapy with mortality, myocardial infarction, and stroke in men with low testosterone levels. JAMA. 2013;310(17):1829–36.
60. Liu F, McCullough LD. Interactions between age, sex, and hormones in experimental ischemic stroke. Neurochem Int. 2012;61(8):1255–65.
61. Kent DM, Buchan AM, Hill MD. The gender effect in stroke thrombolysis: of CASES, controls, and treatment-effect modification. Neurology. 2008;71(14):1080–3.
62. Lorenzano S, Ahmed N, Falcou A, Mikulik R, Tatlisumak T, Roffe C, Wahlgren N, Toni D. Does sex influence the response to intravenous thrombolysis in ischemic stroke?: answers from safe implementation of treatments in Stroke-International Stroke Thrombolysis Register. Stroke. 2013;44(12):3401–6.
63. Hill MD, Kent DM, Hinchey J, Rowley H, Buchan AM, Wechsler LR, Higashida RT, Fischbein NJ, Dillon WP, Gent M, Firszt CM, Schulz GA, Furlan AJ. Sex-based differences in the effect of intra-arterial treatment of stroke: analysis of the PROACT-2 study. Stroke. 2006;37(9):2322–5.
64. Campbell BCV, Donnan GA, Lees KR, Hacke W, Khatri P, Hill MD, Goyal M, Mitchell PJ, Saver JL, Diener HC, Davis SM. Endovascular stent thrombectomy: the new standard of care for large vessel ischaemic stroke. Lancet Neurol. 2015;14(8):846–54.
65. Amiri-Nikpour MR, Nazarbaghi S, Hamdi-Holasou M, Rezaei Y. An open-label evaluator-blinded clinical study of minocycline neuroprotection in ischemic stroke: gender-dependent effect. Acta Neurol Scand. 2015;131(1):45–50.

66. Li J, McCullough LD. Sex differences in minocycline-induced neuroprotection after experimental stroke. J Cereb Blood Flow Metab. 2009;29(4):670–4.
67. Selvamani A, Sathyan P, Miranda RC, Sohrabji F. An antagomir to microRNA Let7f promotes neuroprotection in an ischemic stroke model. PLoS One. 2012;7(2):e32662.
68. Ahnstedt H, McCullough LD, Cipolla MJ. The importance of considering sex differences in translational stroke research. Transl Stroke Res. 2016;7(4):261–73.
69. Chisholm NC, Sohrabji F. Astrocytic response to cerebral ischemia is influenced by sex differences and impaired by aging. Neurobiol Dis. 2016;85:245–53.
70. Morrison HW, Filosa JA. Sex differences in astrocyte and microglia responses immediately following middle cerebral artery occlusion in adult mice. Neuroscience. 2016;339:85–99.
71. Chauhan A, Moser H, McCullough LD. Sex differences in ischaemic stroke: potential cellular mechanisms. Clin Sci (London, England: 1979). 2017;131(7):533–52.
72. Roof RL, Duvdevani R, Stein DG. Progesterone treatment attenuates brain edema following contusion injury in male and female rats. Restor Neurol Neurosci. 1992;4(6):425–7.
73. Stein DG. Brain damage, sex hormones and recovery: a new role for progesterone and estrogen? Trends Neurosci. 2001;24:386–91.
74. Roof RL, Duvdevani R, Heyburn JW, Stein DG. Progesterone rapidly decreases brain edema: treatment delayed up to 24 hours is still effective. Exp Neurol. 1996;138:246–51.
75. Meffre D, Pianos A, Liere P, Eychenne B, Cambourg A, Schumacher M, Stein DG, Guennoun R. Steroid profiling in brain and plasma of male and pseudopregnant female rats after traumatic brain injury: analysis by gas chromatography/mass spectrometry. Endocrinology. 2007;148(5):2505–17.
76. Jiang N, Chopp M, Stein D, Feit H. Progesterone is neuroprotective after transient middle cerebral artery occlusion in male rats. Brain Res. 1996;735:101–7.
77. Gibson CL, Murphy SP. Progesterone enhances functional recovery after middle cerebral artery occlusion in male mice. J Cereb Blood Flow Metab. 2004;24(7):805–13.
78. Liu A, Margaill I, Zhang S, Labombarda F, Coqueran B, Delespierre B, Liere P, Marchand-Leroux C, O'Malley BW, Lydon JP, De Nicola AF, Sitruk-Ware R, Mattern C, Plotkine M, Schumacher M, Guennoun R. Progesterone receptors: a key for neuroprotection in experimental stroke. Endocrinology. 2012;153(8):3747–57.
79. Sutherland BA, Minnerup J, Balami JS, Arba F, Buchan AM, Kleinschnitz C. Neuroprotection for ischaemic stroke: translation from the bench to the bedside. Int J Stroke. 2012;7(5):407–18.
80. Baron JC. Protecting the ischaemic penumbra as an adjunct to thrombectomy for acute stroke. Nat Rev Neurol. 2018;14(6):325–37.
81. Lin YH, Dong J, Tang Y, Ni HY, Zhang Y, Su P, Liang HY, Yao MC, Yuan HJ, Wang DL, Chang L, Wu HY, Luo CX, Zhu DY. Opening a new time window for treatment of stroke by targeting HDAC2. J Neurosci. 2017;37(28):6712–28.
82. Alawieh A, Langley EF, Tomlinson S. Targeted complement inhibition salvages stressed neurons and inhibits neuroinflammation after stroke in mice. Sci Transl Med. 2018;10(441):eaao6459.
83. Bai J, Lyden PD. Revisiting cerebral postischemic reperfusion injury: new insights in understanding reperfusion failure, hemorrhage, and edema. Int J Stroke. 2015;10(2):143–52.
84. Nighoghossian N, Ovize M, Mewton N, Ong E, Cho TH. Cyclosporine A, a potential therapy of ischemic reperfusion injury. A common history for heart and brain. Cerebrovasc Dis. 2016;42(5-6):309–18.
85. Wong R, Renton C, Gibson CL, Murphy SJ, Kendall DA, Bath PM, Progesterone Pre-Clinical Stroke Pooling Project C. Progesterone treatment for experimental stroke: an individual animal meta-analysis. J Cereb Blood Flow Metab. 2013;33(9):1362–72.
86. Gibson CL, Coomber B, Murphy SP. Progesterone is neuroprotective following cerebral ischaemia in reproductively ageing female mice. Brain. 2011;134(Pt 7):2125–33.
87. Wang J, Jiang C, Liu C, Li X, Chen N, Hao Y. Neuroprotective effects of progesterone following stroke in aged rats. Behav Brain Res. 2010;209(1):119–22.
88. Yousuf S, Atif F, Sayeed I, Wang J, Stein DG. Post-stroke infections exacerbate ischemic brain injury in middle-aged rats: immunomodulation and neuroprotection by progesterone. Neuroscience. 2013;239:92–102.

89. Wali B, Ishrat T, Won S, Stein DG, Sayeed I. Progesterone in experimental permanent stroke: a dose-response and therapeutic time-window study. Brain. 2014;137(Pt 2):486–502.
90. Yousuf S, Atif F, Sayeed I, Tang H, Stein DG. Progesterone in transient ischemic stroke: a dose-response study. Psychopharmacology (Berl). 2014;231(17):3313–23.
91. Wali B, Ishrat T, Stein DG, Sayeed I. Progesterone improves long-term functional and histological outcomes after permanent stroke in older rats. Behav Brain Res. 2016;305:46–56.
92. Yousuf S, Sayeed I, Atif F, Tang H, Wang J, Stein DG. Delayed progesterone treatment reduces brain infarction and improves functional outcomes after ischemic stroke: a time-window study in middle-aged rats. J Cereb Blood Flow Metab. 2014;34(2):297–306.
93. Genazzani AR, Petraglia F, Bernardi F, Casarosa E, Salvestroni C, Tonetti A, Nappi RE, Luisi S, Palumbo M, Purdy RH, Luisi M. Circulating levels of allopregnanolone in humans: gender, age, and endocrine influences. J Clin Endocrinol Metab. 1998;83:2099–103.
94. Havlikova H, Hill M, Kancheva L, Vrbikova J, Pouzar V, Cerny I, Kancheva R, Starka L. Serum profiles of free and conjugated neuroactive pregnanolone isomers in nonpregnant women of fertile age. J Clin Endocrinol Metab. 2006;91:3092–9.
95. Byers SL, Wiles MV, Dunn SL, Taft RA. Mouse estrous cycle identification tool and images. PLoS One. 2012;7(4):e35538.
96. Nilsson ME, Vandenput L, Tivesten A, Norlen AK, Lagerquist MK, Windahl SH, Borjesson AE, Farman HH, Poutanen M, Benrick A, Maliqueo M, Stener-Victorin E, Ryberg H, Ohlsson C. Measurement of a comprehensive sex steroid profile in rodent serum by high-sensitive gas chromatography-tandem mass spectrometry. Endocrinology. 2015;156(7):2492–502.
97. Tuckey RC. Progesterone synthesis by the human placenta. Placenta. 2005;26:273–81.
98. Concas A, Mostallino MC, Porcu P, Follesa P, Barbaccia ML, Trabucchi M, Purdy RH, Grisenti P, Biggio G. Role of brain allopregnanolone in the plasticity of gamma-aminobutyric acid type A receptor in rat brain during pregnancy and after delivery. Proc Natl Acad Sci U S A. 1998;95:13284–9.
99. Parizek A, Hill M, Kancheva R, Havlikova H, Kancheva L, Cindr J, Paskova A, Pouzar V, Cerny I, Drbohlav P, Hajek Z, Starka L. Neuroactive pregnanolone isomers during pregnancy. J Clin Endocrinol Metab. 2005;90:395–403.
100. Piekorz RP, Gingras S, Hoffmeyer A, Ihle JN, Weinstein Y. Regulation of progesterone levels during pregnancy and parturition by signal transducer and activator of transcription 5 and 20alpha-hydroxysteroid dehydrogenase. Mol Endocrinol. 2005;19(2):431–40.
101. Kalil B, Leite CM, Carvalho-Lima M, Anselmo-Franci JA. Role of sex steroids in progesterone and corticosterone response to acute restraint stress in rats: sex differences. Stress. 2013;16(4):452–60.
102. Oettel M, Mukhopadhyay AK. Progesterone: the forgotten hormone in men? Aging Male. 2004;7:236–57.
103. Elman I, Breier A. Effects of acute metabolic stress on plasma progesterone and testosterone in male subjects: relationship to pituitary-adrenocortical axis activation. Life Sci. 1997;61:1705–12.
104. Zitzmann M, Erren M, Kamischke A, Simoni M, Nieschlag E. Endogenous progesterone and the exogenous progestin norethisterone enanthate are associated with a proinflammatory profile in healthy men. J Clin Endocrinol Metab. 2005;90:6603–8.
105. Wagner AK, McCullough EH, Niyonkuru C, Ozawa H, Loucks TL, Dobos JA, Brett CA, Santarsieri M, Dixon CE, Berga SL, Fabio A. Acute serum hormone levels: characterization and prognosis after severe traumatic brain injury. J Neurotrauma. 2011;28:871–88.
106. Baulieu EE. Neurosteroids: of the nervous system, by the nervous system, for the nervous system. Recent Prog Horm Res. 1997;52:1–32.
107. Baulieu EE, Robel P, Schumacher M. Neurosteroids: beginning of the story. Int Rev Neurobiol. 2001;46:1–32.
108. Mellon SH, Griffin LD, Compagnone NA. Biosynthesis and action of neurosteroids. Brain Res Rev. 2001;37:3–12.
109. Banks WA. Brain meets body: the blood-brain barrier as an endocrine interface. Endocrinology. 2012;153(9):4111–9.

110. Pardridge WM. shRNA and siRNA delivery to the brain. Adv Drug Deliv Rev. 2007;59(2-3):141–52.
111. Genazzani AR, Stomati M, Morittu A, Bernardi F, Monteleone P, Casarosa E, Gallo R, Salvestroni C, Luisi M. Progesterone, progestagens and the central nervous system. Hum Reprod. 2000;15(Suppl 1):14–27.
112. Do Rego JL, Seong JY, Burel D, Leprince J, Luu-The V, Tsutsui K, Tonon MC, Pelletier G, Vaudry H. Neurosteroid biosynthesis: enzymatic pathways and neuroendocrine regulation by neurotransmitters and neuropeptides. Front Neuroendocrinol. 2009;30:259–301.
113. Brown AR, Mitchell SJ, Peden DR, Herd MB, Seifi M, Swinny JD, Belelli D, Lambert JJ. During postnatal development endogenous neurosteroids influence GABA-ergic neurotransmission of mouse cortical neurons. Neuropharmacology. 2016;103:163–73.
114. Poletti A, Coscarella A, Negri-Cesi P, Colciago A, Celotti F, Martini L. 5 alpha-reductase isozymes in the central nervous system. Steroids. 1998;63(5-6):246–51.
115. Melcangi RC, Poletti A, Cavarretta I, Celotti F, Colciago A, Magnaghi V, Motta M, Negri-Cesi P, Martini L. The 5alpha-reductase in the central nervous system: expression and modes of control. J Steroid Biochem Mol Biol. 1998;65(1-6):295–9.
116. Patte-Mensah C, Li S, Mensah-Nyagan AG. Impact of neuropathic pain on the gene expression and activity of cytochrome P450side-chain-cleavage in sensory neural networks. Cell Mol Life Sci. 2004;61:2274–84.
117. Melcangi RC, Celotti F, Martini L. Progesterone 5-alpha-reduction in neuronal and in different types of glial cell cultures: type 1 and 2 astrocytes and oligodendrocytes. Brain Res. 1994;639:202–6.
118. Rupprecht R, Reul JM, Trapp T, van Steensel B, Wetzel C, Damm K, Zieglgansberger W, Holsboer F. Progesterone receptor-mediated effects of neuroactive steroids. Neuron. 1993;11(3):523–30.
119. Karavolas HJ, Hodges D, O'Brien D. Uptake of (3H)progesterone and (3H)5alpha-dihydroprogesterone by rat tissues in vivo and analysis of accumulated radioactivity: accumulation of 5alpha-dihydroprogesterone by pituitary and hypothalamic tissues. Endocrinology. 1976;98:164–75.
120. Beyer C, Gonzalez-Flores O, Gonzalez-Mariscal G. Ring A reduced progestins potently stimulate estrous behavior in rats: paradoxical effect through the progesterone receptor. Physiol Behav. 1995;58:985–93.
121. Penning TM, Jin Y, Heredia VV, Lewis M. Structure-function relationships in 3alpha-hydroxysteroid dehydrogenases: a comparison of the rat and human isoforms. J Steroid Biochem Mol Biol. 2003;85(2-5):247–55.
122. Belyaeva OV, Chetyrkin SV, Clark AL, Kostereva NV, SantaCruz KS, Chronwall BM, Kedishvili NY. Role of microsomal retinol/sterol dehydrogenase-like short-chain dehydrogenases/reductases in the oxidation and epimerization of 3alpha-hydroxysteroids in human tissues. Endocrinology. 2007;148:2148–56.
123. Penning TM. Human hydroxysteroid dehydrogenases and pre-receptor regulation: insights into inhibitor design and evaluation. J Steroid Biochem Mol Biol. 2011;125: 46–56.
124. Martini L, Melcangi RC, Maggi R. Androgen and progesterone metabolism in the central and peripheral nervous system. J Steroid Biochem Mol Biol. 1993;47:195–205.
125. Agis-Balboa RC, Pinna G, Zhubi A, Maloku E, Veldic M, Costa E, Guidotti A. Characterization of brain neurons that express enzymes mediating neurosteroid biosynthesis. Proc Natl Acad Sci U S A. 2006;103:14602–7.
126. Patte-Mensah C, Penning TM, Mensah-Nyagan AG. Anatomical and cellular localization of neuroactive 5 alpha/3 alpha-reduced steroid-synthesizing enzymes in the spinal cord. J Comp Neurol. 2004;477:286–99.
127. Belelli D, Lambert JJ. Neurosteroids: endogenous regulators of the GABA(A) receptor. Nat Rev Neurosci. 2005;6:565–75.
128. Sieghart W. Allosteric modulation of GABAA receptors via multiple drug-binding sites. Adv Pharmacol. 2015;72:53–96.

129. Majewska MD, Harrison NL, Schwartz RD, Barker JL, Paul SM. Steroid hormone metabolites are barbiturate-like modulators of the GABA receptor. Science. 1986;232:1004–7.
130. Hosie AM, Wilkins ME, da Silva HM, Smart TG. Endogenous neurosteroids regulate GABAA receptors through two discrete transmembrane sites. Nature. 2006;444:486–9.
131. Hosie AM, Wilkins ME, Smart TG. Neurosteroid binding sites on GABA(A) receptors. Pharmacol Ther. 2007;116:7–19.
132. Belelli D, Harrison NL, Maguire J, Macdonald RL, Walker MC, Cope DW. Extrasynaptic GABAA receptors: form, pharmacology, and function. J Neurosci. 2009;29:12757–63.
133. Semyanov A, Walker MC, Kullmann DM, Silver RA. Tonically active GABA A receptors: modulating gain and maintaining the tone. Trends Neurosci. 2004;27:262–9.
134. Farrant M, Nusser Z. Variations on an inhibitory theme: phasic and tonic activation of GABA(A) receptors. Nat Rev Neurosci. 2005;6:215–29.
135. Mihalek RM, Banerjee PK, Korpi ER, Quinlan JJ, Firestone LL, Mi ZP, Lagenaur C, Tretter V, Sieghart W, Anagnostaras SG, Sage JR, Fanselow MS, Guidotti A, Spigelman I, Li Z, DeLorey TM, Olsen RW, Homanics GE. Attenuated sensitivity to neuroactive steroids in gamma-aminobutyrate type A receptor delta subunit knockout mice. Proc Natl Acad Sci U S A. 1999;96:12905–10.
136. Stell BM, Brickley SG, Tang CY, Farrant M, Mody I. Neuroactive steroids reduce neuronal excitability by selectively enhancing tonic inhibition mediated by delta subunit-containing GABAA receptors. Proc Natl Acad Sci U S A. 2003;100:14439–44.
137. Sayeed I, Guo Q, Hoffman SW, Stein DG. Allopregnanolone, a progesterone metabolite, is more effective than progesterone in reducing cortical infarct volume after transient middle cerebral artery occlusion. Ann Emerg Med. 2006;47(4):381–9.
138. Ishrat T, Sayeed I, Atif F, Hua F, Stein DG. Progesterone and allopregnanolone attenuate blood-brain barrier dysfunction following permanent focal ischemia by regulating the expression of matrix metalloproteinases. Exp Neurol. 2010;226(1):183–90.
139. Sternau LL, Lust WD, Ricci AJ, Ratcheson R. Role for gamma-aminobutyric acid in selective vulnerability in gerbils. Stroke. 1989;20(2):281–7.
140. Schwartz-Bloom RD, Sah R. gamma-Aminobutyric acid(A) neurotransmission and cerebral ischemia. J Neurochem. 2001;77(2):353–71.
141. Iwata M, Inoue S, Kawaguchi M, Furuya H. Effects of diazepam and flumazenil on forebrain ischaemia in a rat model of benzodiazepine tolerance. Br J Anaesth. 2012;109(6):935–42.
142. Kastner P, Krust A, Turcotte B, Stropp U, Tora L, Gronemeyer H, Chambon P. Two distinct estrogen-regulated promoters generate transcripts encoding the two functionally different human progesterone receptor forms A and B. EMBO J. 1990;9:1603–14.
143. Kraus WL, Montano MM, Katzenellenbogen BS. Cloning of the rat progesterone receptor gene 5′-region and identification of two functionally distinct promoters. Mol Endocrinol. 1993;7(12):1603–16.
144. Conneely OM, Mulac-Jericevic B, DeMayo F, Lydon JP, O'Malley BW. Reproductive functions of progesterone receptors. Recent Prog Horm Res. 2002;57:339–55.
145. Blaustein JD, Ryer HI, Feder HH. A sex difference in the progestin receptor system of guinea pig brain. Neuroendocrinology. 1980;31:403–9.
146. Rainbow TC, Parsons B, McEwen BS. Sex differences in rat brain oestrogen and progestin receptors. Nature. 1982;300:648–9.
147. Hagan CR, Daniel AR, Dressing GE, Lange CA. Role of phosphorylation in progesterone receptor signaling and specificity. Mol Cell Endocrinol. 2012;357:43–9.
148. Waters EM, Torres-Reveron A, McEwen BS, Milner TA. Ultrastructural localization of extranuclear progestin receptors in the rat hippocampal formation. J Comp Neurol. 2008;511:34–46.
149. Pedram A, Razandi M, Sainson RC, Kim JK, Hughes CC, Levin ER. A conserved mechanism for steroid receptor translocation to the plasma membrane. J Biol Chem. 2007;282(31):22278–88.

150. Thomas P, Pang Y. Membrane progesterone receptors: evidence for neuroprotective, neurosteroid signaling and neuroendocrine functions in neuronal cells. Neuroendocrinology. 2012;96(2):162–71.
151. Wendler A, Albrecht C, Wehling M. Nongenomic actions of aldosterone and progesterone revisited. Steroids. 2012;77(10):1002–6.
152. Guennoun R, Labombarda F, Gonzalez Deniselle MC, Liere P, De Nicola AF, Schumacher M. Progesterone and allopregnanolone in the central nervous system: response to injury and implication for neuroprotection. J Steroid Biochem Mol Biol. 2015;146:48–61.
153. Su C, Cunningham RL, Rybalchenko N, Singh M. Progesterone increases the release of brain-derived neurotrophic factor from glia via progesterone receptor membrane component 1 (Pgrmc1)-dependent ERK5 signaling. Endocrinology. 2012;153(9):4389–400.
154. Nguyen T, Su C, Singh M. Let-7i inhibition enhances progesterone-induced functional recovery in a mouse model of ischemia. Proc Natl Acad Sci U S A. 2018;115(41):E9668–e9677.
155. Pang Y, Dong J, Thomas P. Characterization, neurosteroid binding and brain distribution of human membrane progesterone receptors delta and {epsilon} (mPRdelta and mPR{epsilon}) and mPRdelta involvement in neurosteroid inhibition of apoptosis. Endocrinology. 2013;154(1):283–95.
156. Meffre D, Labombarda F, Delespierre B, Chastre A, De Nicola AF, Stein DG, Schumacher M, Guennoun R. Distribution of membrane progesterone receptor alpha in the male mouse and rat brain and its regulation after traumatic brain injury. Neuroscience. 2013;231:111–24.
157. Thomas P, Pang Y, Dong J, Groenen P, Kelder J, de Vlieg J, Zhu Y, Tubbs C. Steroid and G protein binding characteristics of the seatrout and human progestin membrane receptor alpha subtypes and their evolutionary origins. Endocrinology. 2007;148:705–18.
158. Dubal DB, Rau SW, Shughrue PJ, Zhu H, Yu J, Cashion AB, Suzuki S, Gerhold LM, Bottner MB, Dubal SB, Merchanthaler I, Kindy MS, Wise PM. Differential modulation of estrogen receptors (ERs) in ischemic brain injury: a role for ERalpha in estradiol-mediated protection against delayed cell death. Endocrinology. 2006;147(6):3076–84.
159. Westberry JM, Prewitt AK, Wilson ME. Epigenetic regulation of the estrogen receptor alpha promoter in the cerebral cortex following ischemia in male and female rats. Neuroscience. 2008;152(4):982–9.
160. Wong R, Bath PM, Kendall D, Gibson CL. Progesterone and cerebral ischaemia: the relevance of ageing. J Neuroendocrinol. 2013;25(11):1088–94.
161. Liu F, Yuan R, Benashski SE, McCullough LD. Changes in experimental stroke outcome across the life span. J Cereb Blood Flow Metab. 2009;29(4):792–802.
162. Sitruk-Ware R, Small M, Kumar N, Tsong YY, Sundaram K, Jackanicz T. Nestorone: clinical applications for contraception and HRT. Steroids. 2003;68:907–13.
163. Ilani N, Roth MY, Amory JK, Swerdloff RS, Dart C, Page ST, Bremner WJ, Sitruk-Ware R, Kumar N, Blithe DL, Wang C. A new combination of testosterone and nestorone transdermal gels for male hormonal contraception. J Clin Endocrinol Metab. 2012;97:3476–86.
164. Kumar N, Fagart J, Liere P, Mitchell SJ, Knibb AR, Petit-Topin I, Rame M, El-Etr M, Schumacher M, Lambert JJ, Rafestin-Oblin ME, Sitruk-Ware R. Nestorone(R) as a novel progestin for nonoral contraception: structure-activity relationships and brain metabolism studies. Endocrinology. 2017;158(1):170–82.

Atherogenesis: Estrogen Induction of Polysialylated nCAM (PSA-nCAM) Blocks Monocyte Capture by Vascular Endothelial Cells

15

Frederick Naftolin

Cardiovascular disease (CVD) is the leading cause of death in women, as well as men. However, prior to menopause, women have a lower incidence of CVD than men [1]. This is reversed after the menopause [2]. It has long been known that estrogen treatment of postmenopausal women lowers risk factors for CVD [3–10]. Recent studies have shown that prompt estrogen treatment of postmenopausal women also reduces indicators of CVD, carotid artery intimal-medial thickness (CIMT) [11], and coronary artery calcium (CAC) [12]. Recent studies also show reduced CVD deaths in young estrogen-treated women [13].

Epidemiologic studies show that premature menopause is accompanied by fewer cardiovascular deaths if estrogen replacement is promptly started [4]. A retrospective study showed that Chinese women on MHT for hot flushes, usually starting within a few years of menopause have less atherosclerosis than equally aged, non-treated women [14]. Randomized prospective studies show that women starting MHT within 5 years of the menopause (6 years after the last period) have less CIMT than placebo [10]. And, in the WHI observational study, women on ET have less CAC and cardiac deaths than untreated women of the same age [12, 13].

Primate studies done in Clarkson's laboratory indicated that estrogen blocks atherogenesis in oophorectomized female monkeys and this effect depends on starting the estrogen treatment early, before plaque has formed [15]. This has been born out in studies in women [10, 16].

Thus, evidence supports that estrogen replacement treatment is cardioprotective, but only when begun before significant plaque has formed in the vessels. The mechanism of this action of estrogen is what this chapter is about.

As mentioned above, there is solid evidence that estrogen improves risk factors such as lipids. However, during 4 years of treatment of menopausal women with MHT/ET that lowered lipids and improved other risk factors, our randomized study

F. Naftolin (✉)
Department of Obstetrics and Gynecology, New York University, New York, NY, USA
e-mail: frederick.naftolin@nyumc.org

© International Society of Gynecological Endocrinology 2019
R. D. Brinton et al. (eds.), *Sex Steroids' Effects on Brain, Heart and Vessels*,
ISGE Series, https://doi.org/10.1007/978-3-030-11355-1_15

of the effects of MHT/ET was not able to show a decrease of the CIMT compared to the placebo groups [17]. In light of the evidence that estrogen prevents ASVD, we entertained the possibility that improvement of risk factors is not the only mechanism and that local actions at the vascular level could also play roles in atheroprotection by estrogen.

In previous studies, we had identified possible estrogen action at the level of the interaction of the endothelium and circulatory monocytes. Working with Clarkson and colleagues, we showed that human and monkey artery endothelium expresses the enzyme estrogen synthetase (aromatase) and estrogen receptor immunoreactivity [17]. We had previously shown the expression of aromatase and estrogen receptors by human monocytes/precursors [18]. We combined this information with our understanding of mechanisms involved in the in-migration of circulating monocytes through the immune-brain barrier [19] and their formation into brain macrophages, the microglia [20], to formulate a novel explanation of role of estrogen in the capture of circulating monocytes by the vascular endothelium that initiates atherogenesis [21].

The accumulation of plaque in the vascular wall is initiated by vascular/perivascular inflammation and is characterized by the formation of lipid-laden plaques beneath the endothelium. This involves subendothelial low-density lipoprotein (LDL) accumulation which results in endothelial cell activation and chronic inflammation. Hypertensive pulses may also traumatize blood vessels. Cytokine signals (IL-1, TNFα) from the injured vessel recruit monocytes from the circulation. The activated monocytes adhere to the endothelial cells and penetrate the intimal layer of the vessel as macrophages. The macrophages may become foam cells in the mass termed "plaque" [22–26]. The majority of all deaths from CVD are secondary to infarctions/thromboses caused by deteriorating atherosclerotic vascular plaque or are due to vascular stenosis caused by plaque-based occlusion of vessels [1]. It is increasingly recognized that due to their smaller coronary vessels and other factors, women may be at special risk from the development of plaque, per se, and become symptomatic before there is deterioration and leakage of plaque content so often seen during coronary thrombosis in men [27].

15.1 The Role of Sex Steroids in Blocking Monocyte Tethering and Capture

Cell adhesion is a general phenomenon that is critical to the activities of *all* cells. The molecules P-selectin, vascular cell adhesion molecule 1 (VCAM-1), intercellular adhesion molecule 1 (ICAM-1), neural cell adhesion molecule (nCAM), and P-selectin glycoprotein ligand-1 are molecules that have proven to be important in monocyte recruitment and plaque formation [22–26].

As indicated above, we showed that estrogen receptor and aromatase are present in the vascular endothelium and monocytes that are subject to these signals from inflamed vessels. Therefore, we considered an attack on the nexus of atherogenesis by estrogen could involve blocking the arrest/adhesion of circulating monocytes in

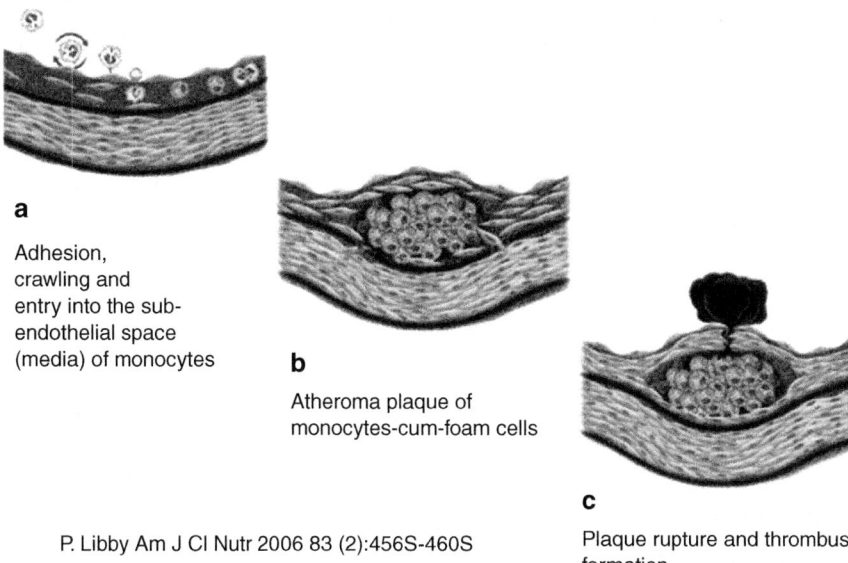

a

Adhesion,
crawling and
entry into the sub-
endothelial space
(media) of monocytes

b

Atheroma plaque of
monocytes-cum-foam cells

c

P. Libby Am J CI Nutr 2006 83 (2):456S-460S

Plaque rupture and thrombus
formation

Fig. 15.1 Libby's depiction of the role of inflammation in the capture and participation of mono-cytes in the development of vascular plaque

response to vascular inflammation (see Fig. 15.1). As part of developing the rationale for this approach, we searched for the molecular means by which estrogen might regulate monocyte availability, especially during periods of vascular inflammation.

15.2 Arresting Circulating Monocytes by Cell-to-Cell Tethering

Prior to monocyte adhesion to endothelial cells, it is necessary to arrest them as they roll past the area of adhesion (Fig. 15.1). One of the means by which organs harmo-nize the movements of adjacent cells is to form molecular bridges between the involved cells [27]. Neural cell adhesion molecule (nCAM) is one of the most widely studied molecules involved in such "molecular tethering." The distal extra-cellular domain of nCAM forms electrostatic bonds with the distal domains of numerous molecules in the glycoprotein family, including nCAM species. The basis for this bonding is the counter-axial complementarity of nCAM distal domains that allows the electrochemical attraction. This may result in tethering one molecule to another, the so-called zippering (Fig. 15.2). While nCAM to nCAM zippering is most widely studied in the central nervous system, it is not limited to the nervous system [28]. For example, zippered distal domains of nCAM molecules protruding from the membranes of rolling monocytes that are in proximity to stationary endo-thelial cells form a multitude of tethers that arrest the monocytes and allow adhesion molecules to reel the monocytes onto the endothelial surface [23–27].

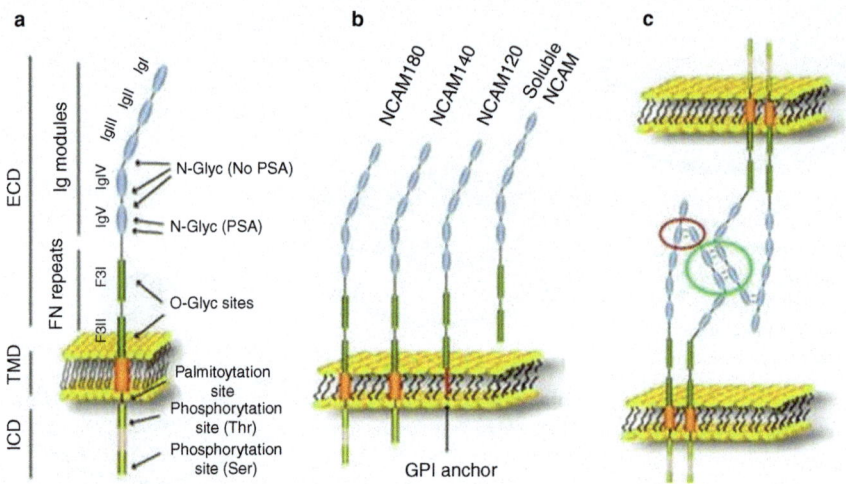

Fig. 15.2 (**a**) The structure on nCAM molecules. (**b**) The four types of nCAM molecules. (**c**) The formation of nCAM to nCAM electrostatic bonds that can result in cell-to-cell tethers. The extracellular domain of nCAM projects away from the cell. The most distal (Ig modules) domain of the nCAM (blue) is constructed so that in ab-axis meetings with other nCAM Ig modules, there is an electrostatic binding (**c**, red and green circles) between adjacent nCAM molecules. If the nCAM molecules are expressed by the luminal endothelium and by a passing monocyte, tethers may form that bind the monocyte to the endothelial cell. Modified from Gascon E, Vutskits L, Kiss JZ (2007) Polysialic acid-neural cell adhesion molecule in brain plasticity: from synapses to integration of new neurons. Brain Res Rev 56:101–18

nCAM zippering is dependent on the proximity of the two involved molecules, addition of space weakens the electrostatic bond. This may be accomplished by post-translational sialylation, the insertion of sugars onto the domain. There are three nCAM sialylases, one for each nCAM species. Addition of the hydrophilic sugars increases the distance between the polysialylated nCAM (PSA-nCAM) molecules, diminishing the ability to form or maintain tethers [28, 29].

15.3 Estrogen Induction of nCAM Sialylation

We showed that nCAM and PSA-nCAM are expressed in human and rodent vascular endothelium, that the enzymes needed to sialylate nCAM are also present, and that their expression appeared to be regulated by estrogen [30]. To assess the role of estrogen, we tested whether cultured human vascular endothelium cells express nCAM and whether estradiol induces polysialylation of that nCAM during the culture of human umbilical vein endothelial cells (HUVEC). There was a strong induction of PSA-nCAM expression, shown in Fig. 15.3. This was blocked by co-incubation of the endothelial cells with the estrogen receptor antagonist (ERA) fulvestrant (Fig. 15.4) [31].

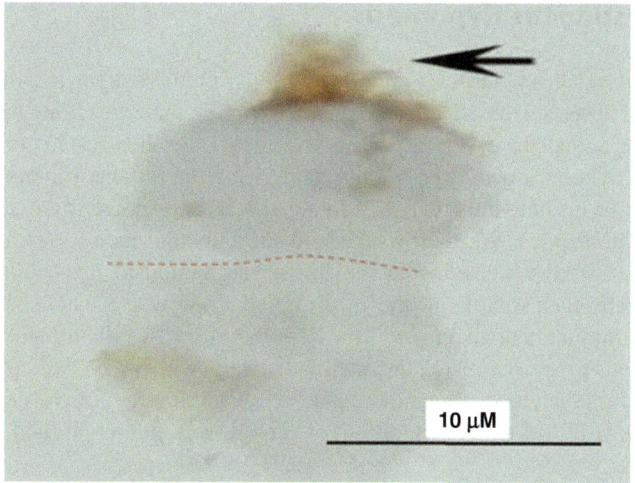

Park H, et al. Reproductive sciences 2010 17:1090-8.

Fig. 15.3 Estradiol-induced polarized expression of PSA-nCAM in the glycocalyx of two human umbilical vein cells. The bottom cell is turned away, so that the polarized PSA-nCAM staining is out of focus

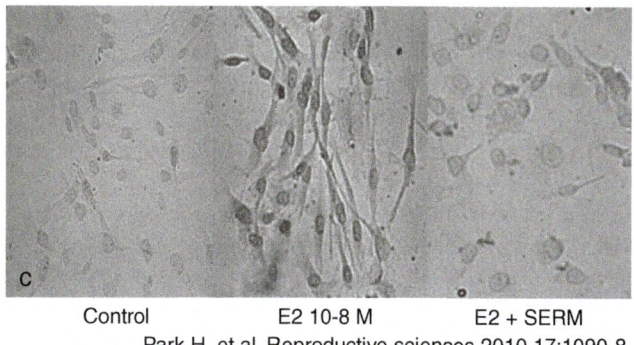

Control   E2 10-8 M   E2 + SERM

Park H, et al. Reproductive sciences 2010 17:1090-8.

Fig. 15.4 Estradiol induces sialylation of human umbilical vein endothelial cells. This is blocked by co-incubation with the SERM fulvestrant. Ir-PSA-nCAM is seen as perinuclear and membrane staining in the center panel

15.4 Our Hypothesis

Based on the above, we proposed that estradiol can, by inducing sialylation of nCAM to form PSA-nCAM, abort electrostatic bonding that is the basis of monocyte to endothelial tethering. This could allow circulating monocytes to pass vascular areas of inflammation without capture, and the lack of captured monocytes would limit the amount of vascular plaque.

15.5   Testing the Hypothesis

We cultured coronary vascular endothelial cells, pretreated them with test compounds, and observed the effects on monocyte capture. After reaching confluence (a "lawn"), we added the test compounds overnight. We then tested for capture of monocytes by pouring a fixed number of green fluorescent protein-expressing human monocytes onto the lawn of endothelial cells and waited for 40 min to allow capture of monocytes. We then washed off the unbound monocytes and, using a fluorescence microscope, counted the monocytes bound to the endothelial cells (Fig. 15.5). In each treatment, the level of induction of PSA-nCAM was documented by immunohistochemistry. To assess the effect of inflammatory cytokines on the system, we co-incubated the endothelial cells with TNFα and compared this with control media alone. Since there was no apparent effect of the co-incubation with TNFα (Fig. 15.6), the addition of TNFα was not continued during the experiments.

15.6   Estrogen-Related Sex Steroids Induce nCAM Sialylation and Curtail the Number of Endothelium-Bound Monocytes

Amounts of estradiol, testosterone, dehydroepiandrosterone (DHEA), and dihydrotestosterone when incubated with cardiovascular endothelial cells from men and women significantly inhibited the binding of macrophages to treated endothelial cells (Figs. 15.6, 15.7, and 15.8). While estradiol generally had the greatest effect, the other steroids were also effective. In these proof of principle experiments, there was no clear sex difference in responses.

The effect of preincubation with estradiol was blocked by co-pretreatment with the estrogen receptor antagonist fulvestrant. In the case of testosterone, the effect on monocyte binding was inhibited by the androgen receptor blocker finasteride. Pretreatment with dehydroepiandrosterone (DHEA) was blocked by trilostane, the enzyme that blocked by conversion of DHEA to androstenedione and thence to estrogen [32].

Fig. 15.5 Experimental design to test the effects of sex steroids on the nexus of atherogenesis (adhesion of human monocytes to endothelial cells)

- Growing a lawn of endothelial cells and treating int with sex steroids ± receptor blocker

- Pore on fluorescent monocytes (activated THP1 cells) for 40 min, wash and count adherent fluorescent cells

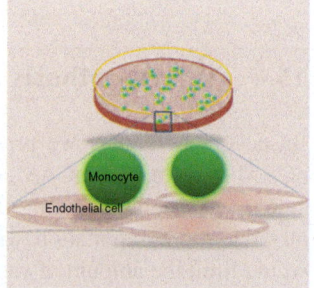

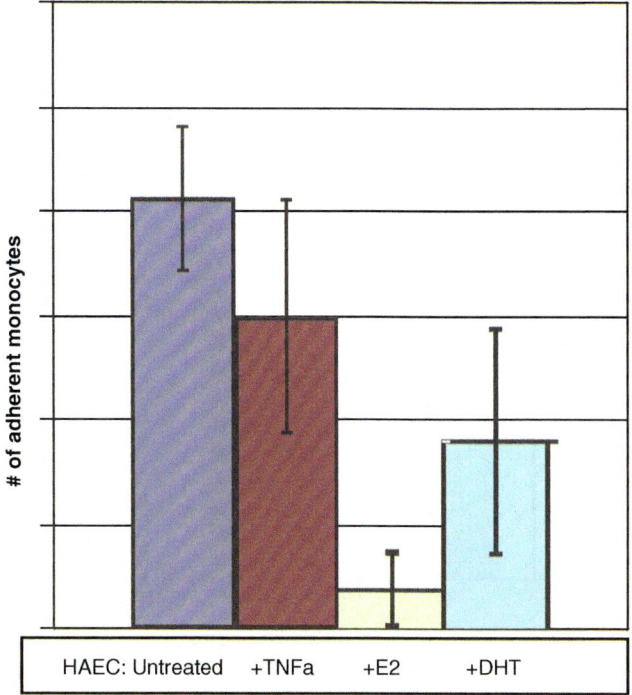

Fig. 15.6 From Curatola et al. [32], with permission. Initial, method-proving incubations including TNF as an inflammatory cytokine. In the absence of an effect of TNFα on the capture of monocytes, further incubations did not include added cytokines. Here we show the action of preincubation of physiological levels of estradiol and dihydrotestosterone (DHT) on monocyte capture. The addition of DHT was to avoid action via the estrogen receptor. The monocyte capture of DHT is commented upon in the discussion

Pretreatment with all steroids was accompanied by increased endothelial cell expression of immunoreactive PSA-nCAM (ir-PSA-NCAM) (Fig. 15.8).

Since DHEA and testosterone are metabolized to estrogen and aromatase and estrogen receptors are expressed in vascular endothelial cells, these results are consistent with an interaction with estrogen receptors being the root cause of blockade of monocyte binding by endothelial cells.

Of interest, the ring A-reduced androgen, dihydrotestosterone, was as effective as the other steroids in inducing polysialylation of nCAM and blocking monocyte binding. While this is compatible with the presence of androgen receptors, there is an alternative explanation that is associated with estrogen receptor action; DHT is metabolized to androstanedione, which binds to estrogen receptors [33–36]. This seems likely since androgen receptor knockout studies showed the inability of DHT-treated vascular endothelial cells to form tubes, which might have been due to the inability of the cells to form nCAM tethers that allowed their three-dimensional formation [37]. Resolution of this possibility will require the co-incubation of the DHT with the ER antagonist SERM, as was done with each of the other steroids.

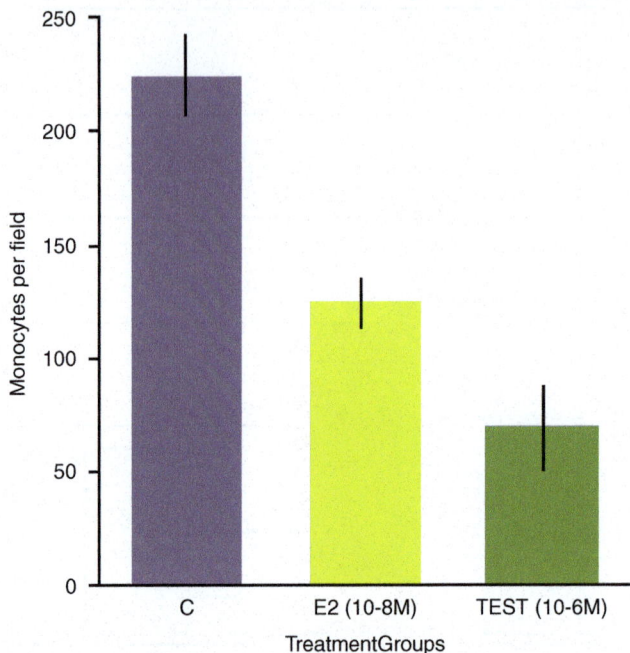

Fig. 15.7 From Curatola et al. [32], with permission, showing the result of incubating monocytes on a lawn of (female) human arterial endothelial cells (HAEC) and washing away the non-adherent cells after 40 min. The antiestrogen SERM fulvestrant blocked the E_2 (estradiol) effect, but not the test (testosterone) effect. All incubations were performed in triplicate and repeated at least twice. Vertical units: number of monocytes per standard field

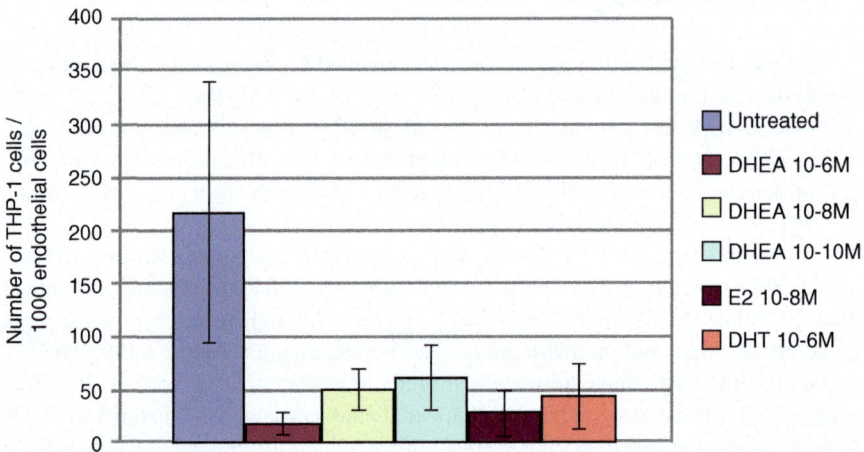

Fig. 15.8 From Curatola et al. [32], with permission, showing the result of incubating monocytes on a lawn of endothelial cells. Dehydroepiandrosterone (DHEA) showed a dose-response effect in blocking the capture of monocytes

In these preliminary studies, preincubation of the endothelial cells with the inflammatory cytokine, tumor necrosis factor alpha (TNFα), did not affect the number of monocytes bound. While there are several possibilities to explain this apparent lack of an inflammatory response by the endothelial cells, the answer may be related to the lack of subintimal stroma in our preparation, as stromal cells are targeted by TNFα [38]. If we are to realize the full potential of sex steroids to affect the capture of circulating leukocytes, further studies should test whether a layer of (vascular) stromal cells beneath the endothelial cell layer responds to TNFα and whether this increases the blockade of monocyte binding induced by estrogen. Alternatively, there may not have been sufficient disturbance of the endothelial cells in our static model [39]. Finally, the monocytes were not pretreated with either the test steroid or the cytokine, which may have stifled the response. Both possibilities will be rectified in future studies.

15.7   Conclusions

In addition to estrogen's well-known positive effects on risk factors for atherogenesis, there is a case for direct effects of estrogen and other sex steroids on the actual process of atherogenesis. We have shown repeatable, dose-related induction of sialylases and PSA-nCAM in human vascular (coronary arterial and umbilical) endothelial cells, and preincubation of human male and female coronary artery endothelial cells with estradiol and other estrogen-associated sex steroids diminished the number of monocytes captured by the endothelium. Estrogen's ability to prevent monocyte adhesion via induction of PSA-nCAM offers a novel molecular and translational explanation for a clinical phenomenon (estrogen-related cardioprotection) that has been observed for decades. The similar effects of other sex steroids on this experimental model may be explained through their relationship with estrogen receptor binding. While more study is required, it appears that breaking the very nexus of atherogenesis, as portrayed by Fig. 15.9, may account for some of the cardioprotective effects of estrogen (Fig. 15.10).

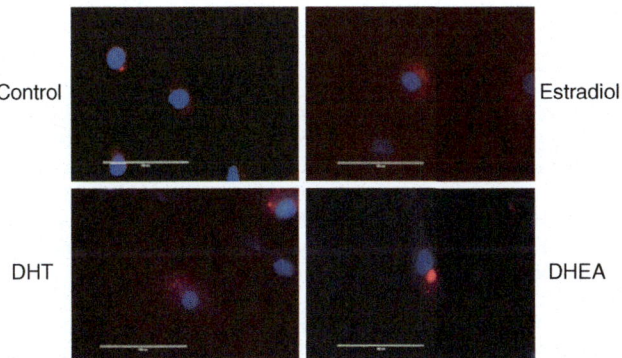

Fig. 15.9 Immunoreactive PSA-nCAM expression by human female coronary artery endothelial cells following 10-h incubation with test substances. Representative micrographs showing density of PSA-nCAM staining in red. The cell nuclei are stained blue with DAPI. From [32], with permission. The line measures 10 μm

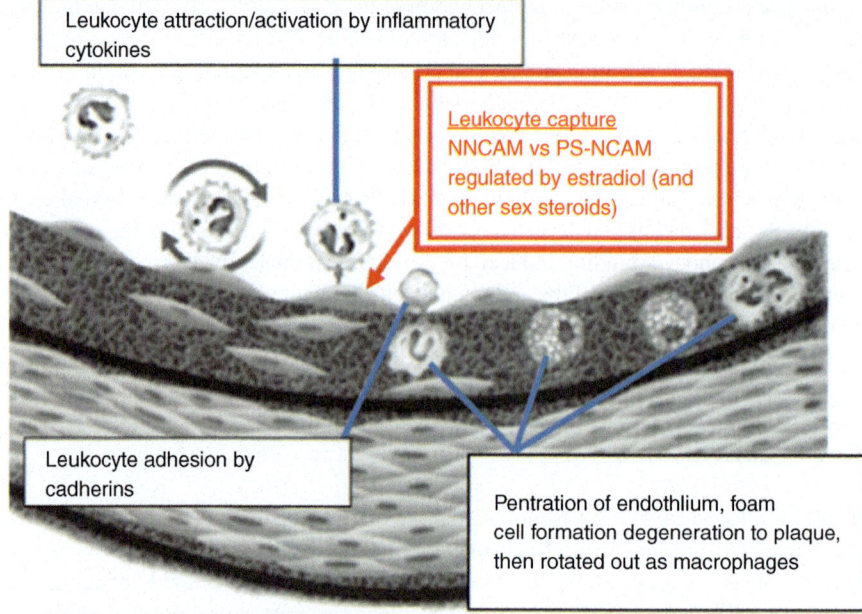

Leukocyte attraction/activation by inflammatory cytokines

Leukocyte capture
NNCAM vs PS-NCAM
regulated by estradiol (and other sex steroids)

Leukocyte adhesion by cadherins

Pentration of endothlium, foam cell formation degeneration to plaque, then rotated out as macrophages

P. Libby Am J Cl Nutr 2006 83 (2):456S-460S

Fig. 15.10 The sex steroid regulated nexus at which the capture and processing of circulating monocytes for the development of vascular plaque. Modified from Libby, with permission

Acknowledgments Support—NIH HL100769. Helpful conversations with Drs. Gil Mor and Andrei Kindzelski are gratefully acknowledged.

Support NIH HL 796100

Conflicts: None

References

1. Mendelsohn ME, Karas RH. Molecular and cellular basis of cardiovascular gender differences. Science. 2005;308(5728):1583–7.
2. Tunstall-Pedoe H. Myth and paradox of coronary risk and the menopause. Lancet. 1998;351:1425–7.
3. Colditz GA, Willet WC, Stampfer MJ, Rosner B, Speizer FE, Hennekens CH. Menopause and the risk of coronary heart disease in women. N Engl J Med. 1987;316:1105–10.
4. Salpeter SR, Cheng J, Thabane L, Buckley NS, Salpeter EE. Bayesian meta-analysis of hormone therapy and mortality in younger postmenopausal women. Am J Med. 2009;122(11):1016–22.
5. Kalantaridou SN, Naka KK, Papanikolaou E, Kazakos N, Kravariti M, Calis KA, Paraskevaidis EA, Sideris DA, Tsatsoulis A, Chrousos GP, Michalis LK. Impaired endothelial function in young women with premature ovarian failure: normalization with hormone therapy. J Clin Endocrinol Metab. 2004;89:3907–13.
6. Perez-Lopez FR, Chedraui P, Gilbert JJ, Perez-Roncero G. Cardiovascular risk in menopausal women and prevalent related co-morbid conditions: facing the post-Women's health initiative era. Fertil Steril. 2009;92:1171–86.
7. Stevenson JC, Crook D, Godsland IF. Influence of age and menopause on serum lipids and lipoproteins in healthy women. Atherosclerosis. 1993;98:83–90.

8. Rosenberg L, Hennekens CH, Rosner B, Belanger C, Rothman KJ, Speizer FE. Early menopause and the risk of myocardial infarction. Am J Obstet Gynecol. 1981;139(1):47–51.
9. Grodstein F, Manson JE, Colditz GA, Willett WC, Stampfer MJ. A prospective, observational study of postmenopausal hormone therapy and primary prevention of cardiovascular disease. Ann Intern Med. 2000;133(12):933–41.
10. Manson JE. Postmenopausal hormone therapy and atherosclerotic disease. Am Heart J. 1994;128(6 Pt 2):1337–43.
11. Hodis HN, Mack WJ, Shoupe D, et al. Testing the menopausal hormone therapy timing hypothesis: the Early vs Late Intervention Trial with Estradiol. Circulation. 2014;130:A13283.
12. Manson JE, Allison MA, Rossouw JE, Carr JJ, Langer RD, Hsia J, Kuller LH, Cochrane BB, Hunt JR, Ludlam SE, Pettinger MB, Gass M, Margolis KL, Nathan L, Ockene JK, Prentice RL, Robbins J, Stefanick ML. Estrogen therapy and coronary artery calcification. N Engl J Med. 2007;256:2591–602.
13. Poornima IG, Mackey RH, Allison MA, Manson JE, Carr JJ, LaMonte MJ, Chang Y, Kuller LH, WHI and WHI-CAC Study Investigators. Coronary artery calcification (CAC) and posttrial cardiovascular events and mortality within the women's health initiative (WHI) estrogen-alone trial. J Am Heart Assoc. 2017;6(11):e006887.
14. Ge QS, Tian QJ, Tseng H, Naftolin F. Development of low-dose reproductive hormone therapies in China. Gynecol Endocrinol. 2006;22:636–45.
15. Clarkson TB, Meléndez GC, Appt SE. Timing hypothesis for postmenopausal hormone therapy: its origin, current status, and future. Menopause. 2013;20:342–53.
16. Choi S, Steinberg E, Lee H, Naftalin F. The Timing Hypothesis remains a valid explanation of different cardioprotective effects of menopausal hormone treatment. Menopause. 2011;18(2):230–6.
17. Harman SM, Black DM, Naftolin F, et al. Arterial imaging outcomes and cardiovascular risk factors in recently menopausal women in the kronos early estrogen prevention study (KEEPS): a randomized controlled trial. Ann Intern Med. 2014;161(4):249–60.
18. Diano S, Horvath TL, Mor G, Register T, Adams M, Harada N, Naftolin F. Aromatase and estrogen receptor immunoreactivity in the coronary arteries of monkeys and human subjects. Menopause. 1999;6(1):21–8.
19. Bechmann I, Goldmann J, Kovac AD, Kwidzinski E, Simbürger E, Naftolin F, Dirnagl U, Nitsch R, Priller J. Circulating monocytic cells infiltrate layers of anterograde axonal degeneration where they transform into microglia. FASEB J. 2005;19(6):647–9.
20. Mor G, Nilsen J, Horvath T, Bechmann I, Brown S, Garcia-Segura LM, Naftolin F. Estrogen and microglia: a regulatory system that affects the brain. J Neurobiol. 1999;40(4):484–96.
21. Naftolin F, Mehr H, Fadiel A. Sex steroids block the initiation of atherosclerosis. Reprod Sci. 2016;23(12):1620–5.
22. Berliner JA, Territo MC, Sevanian A, et al. Minimally modified low density lipoprotein stimulates monocyte endothelial interactions. J Clin Invest. 1990;85:1260–6.
23. Berliner JA, Navab M, Fogelman AM, et al. Atherosclerosis: basic mechanisms. Oxidation, inflammation, and genetics. Circulation. 1995;91(9):2488–96.
24. Dong ZM, Chapman SM, Brown AA, Frenette PS, Hynes RO, Wagner DD. The combined role of P- and E-selectins in atherosclerosis. J Clin Invest. 1998;102:145–52.
25. Galkina E, Ley E. Vascular adhesion molecules in atherosclerosis. Atherioscler Thromb Vas Biol. 2007;27(11):2292–301.
26. Collins RG, Velji R, Guevara NV, Hicks MJ, Chan L, Beaudet AL. P-Selectin or intercellular adhesion molecule (ICAM)-1 deficiency substantially protects against atherosclerosis in apolipoprotein E- deficient mice. J Exp Med. 2000;191:189–94.
27. Garcia M, Miller VM, Gulati M, Hayes SN, Manson JE, Wenger NK, et al. Focused cardiovascular care for women: the need and role in clinical practice. Mayo Clin Proc. 2016;91:226–40.
28. Gascon E, Vutskits L, Kiss JZ. Polysialic acid-neural cell adhesion molecule in brain plasticity: from synapses to integration of new neurons. Brain Res Rev. 2007;56:101–18.

29. Rougon G. Structure, metabolism and cell biology of polysialic acids. Eur J Cell Biol. 1993;61(2):197–207.
30. Tan O, Fadiel A, Chang A, Demir N, Jeffrey R, Horvath T, Garcia-Segura LM, Naftolin F. Estrogens regulate posttranslational modification of neural cell adhesion molecule during the estrogen-induced gonadotropin surge. Endocrinology. 2009;150(6):2783–90.
31. Park H, Pagan L, Tan O, Fadiel A, Demir N, Huang K, Mittal K, Naftolin F. Estradiol regulates expression of polysialylated neural cell adhesion molecule by human vascular endothelial cells. Reprod Sci. 2010;17:1090–8.
32. Curatola AM, Huang K, Naftolin F. Dehydroepiandrosterone (DHEA) inhibition of monocyte binding by vascular endothelium is associated with sialylation of neural cell adhesion molecule. Reprod Sci. 2012;19:86–91.
33. Horst HJ, Dennis M, Kaufmann J, Voigt KD. In vivo uptake and metabolism of 3-h-5alpha-androstane-3alpha,17beta-diol and of 3-h-5alpha-androstane-3beta,17beta-diol by human prostatic hypertrophy. Acta Endocrinol. 1975;79(2):394–402.
34. Garcia M, Greene G, Rochefort H, Jensen EV. Effect of antibodies to estrogen receptor on the binding of 3H-labeled antiestrogens and androstanediol in the uterus. Endocrinology. 1982;110(4):1355–61.
35. Kuiper GG, Carlsson B, Grandien K, et al. Comparison of the ligand binding specificity and transcript tissue distribution of estrogen receptors. Endocrinology. 1997;138:863–70.
36. Frye CA, Ryan A, Rhodes M. Antiseizure effects of 3 alpha-androstanediol and/or 17beta-estradiol may involve actions at estrogen receptor beta. Epilepsy Behav. 2009;16(3):418–22.
37. Torres-Estay V, Carreño DV, Fuenzalida P, Watts A, San Francisco IF, Montecinos VP, Sotomayor PC, Ebos J, Smith GJ, Godoy AS. Androgens modulate male-derived endothelial cell homeostasis using androgen receptor-dependent and receptor-independent mechanisms. Angiogenesis. 2017;20(1):25–38.
38. Cardenas C, Alvero AB, Yun BS, Mor G. Redefining the origin and evolution of ovarian cancer: a hormonal connection. Endocr Relat Cancer. 2016;23(9):R411–22.
39. van Gils JM, Zwaginga JJ, Hordijk PL. Molecular and functional interactions among monocytes, platelets, and endothelial cells and their relevance for cardiovascular diseases. J Leukoc Biol. 2009;85(2):195–204.

Cardiovascular Risk in Climacteric Women: When to Begin the Hormone Treatment?

16

Néstor Siseles, Pamela Gutiérrez, Maria Alejandra Schüle, and Nilson Roberto de Melo

16.1 Introduction

Cardiovascular disease (CVD) is the main cause of death worldwide. More people die of CVD than of any other causes.

In both sexes and at any age, the risk of developing a cardiovascular disease is influenced by numerous factors, such as plasma concentration of lipids and lipoproteins,

N. Siseles (✉)
University of Buenos Aires (UBA), Buenos Aires, Argentina

Latin American Federation of the Societies of Climacteric and Menopause (FLASCYM), San Jose, Costa Rica

International Society of Gynecological Endocrinology (ISGE), Pisa, Italy

National Academy of Medicine of the Republic of Uruguay, Montevideo, Uruguay

International Menopause Society (IMS), Cornwall, UK

P. Gutiérrez
Argentine Society of Menopause (AAPEC), Buenos Aires, Argentina

M. A. Schüle
Argentine Society of Menopause (AAPEC), Buenos Aires, Argentina

Menopause Section, Cordoba Society of Obst/Gynec (SOGC), Cordoba, Cordoba, Argentina

N. R. de Melo
Latin American Federation of the Societies of Climacteric and Menopause (FLASCYM), San Jose, Costa Rica

International Society of Gynecological Endocrinology (ISGE), Pisa, Italy

Brazilian Federation of Societies of Gynecology and Obstetrics (FEBRASGO), Sala, Brazil

Latin American Federation of Societies of Obstetrics and Gynecology (FLASOG), San Jose, Costa Rica

Brazilian Society of Human Reproduction (SBRH), Sala, Brazil

Ibero American Society of Osteology and Mineral Metabolism (SIBOMM), Lisbon, Portugal

© International Society of Gynecological Endocrinology 2019
R. D. Brinton et al. (eds.), *Sex Steroids' Effects on Brain, Heart and Vessels*, ISGE Series, https://doi.org/10.1007/978-3-030-11355-1_16

uric acid and fibrinogen, carbohydrate intolerance or diabetes mellitus, obesity, hypertension, family history, and habits such as smoking and a sedentary lifestyle.

In women, postmenopause further increases the relative risk of a cardiovascular disease.

Prevention is achieved through an early reduction in risk factors and changes in lifestyle, weight, and blood pressure. With this end in view, it is essential that gynecologists and cardiologists work together as a team [1].

Addressing the menopausal woman's cardiovascular health, JoAnn Manson [2] stressed the need for personalized medicine to allow the identification of appropriate candidates for menopausal hormone therapy (MHT).

She maintained that biological and/or clinical characteristics could modify the response to MHT and, therefore, that some women are more suitable candidates than others to receive the treatment. Hence, it is important to personalize the optimal dose, the formula, and the administration route. In addition, it is essential to determine the MHT effects on the cardiovascular disease early on, assess whether there is a particular group of women whose risk of CVD may increase or diminish with therapy, and clarify the differences between the research protocols according to the MHT administration route in relation to the cardiovascular system.

16.2 Basic Research Work

In their basic investigation using animal models with Monas, Clarkson et al. [3] demonstrated, as shown in Fig. 16.1, the effect of estrogens on coronary artery disease according to time of MHT initiation.

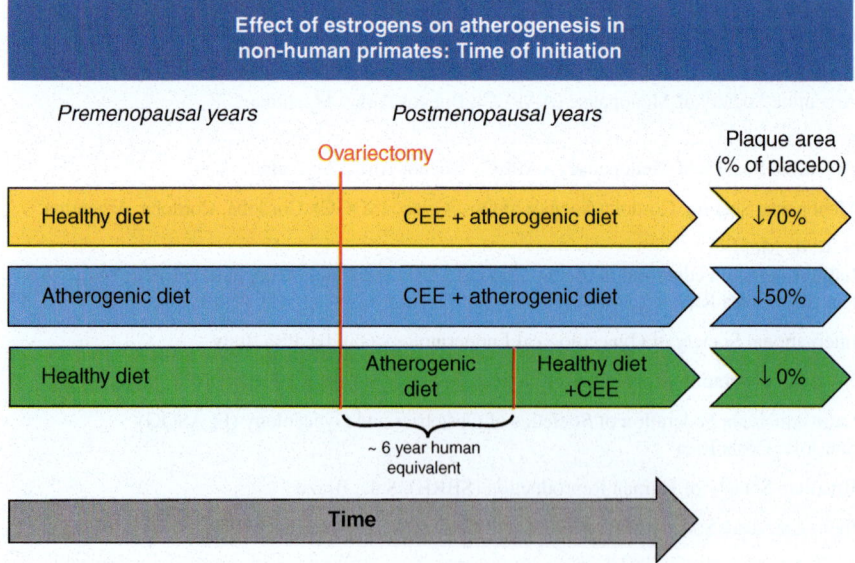

Fig. 16.1 Cardiovascular and metabolic risks and benefits. Adapted from Clarkson TB. *Menopause*. 2013 Mar;20(3):342–53

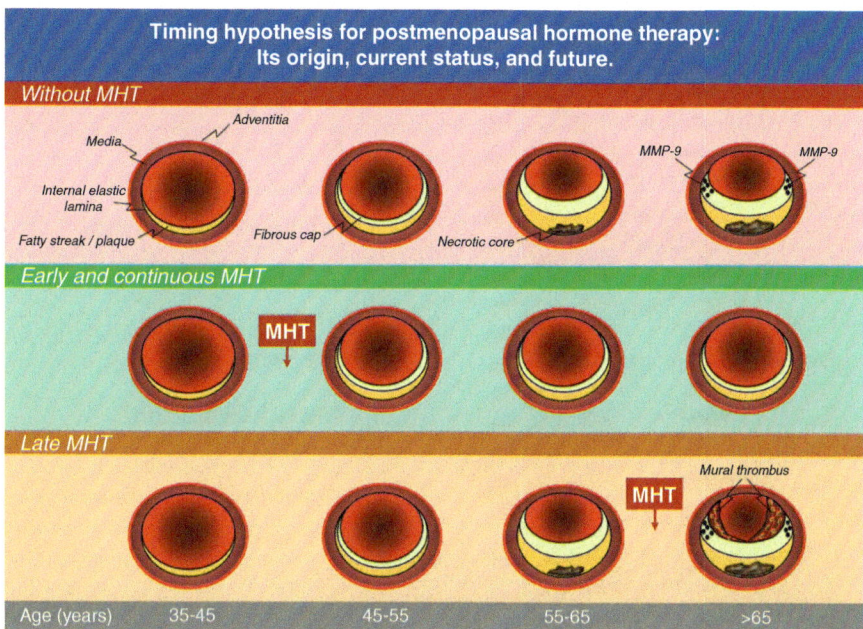

Fig. 16.2 Timing hypothesis for postmenopausal hormone therapy: its origin, current status, and future

The findings indicate the importance of initiating MHT immediately after menopause to allow for the removal of atheromatous plaques from a larger area.

In these animal models, according to the graph in Fig. 16.2, it can be seen that if MHT is undergone early on and continuously, the atheromatous plaques do not increase, whereas if the treatment initiates later on, progression is not only unhindered, but it also has a harmful effect. This is essentially due to estrogen-induced enzyme stimulation of matrix metalloproteases, which destabilizes the plaques and, therefore, poses a risk of embolism and its consequences (Fig. 16.2).

Mendelsohn et al. [4] reported the effect of estrogens (E2) on arteries in early menopause in comparison with late menopause as can be seen in Fig. 16.3.

It is clearly demonstrated that, in early menopause, estrogens produce an increase in vasodilation, a reduction in inflammatory factors, and a slowdown in the progression of the atherosclerotic lesion. On the other hand, in late menopause, estrogens can be seen to have the reverse effect, that is, a decrease in vasodilation, an increase in inflammatory factors, and greater instability in the atherosclerotic plaques (Fig. 16.3).

16.3   Clinical Trials

What do randomized controlled clinical trials, such as the Women's Health Initiative (WHI), show us?

In WHI, 64% of the enrolled women were older adults with more than 10 years of menopause. Furthermore, over 36% were hypertensive, 50% had been smokers, and most were obese, all of which features are risk factors for CVD [5].

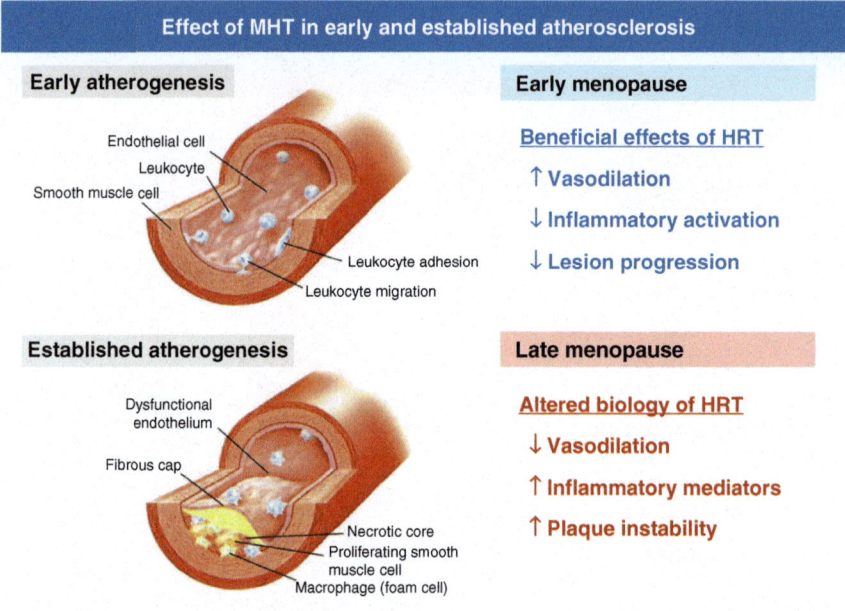

Fig. 16.3 Effect of MHT in early and established atherosclerosis

This is the reason WHI is not an ideal study for assessing MHT and primary prevention of CVD.

Contrariwise, observational studies, such as the cohort study of nurses [6], and randomized clinical studies, such as KEEPS [7] and ELITE [8, 9], recruited younger women with a healthier and more intact vascular endothelium, more favorably responsive to estrogen action.

Among the randomized controlled clinical trials of *secondary prevention of CVD and MHT*, that is, studies including patients with a history of CVD, we found HERS [10] and ERA [11]; we should also include WHI [5]. Though the latter was initially considered a study of primary prevention, in fact, it should not have been, given the aforementioned characteristics of its population.

Among the randomized controlled clinical trials of *primary prevention of CVD and MHT*, we found KEEPS [7], ELITE [8], and the DANISH STUDY [12]. We also included the observational cohort study of nurses in this group [6].

Taylor and Manson suggested a complex interplay of vasomotor symptoms, MHT, and cardiovascular risk [13].

The results of the stratified secondary analysis of WHI show that conjugated equine estrogens (CEE) alone may be associated with a diminished risk of CVD in women in the 50–59 age range.

In Table 16.1 and in Graph 16.1, Rossouw et al. [14] point out the risks as well as the metabolic and cardiovascular benefits of MHT according to age and time since menopause.

Table 16.1 Cardiovascular and metabolic risks and benefits

CHD events by age and time since menopause in the WHI studies

	CEE	CEE/MPA
	RR (CI)	RR (CI)
Age (year)		
50–59	0.63 (0.36–1.09)	1.29 (0.79–2.12)
60–69	0.94 (0.71–1.24)	1.03 (0.74–1.43)
70–79	1.13 (0.82–1.54)	1.48 (104–2.11)
p value for trend	0.12	0.70
Time since menopause (year)		
<10	0.48 (0.20–1.17)	0.88 (0.54–1.43)
10–19	0.96 (0.64–1.44)	1.23 (0.85–1.77)
≥20	1.12 (0.86–1.46)	1.66 (1.14–2.41)
p value for trend	0.15	0.05

Adapted from Rossouw JE, et al. *JAMA*. 2008;299:1426

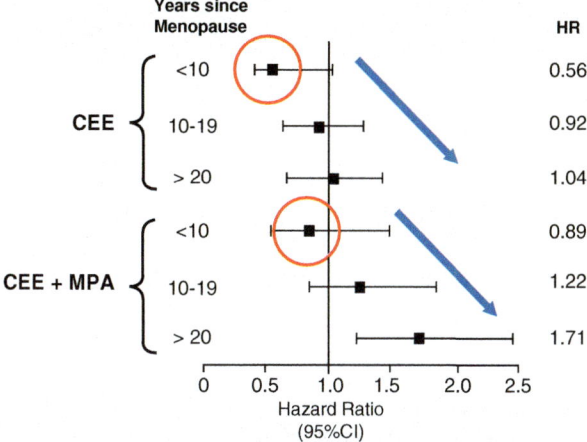

Graph 16.1 Effect of estrogens on atherogenesis in non-human primates: time of initiation

It can be seen that women did not have an increase in cardiovascular risk if MHT was initiated within 10 years of menopause and if they were under 60 years of age (RR 0.48 [CI 0.20–1.17] for CEE and RR 0.88 [CI 0.54–1.43] for CEE and medroxyprogesterone acetate [MPA]).

Santen et al. [15] at a wide-ranging consensus with the participation of endocrinologists, gynecologists, basic and clinical researchers, etc. concluded that basic sciences, animal models, and observational studies support the hypothesis that MHT prevents atherosclerosis and reduces coronary events. Additionally, the analysis of subgroups suggests that the little benefit or the small increase in risk seen in CVDs in the WHI is the result of MHT use by elderly women or postmenopausal women.

A group of researchers of the WHI study [16], most of whom were epidemiologists, wanted to determine whether the effects of CEE, used alone by a group of female volunteers with a previous hysterectomy, would remain after the end of the treatment. To this end, they obtained a written statement of informed consent from 7645 women who had received CEE or placebo and followed them up until August 2009 (totaling 75 months), which means an analysis spanning 10.7 years of follow-up.

The age-stratified results are of considerable interest. The cohort was divided into three age groups: 50–59, 60–69, and 70–79 years. It should be emphasized that taking CEE is much more favorable to younger than to older women. For the former, with the exception of those taking placebo, it meant fewer CVDs and acute myocardial infarctions (AMI), fewer breast cancers, fewer mortalities, and fewer events contributing to the global index of chronic diseases. These data, when translated into absolute numbers, indicate that for every 10,000 women under 60 receiving CEE, there is an expected fallout of 12 AMIs, 13 deaths, and 18 events lowering the global index.

In 2012, Hodis et al. [17] published a study emphasizing the hypothesis that there is a time for preventing coronary disease with HT and they reached the conclusion that an early rather than a later prescription conditions the beneficial effects of HT. They further stressed that to maximize the beneficial effects of MHT on CVD and minimize risks, treatment should start during the *"window of opportunity*," that is, before age 60 and/or with less than 10 years of menopause and continue for 6 years or more.

16.4   Clinical Trials in Primary Prevention of CVD

The recent randomized controlled clinical trials in primary prevention are the following:

1. *ELITE* (Early vs. Late Intervention Trial with Estradiol) [8]
2. *KEEPS* (Kronos Early Estrogen Prevention Study) [7]
3. *DOPS* (Danish Osteoporosis Prevention Study) [12]

16.4.1 ELITE (Early vs. Late Intervention Trial with Estradiol) [8]

The ELITE study, whose chief researcher was Howard Hodis, enrolled 643 women. The inclusion criteria and the design were as follows:

- Women <6 or >10 years since menopause
- Serum estradiol <25 pg/ml
- Amenorrhea >6 months
- Oral estradiol (1 mg/day) or placebo with 4% vaginal progesterone gel or placebo for 10 days/month
- Assessment of the carotid intima-media thickness and of coronary calcification

The hypothesis being tested was whether 17β-estradiol could reduce atherosclerosis progression with therapy initiating in the immediate postmenopausal period when the endothelium is still healthy as opposed to a later initiation when the endothelium is unresponsive. Ultrasonography enables the measurement of the changes taking place in carotid thickness, and cardiac computed tomography (CCT) quantifies coronary artery calcium and arterial lesions.

The ELITE was specifically designed to test the hypothesis of "time of initiation" of MHT in relation to atherosclerotic progression and cognitive changes in postmenopause. It was a double-blind, placebo-controlled study in which women were randomized according to their time of menopause (<6 years, $n = 271$ or >10 years, $n = 370$) prior to enrollment in the study. The first results with respect to atherosclerosis pertained to the progression of the carotid intima-media thickness following 5–6 years of 1 mg/day of oral 17β-estradiol with or without 4% vaginal progesterone gel in contrast with placebo.

The second results relative to atherosclerosis included the CCT scans with or without contrast enhancement taken of the participants who completed the study.

In 2016, the final results of the ELITE studies were published [9]. They emphasized that estradiol use was associated with a slower progression of subclinical atherosclerosis than placebo (measured as CIMT) when MHT started within 6 postmenopausal years, but not when it began 10 or more years after menopause.

Estradiol had no significant effect on atherosclerosis as measured by CCT in any of the groups of postmenopausal women.

The ELITE study provided evidence substantiating the hypothesis that multiple benefits are obtainable when MHT begins around the onset of menopause (*"time hypothesis"* or *"window of opportunity"*) and that MHT does not increase the cardiovascular risk in healthy and recently menopausal women [9].

The authors maintain that further evidence is needed to support the relationship between MHT duration and cardiovascular events. They also stress that more studies of micronized natural progesterone and of synthetic progestins are necessary.

16.4.2 KEEPS (Kronos Early Estrogen Prevention Study) [7]

The KEEPS study is another study of primary prevention, whose working hypothesis was that there is a *"window of opportunity"* in early menopause for hormone therapy to have a cardioprotective effect.

The study had the following objectives:

- To determine the effects of MHT started by 737 recently menopausal women (mean age: 52 years) on atherosclerotic progression
- To compare the effects of CEE via the oral route (OR) and of E2 via the transdermal route (TD) with placebo in relation to risk factors for CVD and venous thromboembolism (VTE)
- To assess the safety of micronized natural progesterone

The KEEPS found that, in the treatment groups, neither the oral route nor the transdermal route affected arterial pressure in contrast with the high CEE doses used in the WHI. The oral route was associated with an increase in HDL-chol and a decrease in LDL-chol, albeit with a rise in TG. The transdermal route was neutral relative to the biomarkers with the additional advantage that it improved sensitivity to insulin (insulin resistance decreased) as calculated by HOMA-IR [7].

During the 48 months of hormone replacement therapy (HRT) vs. placebo, there were no effects on atherosclerosis progression as measured by carotid ultrasound and there was a tendency toward diminished accumulation of coronary calcium as quantified by CCT.

The conclusion was that HRT with the doses used in the population of healthy recently menopausal women neither slows down nor speeds up atherosclerosis progression as assessed by imaging. The study showed the favorable effects of MHT in recently menopausal women. The need for individualizing decision-making with respect to MHT is stressed, given that the oral and the transdermal routes have different effects and different women have different symptom profiles and treatment priorities [7].

16.4.3 DOPS (Danish Osteoporosis Prevention Study) (Effect of Hormone Replacement Therapy on Cardiovascular Events in Recently Menopausal Women: Randomized Trial) [12]

The DOPS is a study of 1006 healthy recently menopausal women aged 45–58 years, 502 of whom received HRT. These were divided into two groups, as follows: Group 1, 2/1 mg of 17β E2 + 1 mg of norethisterone acetate (NETA), 10 days, and Group 2, 2 mg of E2/day (hysterectomized); and 504 comprised the control group.

The objective was to evaluate the long-term effect of MHT on CVD in recently menopausal women, and the endpoints were mortality, heart failure, and AMI.

This study is considered the first randomized controlled clinical trial of healthy women treated in immediate postmenopause with 17β E2 and NETA, and it is the only one with 10 years of randomized treatment. In addition, the women were followed up for 6 more years after the end of therapy [12].

The findings suggest that starting MHT in early menopause reduces the risk of a combined endpoint of mortality, AMI, and heart failure. Early initiation of MHT and its prolonged use did not increase the risk of breast cancer or cerebrovascular accident (CVA).

16.5 The International Menopause Society (IMS) Comments on the Danish Study [12]

Commenting on DOPS, Prof. Howard Hodis said it was the only randomized controlled study (RCT) designed for the long term and which included women close to menopause for the MHT. He added that it provided evidence that the preventive benefits surpassed the risks and that the study confirmed the data accumulated in the last 50 years indicating that MHT reduces CVD and mortality when prescribed for women in immediate postmenopause.

He went on to say that the study produced additional evidence to contradict the concept that "a lower dose and for the shortest possible time" is preferable. This postulate, which never had a scientific basis, can keep women from obtaining the benefits associated with long-term use of MHT: a reduction in cardiovascular diseases, bone fractures, and total mortality [12].

Prof. John Stevenson remarked that the study, which had a 16-year follow-up, had no significant adverse events. This is evidence that MHT, when prescribed for women around the onset of menopause, in the long term produces consistent benefits as demonstrated by other studies. The importance of this study is its long duration, its initiation in early menopause, and its therapy individualization [12].

16.6   Consensus on MHT and CVD

In 2012, experts from the most representative societies related to menopause (the American Society for Reproductive Medicine, the Asia Pacific Menopause Federation, the Endocrine Society, the European Menopause and Andropause Society, the International Menopause Society, the International Osteoporosis Foundation, and the North American Menopause Society) got together and wrote a short and simple document about the points of consensus on MHT.

This Global Consensus Statement on Menopausal Hormone Therapy was published in specialty journals such as Maturitas [18] and the most important CVD-related points are the following:

– The RCT and observational studies, along with meta-analyses, show that estrogens, as those used in MHT, may reduce CVDs and the causes of mortality in women younger than 60 and with less than 10 years of menopause.
– The data on estrogens + progestogens in this population show a similar tendency, but some RCTs did not find a significant increase or decrease in CVDs.

In 2016, a revision of this consensus was published with the inclusion of FLASCYM (Federación Latinoamericana de Sociedades de Climaterio y Menopausia) [19] aiming to update and broaden the previous consensus points.

It corroborates MHT, including tibolone and the association of conjugated equine estrogens (CEEs) with a SERM (bazedoxifene), as the most effective therapy for treating vasomotor symptoms associated with menopause. However, the benefits outdo the risks when women start therapy before age 60 or with less than 10 years of menopause.

It emphasizes the difference between ET and combined MHT, the difference in risk of VTE and ischemic stroke between the oral and transdermal routes, and the fact that MHT should be individualized and its duration should be a function of treatment objectives and safety issues.

16.7 Final Considerations

- In the menopausal transition, the risk of a CVD increases.
- Hormonal changes increase the vulnerability of the cardiovascular system.
- The gynecologist is the primary care physician for:
  - Identifying the risk factors for CVD
  - Educating women to age in a healthy way
  - Treating or preventing the progression of emerging CVDs
- The MHT poses no danger to the cardiovascular system; on the contrary, if it is given to the right woman and at the right time, it may reduce the risk of CVD: the *"window of opportunity"* should be emphasized.
- Every woman is unique and has her own risk profile; thus, MHT should be tailored to her and her preferences, adjusting to the responses.
- If followed, these recommendations should lead to a better quality of life and increase the life expectancy of our patients.

References

1. Collins P, et al. Management of cardiovascular risk in the peri-menopausal woman: a consensus statement of European cardiologists and gynaecologists. Eur Heart J. 2007;28:2028–40. ISGE Congress, Florence, 2016.
2. Manson JE. The role of personalized medicine in identifying appropriate candidates for menopausal estrogen therapy. Metabolism. 2013;62(Suppl 1):S15–9.
3. Clarkson TB, et al. Timing hypothesis for postmenopausal hormone therapy: its origin, current status, and future. Menopause. 2013;20(3):342–53.
4. Mendelsohn ME, Karas RH. Molecular and cellular basis of cardiovascular gender differences. Science. 2005;308:1583–7.
5. WHI. Writing group for the women's health initiative investigators risks and benefits of estrogen plus progestin in healthy postmenopausal women. JAMA. 2002;288:321–33.
6. Grodstein F, et al. A prospective observational study of postmenopausal hormone therapy and primary prevention of cardiovascular disease. Ann Intern Med. 2000;133:933–41.
7. Harman M et al. NAMS 23rd Annual Meeting, 3–6 October 2012.
8. Hodis HN, et al. The early versus late intervention trial with estradiol: a randomized trial to test the timing. NAMS Annual Meeting, October 8, 2013.
9. Hodis HN, et al. Vascular effects of early vs late postmenopausal treatment with estradiol. N Engl J Med. 2016;374:1221–31.
10. Hulley S, et al. Randomized trial of estrogen plus progestin for secondary prevention of coronary heart disease in postmenopausal women. Heart and Estrogen/progestin Replacement Study (HERS Research Group). JAMA. 1998;280:605–13.
11. Lakoski S, et al. Interleukin-10 concentration and coronary heart disease (CHD). Event risk in the estrogen replacement and atherosclerosis (ERA) study. Atherosclerosis. 2008;197:443–7.
12. Schierbeck LL, et al. Effect of hormone replacement therapy on cardiovascular events in recently menopausal women: randomised trial (Danish Study). BMJ. 2012;345:e6409.
13. Taylor H, Manson JAE. Update in hormone therapy use in menopause. J Clin Endocrinol Metabol. 2011;96:255–64.
14. Rossouw JE, et al. Postmenopausal hormone therapy and risk of cardiovascular disease by age and years since menopause. JAMA. 2008;299:1426. 297:1465–1477.

15. Santen RJ, et al. Scientific statement: postmenopausal hormone therapy. J Clin Endocrinol Metab. 2010;95(Suppl 1):S7–S66.
16. La Croix A, et al. Health outcomes after stopping conjugated equine estrogens among post-menopausal women with prior hysterectomy. JAMA. 2011;305(13):1305–14.
17. Hodis NH, et al. The timing hypothesis for coronary heart disease prevention with hormone therapy: past, present and future in perspective. Climacteric. 2012;15(3):217–21.
18. de Villiers TJ, et al. Global Consensus Statement on menopausal hormone therapy. Maturitas. 2013;74:391–2.
19. de Villiers TJ, et al. Revised Global Consensus Statement on menopausal hormone therapy. Maturitas. 2016;91:153–5.

HRT for the Primary Prevention of Coronary Heart Disease

17

John C. Stevenson

17.1 Introduction

Coronary heart disease (CHD) is a leading cause of death in women. Many risk factors for CHD are common to both men and women [1], and treatment of conditions such as diabetes mellitus, hypertension and abdominal obesity will contribute to the primary prevention of CHD. Of the lifestyle factors, smoking is the most important as it has now been shown that even one cigarette per day is associated with a major increase in cardiovascular disease [2]. The loss of ovarian function at the menopause leads to an increase in CHD [3], and this chapter will examine the effects of hormone replacement therapy (HRT) in the primary prevention of CHD.

17.2 Metabolic Effects of HRT

Low-density lipoprotein (LDL) cholesterol is a proven causal factor of atherosclerosis [4], and estrogen replacement results in a decrease in total and LDL cholesterol [5]. High density lipoprotein (HDL) cholesterol is associated with a reduction in CHD particularly in postmenopausal women [6], and estrogen also induces an increase in HDL cholesterol [5]. These effects are greater with oral than with transdermal estrogen. Triglycerides are an independent risk factor for CHD, more so in women than in men [7]. Triglycerides are increased with oral estrogen but decreased with transdermal estrogen administration [5]. Estrogen effects on lipids and lipoproteins may be modified by progestogen administration. Androgenic progestogens such as norethisterone acetate (NETA) and medroxyprogesterone acetate (MPA) can blunt the increase in HDL but may also blunt the increase in triglycerides induced by

J. C. Stevenson (✉)
National Heart & Lung Institute, Imperial College London, Royal Brompton Hospital, London, UK
e-mail: j.stevenson@imperial.ac.uk

© International Society of Gynecological Endocrinology 2019
R. D. Brinton et al. (eds.), *Sex Steroids' Effects on Brain, Heart and Vessels*,
ISGE Series, https://doi.org/10.1007/978-3-030-11355-1_17

oral estrogens [5]. This is also seen to a lesser extent when bazedoxifene is used in place of a progestogen [8]. Non-androgenic progestogens such as micronized progesterone and dydrogesterone do not impede the increase in HDL [9]. Elevated lipoprotein (a) is another independent risk factor for CHD [10], and its levels are reduced by HRT [9, 11]. Thus overall HRT has a favourable impact on lipids and lipoproteins, but the types of hormones and routes of administration can be tailored to achieve the best effects according to the individual's lipid profile.

Insulin resistance is another important metabolic risk factor for CHD [12]. Oral oestradiol improves glucose tolerance and reduces insulin resistance more than transdermal oestradiol [13]. High-dose, but not low-dose, conjugated equine estrogens can impair glucose tolerance. These effects on glucose and insulin metabolism can be modified by the addition of progestogens. Androgenic progestogens such as NETA [13] and MPA [14] increase insulin resistance, whilst non-androgenic progestogens such as micronized oral progesterone [15] and dydrogesterone [16] are neutral in this respect.

Increased central fat and abdominal obesity are directly related to the development of cardiovascular disease [17]. HRT reduces the central deposition of body fat [18], thus reversing the effect of menopause on body fat distribution. Oral estrogens increase coagulation activation and are associated with a transient increase in venous thromboembolism (VTE) [19]. This is avoided with the use of transdermal estrogen [20] and possibly reduced with low-dose oral estrogen.

17.3 Vascular Effects of HRT

Estrogen induces vasodilatation by a number of different mechanisms. It acts directly on the vascular endothelium to increase nitric oxide synthase levels and hence the production of nitric oxide (NO), a potent vasodilator [21]. NO is involved in the regulation of blood pressure, platelet function, inhibition of vascular smooth muscle proliferation and expression of adhesion molecules. Estrogen reduces the release of the potent vasoconstrictor, endothelin-1 [22]. It also inhibits calcium channels and activates BKCa channels, both of which are vasodilatory [23]. Estrogen reduces angiotensin-converting enzyme activity [24] and is usually associated with small decreases in blood pressure. The addition of drospirenone, a progestogen with antimineralocorticoid effects, results in a further decrease in blood pressure [25]. Estrogen has a dose-dependent effect on matrix metalloproteinases (MMPs) which are involved with vascular remodelling [26]. Thus high-dose estrogen can induce a large increase in MMPs which could potentially destabilise atheromatous plaques, but at lower doses the smaller increase in MMPs may normalise the remodelling processes and potentially reduce atheroma formation.

17.4 HRT Effects on CHD Incidence

Many observational studies have shown that postmenopausal HRT use is associated with a 40–50% reduction in cardiovascular outcomes, primarily CHD events. This is well illustrated by the Nurses' Health Study where a reduction in coronary events was seen soon after initiation of therapy and persisted for up to 10 years of use [27]. There is also good evidence that HRT use is associated with reduced CHD mortality. In a study of over 90,000 women, those initiating HRT below age 60 years showed a significant reduction in CHD death, whereas in those initiating HRT above age 60 years, the reduction was non-significant [28]. To compliment this finding, another study using Finnish national registry data examined the effects of stopping HRT on cardiovascular outcomes [29]. The standardised mortality ratios of 330,000 postmenopausal women who discontinued HRT were compared with those expected for the general population. A significant increase in mortality was seen during the first year after HRT cessation, but thereafter returned to that expected. When the standard mortality ratios of these women who ceased HRT use was compared with those of women continuing HRT rather than the general population, the mortality was higher during the first year following HRT cessation and was still significantly increased beyond the first year. This is probably due to the continuing CHD benefit of HRT for those remaining on the treatment. What is not known from the registry data is whether the women discontinuing HRT did so abruptly or gradually. This issue is clearly very important and has yet to be addressed, but it seems biologically more likely that sudden cessation of HRT would have a more adverse outcome.

17.5 HRT Effects on CHD Surrogates

Numerous studies looking at the effects of HRT on surrogate outcomes for CHD have been conducted. A series of studies of cynomolgus macaques gave rise to the concept of the timing hypothesis or window of opportunity for CHD prevention. In an initial study [30], monkeys were given a normal diet, made surgically menopausal and then given an atherogenic diet and randomised to either conjugated equine estrogens or placebo. At the end of the study, the amount of atheromatous plaque was reduced by 70% in the estrogen group compared with placebo. In a second study [31], the monkeys were put on an atherogenic diet to induce atheroma formation before being made surgically menopausal. They continued on the atherogenic diet and were randomised to either conjugated equine estrogens or placebo. At the end of this study, the estrogen group still had 50% less atheromatous plaque than the placebo group. In a third study [32], the monkeys were made surgically menopausal and put onto an atherogenic diet, but there was then a delay of the equivalent of 6 human years before being randomised to conjugated equine estrogens or placebo. At the end of this study, there was no difference in atheromatous plaque between the estrogen and placebo groups. These studies suggested that intervention with HRT fairly soon after the menopause is needed to get CHD benefit. There are human studies which support this timing hypothesis. A clinical trial of healthy women in the early postmenopausal period showed less progression of atheroma as assessed by ultrasound measurement of carotid artery intima-media thickness in those randomised to oral oestradiol compared with placebo [33]. In the ELITE trial comprising almost 650 healthy postmenopausal women treated for around 6 years, oral oestradiol 1 mg daily reduced carotid artery atheroma progression if initiated within 6 years of the onset of menopause, whilst no such effect was seen in those initiating treatment beyond

10 years postmenopause [34]. However, no effect was seen on coronary artery calcium scores. The KEEPS trial enrolled over 700 women within 3 years of menopause onset and randomised them to either conjugated equine estrogens 0.45 mg daily, transdermal oestradiol 50 µg or placebo [35]. After 4 years, there was no difference between the groups in terms of carotid artery intima-media thickness changes or those of coronary artery calcification scores. It has been suggested that the women were too healthy to show any change in atheroma development.

A highly accurate epigenetic marker of ageing has been studied in large populations of women to assess the effects of menopause [36]. It was found that HRT use was associated with a lower epigenetic age compared with non-users. Recently a cross-sectional study has been conducted in postmenopausal women looking at cardiac structure and function, which are markers of subclinical cardiovascular disease [37]. Postmenopausal women participating in the UK Biobank who were free of known cardiovascular disease and had undergone cardiac magnetic resonance imaging were included. Five hundred and thirteen women had used HRT for 3 or more years, whilst 1091 women were non-users. The groups were of similar age at menopause. The HRT users had significantly smaller left ventricle and left atrium volumes, which have been linked to favourable cardiovascular outcomes.

17.6   HRT Effects on CHD Clinical Endpoints

Several randomised clinical trials have been conducted for both primary and secondary prevention of CHD events. The secondary prevention trials have not shown any significant reduction in coronary outcomes, but in all of these studies, the doses of estrogen used were inappropriately high for the age of the populations [38]. It remains possible that different types of hormones, doses and routes of administration could have different outcomes. The largest primary prevention randomised clinical trial was the Women's Health Initiative (WHI) [39]. 16,608 postmenopausal women, mean age 63 years, were randomised to conjugated equine estrogens 0.625 mg plus MPA 2.5 mg daily or placebo. After 5.6 years of intervention, there was no overall benefit for CHD events with the HRT. In the WHI estrogen alone arm, 10,739 hysterectomised women, mean age 63 years, received conjugated equine estrogens 0.625 mg alone or placebo. After 7.2 years of intervention, there was no significant difference between estrogen and placebo groups in the primary outcome of myocardial infarction or coronary death. However, there was a significant reduction in coronary interventions and in a composite CHD outcome in those initiating estrogen treatment below age 60 years compared with placebo, and these women were subsequently shown to have less coronary atheroma than those who had taken placebo [40]. Furthermore, with long-term follow-up post-intervention in those women initiating estrogen alone treatment below age 60 years, there was a significant reduction in CHD events compared with placebo [39]. The Danish Osteoporosis Prevention Study (DOPS) was a 10 year prospective clinical trial of over 1000 women in the early postmenopause which randomised healthy women to oral oestradiol 2 mg daily plus NETA if non-hysterectomised, or to no treatment [41]. There was an additional 6 year observational post-trial follow-up.

Women on HRT had a significant reduction of a composite endpoint of myocardial infarction, death or hospital admission with heart failure, although the number of events was small because of the relatively young age of the participants. A meta-analysis of 23 randomised clinical trials of HRT versus placebo or no treatment included over 39,000 women [42]. Those initiating HRT below age 60 years or within 10 years of menopause had a one-third reduction in the endpoint of myocardial infarction or death. Those initiating HRT above age 60 years or beyond 10 years of menopause had an increase in events during the first year but then showed a 20% reduction after 2 years. A more recent meta-analysis of 19 randomised clinical trials of HRT versus placebo or no treatment included over 49,000 women [43]. Those initiating HRT within 10 years of menopause had a 50% reduction in the endpoint of myocardial infarction or death, whilst there was no significant change in those initiating HRT beyond 10 years postmenopause. The optimal duration of HRT use for CHD prevention remains to be determined, but need not necessarily be lifelong. Women who took part in randomised placebo-controlled trials of HRT for prevention of postmenopausal bone loss in the early postmenopause and subsequently had no further treatment were followed for up to 15 years [44]. Those women who had been randomised to HRT and took it for 2–3 years had significantly less aortic calcification and cardiovascular death subsequently than those randomised to placebo.

17.7 HRT and Safety Issues

Finally, there is growing evidence for the safety of HRT. In the DOPS trial there was no increase in adverse outcomes with HRT, including stroke, VTE and all cancers including breast cancer, during the 16 years of intervention plus observational follow-up [41]. A Bayesian meta-analysis of HRT and all-cause mortality in women below age 60 years participating in randomised trials of HRT included 16,000 women from 19 trials [45]. There was a significant reduction in mortality in HRT users of around 25%. A Cochrane review showed a reduction in all-cause mortality of 30% in women initiating HRT within 10 years of the onset of menopause [43]. For all ages, there was a neutral effect (RR 1.0, CI 0.89–1.12). These findings are also reflected by the 18-year follow-up of the WHI trials [46]. For all ages there was a neutral effect on all-cause mortality in both the estrogen-progestogen and estrogen alone arms (pooled treatment arms HR 0.99, CI 0.94–1.03). For women initiating estrogen alone treatment below age 60 years, there was a significant reduction of 21% in all-cause mortality (HR 0.79, CI 0.64–0.96). A treatment that reduces the chance of dying can hardly be regarded as unsafe!

17.8 Conclusions

HRT has well-established effects on metabolic risk factors for CHD. There are mainly beneficial changes in lipids and lipoproteins, glucose and insulin metabolism, body fat distribution and arterial function. These changes should result in decreases in CHD. However, a number of factors need to be considered if HRT is to be of benefit. The age at initiation of HRT is very important. Although the greatest benefits of CHD event reduction are seen in those initiating treatment close to the onset of menopause, initiating HRT at later ages does not necessarily result in overall CHD harm. Many of the cardiovascular effects of estrogen are dose-dependent, and the appropriate dose at initiation must be chosen for the age of the women, the older the woman the lower the dose. Had lower starting doses been used in the older women in some of the clinical trials, it is possible that cardiovascular harm would have been avoided and perhaps cardiovascular benefit could have been seen. The route of administration of HRT could be important, particularly in terms of atherothrombotic events. Nonoral estrogen administration has less adverse effects on coagulation activation compared with oral administration, although this could in part also be related to dosage. There may be differences in CHD outcomes according to the type of progestogen used in HRT. Androgenic progestogens can have adverse metabolic and vascular effects which are not seen with non-androgenic progestogens. The totality of current data suggests that HRT is beneficial for the primary prevention of CHD in postmenopausal women. Doses of hormones at initiation should be appropriate for the age of the woman, whilst the types of hormones and their route of administration also need to be considered to optimise the treatment for the individual.

References

1. Yusuf S, Hawken S, Ounpuu S, et al. Effect of potentially modifiable risk factors associated with myocardial infarction in 52 countries (the INTERHEART study): case-control study. Lancet. 2004;364:937–52.
2. Hackshaw A, Morris JK, Boniface S, Tang JL, Milenkovic D. Low cigarette consumption and risk of coronary heart disease and stroke: meta-analysis of 141 cohort studies in 55 study reports. Br Med J. 2018;360:j5855.
3. Lokkegaard E, Jovanovic Z, Heitmann BE, et al. The association between early menopause and risk of ischaemic heart disease: influence of hormone therapy. Maturitas. 2006;53:226–33.
4. Ference BA, Ginsberg HN, Graham I, et al. Lipoproteins cause atherosclerotic cardiovascular disease. 1, Evidence from genetic, epidemiologic and clinical studies. A consensus statement from the European Atherosclerosis Society Consensus Panel. Eur Heart J. 2017;38:2450–72.
5. Godsland IF. Effects of postmenopausal hormone replacement therapy on lipid, lipoprotein, and apolipoprotein (a) concentrations: analysis of studies published from 1974–2000. Fertil Steril. 2001;75:898–915.
6. Eapen DJ, Kalra GL, Rifai L, Eapen CA, Merchant N, Khan BV. Raising HDL cholesterol in women. Int J Womens Health. 2009;1:181–91.
7. McBride P. Triglycerides and risk for coronary artery disease. Curr Atheroscler Rep. 2008;10:386–90.
8. Stevenson JC, Pan K, Ryan KA, Chines AC, Mirkin S. A pooled analysis of the effects of conjugated estrogens/bazedoxifene on lipid parameters in postmenopausal women from the selective estrogens, menopause, and response to therapy (SMART) trials. J Clin Endocrinol Metab. 2015;100:2329–38.
9. Stevenson JC, Rioux JE, Komer L, Gelfand M. 1 and 2 mg 17β-estradiol combined with sequential dydrogesterone have similar effects on the serum lipid profile of postmenopausal women. Climacteric. 2005;8:352–9.

10. Danesh J, Collins R, Peto R. Lipoprotein (a) and coronary heart disease. Meta-analysis of prospective studies. Circulation. 2000;102:1082–5.
11. Anagnostis P, Galanis P, Chatzistergiou V, et al. The effect of hormone replacement therapy and tibolone on lipoprotein (a) concentrations in postmenopausal women: a systematic review and meta-analysis. Maturitas. 2017;99:27–36.
12. Reaven G. Insulin resistance and coronary heart disease in nondiabetic individuals. Arterioscler Thromb Vasc Biol. 2012;32:1754–9.
13. Spencer CP, Godsland IF, Cooper AJ, Ross D, Whitehead MI, Stevenson JC. Effects of oral and transdermal 17 β-estradiol with cyclical oral norethindrone acetate on insulin sensitivity, secretion, and elimination in postmenopausal women. Metabolism. 2000;49:742–7.
14. Shadoan MK, Kavanagh K, Zhang L, Anthony MS, Wagner JD. Addition of medroxyprogesterone acetate to conjugated equine estrogens results in insulin resistance in adipose tissue. Metabolism. 2007;56:830–7.
15. Casanova G, Spritzer PM. Effects of micronized progesterone added to non-oral estradiol on lipids and cardiovascular risk factors in early postmenopause: a clinical trial. Lipids Health Dis. 2012;11:133.
16. Manassiev NA, Godsland IF, Crook D, et al. Effect of postmenopausal oestradiol and dydrogesterone therapy on lipoproteins and insulin sensitivity, secretion and elimination in hysterectomised women. Maturitas. 2002;42:233–42.
17. Donahue RP, Abbott RD, Bloom E, Reed DM, Yano K. Central obesity and coronary heart disease. Lancet. 1987;1:821–4.
18. Gambacciani M, Ciaponi M, Cappagli B, et al. Body weight, body fat distribution, and hormonal replacement therapy in early postmenopausal women. J Clin Endocrinol Metab. 1997;82:414–7.
19. Oger E, Scarabin P-Y. Assessment of the risk for venous thromboembolism among users of hormone replacement therapy. Drugs Aging. 1999;14:55–61.
20. Scarabin P-Y, Oger E, Plu-Bureau G. Differential association of oral and transdermal oestrogen-replacement therapy with venous thromboembolism risk. Lancet. 2003;362:428–32.
21. Wingrove CS, Garr E, Pickar JH, Dey M, Stevenson JC. Effects of equine oestrogens on markers of vasoactive function in human coronary artery endothelial cells. Mol Cell Endocrinol. 1999;150:33–7.
22. Wingrove CS, Stevenson JC. 17β-oestradiol inhibits stimulated endothelin release in human vascular endothelial cells. Eur J Endocrinol. 1997;137:205–8.
23. Stevenson JC, Gerval MO. The influence of sex steroids on affairs of the heart. In: Genazzani AR, Brincat M, editors. Frontiers in gynecological endocrinology Volume 1. From symptoms to therapies. Heidelberg: Springer; 2014. p. 225–31.
24. Proudler AJ, Cooper A, Whitehead MI, Stevenson JC. Effect of oestrogen-only and oestrogen-progestogen replacement therapy upon circulating angiotensin I-converting enzyme activity in postmenopausal women. Clin Endocrinol. 2003;58:30–5.
25. Archer DF, Thorneycroft IH, Foegh M, et al. Long term safety of drospirenone-estradiol for hormone therapy: a randomized, double-blind, multicenter trial. Menopause. 2005;12:716–27.
26. Wingrove CS, Garr E, Godsland IF, Stevenson JC. 17 β-Oestradiol enhances release of matrix metalloproteinase-2 from human vascular smooth muscle cells. Biochim Biophys Acta. 1998;1406:169–74.
27. Grodstein F, Manson JE, Colditz GA, et al. A prospective, observational study of postmenopausal hormone therapy and primary prevention of cardiovascular disease. Ann Intern Med. 2000;133:933–41.
28. Tuomikoski P, Lyytinen H, Korhonen P, et al. Coronary heart disease mortality and hormone therapy before and after the Women's Health Initiative. Obstet Gynecol. 2014;124:947–53.
29. Mikkola TS, Tuomikoski P, Lyytinen H, et al. Increased cardiovascular mortality risk in women discontinuing postmenopausal hormone therapy. J Clin Endocrinol Metab. 2015;100:4588–94.
30. Clarkson TB, Anthony MS, Jerome CP. Lack of effect of raloxifene on coronary artery atherosclerosis of postmenopausal monkeys. J Clin Endocrinol Metab. 1998;83:721–6.

31. Clarkson TB, Morgan TM. Inhibition of postmenopausal atherosclerosis progression: a comparison of the effects of conjugated equine estrogens and soy phytoestrogens. J Clin Endocrinol Metab. 2001;86:41–7.
32. Williams JK, Anthony MS, Honore EK, et al. Regression of atherosclerosis in female monkeys. Arterioscler Thromb Vasc Biol. 1995;15:827–36.
33. Hodis HN, Mack WJ, Lobo RA, et al. Estrogen in the prevention of atherosclerosis. A randomized, double-blind, placebo-controlled trial. Ann Intern Med. 2001;135:939–53.
34. Hodis HN, Mack WJ, Henderson VW, et al. Vascular effects of early versus late postmenopausal treatment with estradiol. N Engl J Med. 2016;374:1221–31.
35. Harman SM. Effects of oral conjugated estrogen or transdermal estradiol plus oral progesterone treatment on common carotid artery intima media thickness (CIMT) & coronary artery calcium (CAC) in menopausal women: initial results from the Kronos Early Estrogen Prevention Study (KEEPS). North American Menopause Society Annual Meeting, 2012.
36. Levine ME, Lu AT, Chen BH, et al. Menopause accelerates biological aging. Proc Natl Acad Sci U S A. 2016;113:9327–32.
37. Sanghvi MM, Aung N, Cooper JA, et al. The impact of menopausal hormone therapy (MHT) on cardiac structure and function: insights from the UK Biobank imaging enhancement study. PLoS One. 2018;13(3):e0194015.
38. Stevenson JC, Flather M, Collins P. Coronary heart disease in women. N Engl J Med. 2000;343:1891.
39. Manson JE, Chlebowski RT, Stefanick ML, et al. Menopausal hormonal therapy and health outcomes during the intervention and poststopping phases of the Women's Health Initiative randomized trials. JAMA. 2013;310:1353–68.
40. Manson JE, Allison MA, Rossouw JE, et al. Estrogen therapy and coronary-artery calcification. N Engl J Med. 2007;356:2591–602.
41. Schierbeck LL, Rejnmark L, Tofteng CL, et al. Effect of hormone replacement therapy on cardiovascular events in recently postmenopausal women: randomized trial. Br Med J. 2012;345:e6409.
42. Salpeter SR, Walsh JME, Greyber E, Salpeter EE. Coronary heart disease events associated with hormone therapy in younger and older women. J Gen Intern Med. 2006;21:363–6.
43. HMP B, Hartley L, Eisinga A, et al. Hormone therapy for preventing cardiovascular disease in postmenopausal women. Cochrane Database Syst Rev. 2015;4:CD002229.
44. Alexandersen P, Tanko LB, Bagger YZ, et al. The long term impact of 2–3 years of hormone replacement therapy on cardiovascular mortality and atherosclerosis in healthy women. Climacteric. 2006;9:108–18.
45. Salpeter SR, Cheng J, Thabane L, Buckley NS, Salpeter EE. Bayesian meta-analysis of hormone therapy and mortality in younger postmenopausal women. Am J Med. 2009;122:1016–22.
46. Manson JE, Aragald AK, Rossouw JE, et al. Menopausal Hormone Therapy and long-term all-cause and cause-specific mortality. The Women's Health Initiative randomized trials. JAMA. 2017;318:927–38.

Symptoms and Hormones: Fine-Tuning Atherosclerotic Risk?

18

Juan José Hidalgo-Mora, Darya Dudenko, Sandra Ruiz-Vega, and Antonio Cano

18.1 Introduction

The drastic reduction in the circulating levels of estrogens along the menopausal transition triggers a list of symptoms, where hot flashes (HF) constitute a frequently reported episode. Women describe hot flashes as a sudden feeling of heat affecting the upper body, trunk, head, and neck and spreading upwards or, less frequently, downwards. The whole phenomenon is described as a heat wave, which is accompanied by sweating and reddening of the skin, and that persists for short intervals, of minutes or even seconds. HF present during day and night and, when intense enough, affect the quality of sleep and provoke frequent waking-up episodes.

The prevalence of HF changes as a function of a series of variables, including the ethnic origin, climate, diet, the attitude to women's role regarding reproduction, etc. (for a review, see [1]). Also, the intensity varies, with some women reporting only night sweats or very slight forms, which do not alter the quality of life.

One interesting feature of HF is the accompanying vascular reactivity, which has been taken by investigators to use the more general and descriptive designation of vasomotor symptoms (VMS). Indeed, HF develop an initial vasodilation, occurring as a response to the heat wave, and are followed by subsequent vasoconstriction. These changes have been connected by some authors with altered function of the autonomic nervous system and associated with metabolic dysfunctions [2]. Accordingly, the question has been raised of whether a link might exist between susceptibility to VMS and the risk for cardiovascular disease (CVD).

The connections between HF and CVD, two apparently different categories, might be based in the well-known association between endothelial dysfunction and atherosclerotic risk, as shown in the 1980s and 1990s of the past century [3]. Based on those assumptions, pioneering work by British investigators showed that women

J. J. Hidalgo-Mora · D. Dudenko · S. Ruiz-Vega · A. Cano (✉)
Service of Obstetrics and Gynecology, Hospital Clínico Universitario, Valencia, Spain
e-mail: antonio.cano@uv.es

© International Society of Gynecological Endocrinology 2019
R. D. Brinton et al. (eds.), *Sex Steroids' Effects on Brain, Heart and Vessels*,
ISGE Series, https://doi.org/10.1007/978-3-030-11355-1_18

suffering VMS had altered vasomotor responses, specifically diminished response to cold [4, 5], and increased blood flow in the upper limb during flushing episodes [6]. In a more recent study, Sassarini et al. found that subcutaneous vessels of women who flushed had a greater response to both endothelium-dependent and endothelium-independent vasodilator stimuli [7] than matched controls. Of specific interest, flushers had lower levels of high-density lipoprotein cholesterol (HDL-C) and apoA1 and higher levels of intercellular adhesion molecule-1 (ICAM-1). These changes have contributed to the conception that HF might be related with cardiovascular risk. Those changes might have an impact in cardiovascular risk and, secondarily, in other systems in the body.

18.2   Central Nervous System and HF

Women with HF do not appear to have lower levels of circulating estrogens than asymptomatic postmenopausal women, although the issue has not been adequately investigated. The main limiting factor is methodological, because very sensitive technology is required to adequately discriminate estrogen concentration when it is already low. In any case, and whichever the conditioning factor, the increased blood flow in the skin of women with HF involves neural mechanisms, either the reduction of the sympathetic-dependent constrictor action or the increase in the sympathetic cholinergic-dependent vasodilator activity.

There are abundant data suggesting that the narrowing of the thermoneutral zone in symptomatic women is associated with increased central noradrenergic activation. For example, neurons in the arcuate nucleus of symptomatic women are hypertrophied and show an increased expression of neurokinin B and kisspeptin (Fig. 18.1). The changes have been observed in female monkeys subjected to ovariectomy (for a review, see [8]). These neurons are involved in the regulation of GnRH pulses as well as in the induction of puberty.

It is of interest that work with rodent models has shown that projections of these neurons extend to the median preoptic nucleus, a crucial element in the CNS pathway regulating heat dissipation. All those neurons express the neurokinin-3 receptor (NK$_3$R), which has been shown a role in the HF phenotype. Indeed, a recent clinical trial has made evident that women treated with an antagonist to the NK$_3$R experiment a reduction in the number and severity of HF [9].

18.3   HF and Risk of Cardiovascular Disease

The link between vascular tone and atherosclerosis initiation and progression has raised questions about an association between HF and cardiovascular risk. The studies showing a differential response of vascular reactivity in women with HF [4, 6, 7], added to alterations in the lipidogram and higher levels of ICAM-1, have fed the hypothesis of a higher cardiovascular risk in women with HF. Subsequent cross-sectional American studies, like the *Study of Women's Health Across the Nation*

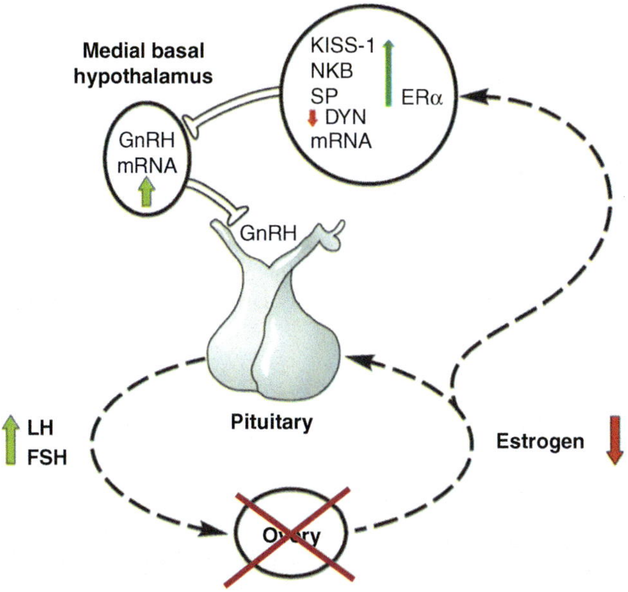

Fig. 18.1 There is hypertrophy of neurons expressing KiSS-1, NKB, substance P, dynorphin, and ERa mRNA in the infundibular nucleus concomitant with the decline of estrogens during menopause. Kisspeptin and NKB stimulate GnRH gene expression. With permission from Rance N. Peptides 2009; 30:111. Permission conveyed through Copyright Clearance Center, Inc.

(SWAN), have confirmed association of VMS with established cardiovascular risk factors, like altered lipidogram or hypertension [10, 11].

Meanwhile, post hoc analyses from other American studies, like the *Women's Health Initiative* (WHI) and the *Heart and Estrogen/Progestin Replacement Study* (HERS), showed that the association between hormone therapy (HT) and risk for CVD was modified not only by age but also by HF [12, 13]. Since then, several groups of investigators have increased their interest into the topic and have provided a wealth of extremely valuable data.

In a cross-sectional study, Lambrinoudaki et al. found that the carotid intima-media thickness (IMT), a recognized biomarker of atherosclerosis, was increased in women with HF as compared with matched controls of women with no or mild HF. The association was independent from well-known cardiovascular risk factors or circulating estrogen levels [14].

The SWAN study, which includes women who have been followed longitudinally for several years, has provided a wealth of interesting data. Subclinical parameters, including vascular reactivity or atherosclerosis imaging at the carotid (IMT) or the coronary (coronary artery calcium, CAC), have been explored and contrasted with the HF phenotype. Both cross-sectional and longitudinal studies, led by the group of R Thurston at the University of Pittsburg, have confirmed the association of VMS with subclinical atherosclerosis indicators (for a review, see [15]). Furthermore, longitudinal studies have disclosed that duration of VMS was more clearly determining the association with CVD risk indicators, the association being then replicated in other big cardiovascular studies, like the *Women's Ischemia Syndrome Evaluation* (WISE) [16]. These data are consistent with studies that along the latter years have shown an association between the fall in estrogens and initial steps of atherosclerosis, such as endothelial function parameters [17].

In a more sophisticated step, Thurston and cols have prospectively followed a group of 300 non-smoking midlife women in the MsHeart Study. VMS were recorded with the use of electronic digital diaries and physiologic monitoring with appropriate sensors. The study confirmed that VMS were related with IMT values and plaque identification, and that the association was above traditional CV risk factors or circulating estrogens [18].

18.4 Conclusion

Evidence in favor of VMS as marker of cardiovascular vulnerability accumulates as a result of studies from different groups. Despite so, the key question of the pathophysiological link remains elusive. Some data suggest that it is the VMS during the early menopause that seem determinant. This hypothesis agrees with recent data giving relevance to the lipid changes during the initiation of menopause transition as a key determinant variable for later IMT increase [19]. The assumption might be that, if the menopausal transition seems a vulnerability window, and changes in lipids and other cardiovascular risk factors seem to occur in association with VMS during that period, a potential link might exist. Parallel to lipid changes, some studies have found that alterations in the control mechanisms in the autonomic nervous system, with increased sympathetic or reduced parasympathetic control of heart rate variability, occur during HF. Those changes in the autonomic system have been linked with cardiovascular risk [20]. But, still, the association of VMS with those lipid or nervous system changes is not clearly understood.

Another option might consider the sequence of altered vascular wall reactivity leading to atherosclerosis, an interpretation already maintained for years to explain the estrogenic protective role. There are abundant data showing the association of VMS with vascular reactivity dysfunctions, but, still, more consolidated evidence is required.

References

1. Llaneza P. Clinical symptoms and quality of life: hot flashes and mood. In: Menopause, a comprehensive approach. New York, NY: Springer; 2017.
2. Archer DF, Sturdee DW, Baber R, de Villiers TJ, Pines A, Freedman RR, Gompel A, Hickey M, Hunter MS, Lobo RA, Lumsden MA, MacLennan AH, Maki P, Palacios S, Shah D, Villaseca P, Warren M. Menopausal hot flushes and night sweats: where are we now? Climacteric. 2011;14(5):515–28.
3. Ross R. Atherosclerosis--an inflammatory disease. N Engl J Med. 1999;340(2):115–26.

4. Rees MC, Barlow DH. Absence of sustained reflex vasoconstriction in women with menopausal flushes. Hum Reprod. 1988;3(7):823–5.
5. Brockie JA, Barlow DH, Rees MC. Menopausal flush symptomatology and sustained reflex vasoconstriction. Hum Reprod. 1991;6(4):472–4.
6. Ginsburg J, Hardiman P, O'Reilly B. Peripheral blood flow in menopausal women who have hot flushes and in those who do not. BMJ. 1989;298(6686):1488–90.
7. Sassarini J, Fox H, Ferrell W, Sattar N, Lumsden MA. Vascular function and cardiovascular risk factors in women with severe flushing. Clin Endocrinol (Oxf). 2011;74(1):97–103.
8. Rance NE, Dacks PA, Mittelman-Smith MA, Romanovsky AA, Krajewski-Hall SJ. Modulation of body temperature and LH secretion by hypothalamic KNDy (kisspeptin, neurokinin B and dynorphin) neurons: a novel hypothesis on the mechanism of hot flushes. Front Neuroendocrinol. 2013;34(3):211–27.
9. Prague JK, Roberts RE, Comninos AN, Clarke S, Jayasena CN, Nash Z, Doyle C, Papadopoulou DA, Bloom SR, Mohideen P, Panay N, Hunter MS, Veldhuis JD, Webber LC, Huson L, Dhillo WS. Neurokinin 3 receptor antagonism as a novel treatment for menopausal hot flushes: a phase 2, randomised, double-blind, placebo-controlled trial. Lancet. 2017;389(10081):1809–20.
10. Thurston RC, El Khoudary SR, Sutton-Tyrrell K, Crandall CJ, Gold EB, Sternfeld B, Joffe H, Selzer F, Matthews KA. Vasomotor symptoms and lipid profiles in women transitioning through menopause. Obstet Gynecol. 2012;119(4):753–61.
11. Jackson EA, El Khoudary SR, Crawford SL, Matthews K, Joffe H, Chae C, Thurston RC. Hot flash frequency and blood pressure: data from the study of women's health across the nation. J Womens Health (Larchmt). 2016;25(12):1204–9.
12. Rossouw JE, Prentice RL, Manson JE, Wu L, Barad D, Barnabei VM, Ko M, LaCroix AZ, Margolis KL, Stefanick ML. Postmenopausal hormone therapy and risk of cardiovascular disease by age and years since menopause. JAMA. 2007;297(13):1465–77.
13. Huang AJ, Sawaya GF, Vittinghoff E, Lin F, Grady D. Hot flushes, coronary heart disease, and hormone therapy in postmenopausal women. Menopause. 2009;16(4):639–43.
14. Lambrinoudaki I, Augoulea A, Armeni E, Rizos D, Alexandrou A, Creatsa M, Kazani M, Georgiopoulos G, Livada A, Exarchakou A, Stamatelopoulos K. Menopausal symptoms are associated with subclinical atherosclerosis in healthy recently postmenopausal women. Climacteric. 2012;15(4):350–7.
15. Thurston RC. Vasomotor symptoms: natural history, physiology, and links with cardiovascular health. Climacteric. 2018;2:1–5.
16. Thurston RC, Johnson BD, Shufelt CL, Braunstein GD, Berga SL, Stanczyk FZ, Pepine CJ, Bittner V, Reis SE, Thompson DV, Kelsey SF, Sopko G, Bairey Merz CN. Menopausal symptoms and cardiovascular disease mortality in the Women's Ischemia Syndrome Evaluation (WISE). Menopause. 2017;24(2):126–32.
17. Bechlioulis A, Kalantaridou SN, Naka KK, Chatzikyriakidou A, Calis KA, Makrigiannakis A, Papanikolaou O, Kaponis A, Katsouras C, Georgiou I, Chrousos GP, Michalis LK. Endothelial function, but not carotid intima-media thickness, is affected early in menopause and is associated with severity of hot flushes. J Clin Endocrinol Metab. 2010;95(3):1199–206.
18. Thurston RC, Chang Y, Barinas-Mitchell E, Jennings JR, Landsittel DP, Santoro N, von Känel R, Matthews KA. Menopausal hot flashes and carotid intima media thickness among midlife women. Stroke. 2016;47(12):2910–5.
19. Matthews KA, El Khoudary SR, Brooks MM, Derby CA, Harlow SD, Barinas-Mitchell EJ, Thurston RC. Lipid changes around the final menstrual period predict carotid subclinical disease in postmenopausal women. Stroke. 2017;48(1):70–6.
20. Thurston RC, Christie IC, Matthews KA. Hot flashes and cardiac vagal control: a link to cardiovascular risk? Menopause. 2010;17(3):456–61.

Cardiovascular Mortality Risk and HRT

19

Tomi S. Mikkola

19.1 New Evidence to Support the Benefit of HRT in Mortality Risk

Observational studies consistently show that women who choose to use HRT have reduced overall mortality risk compared to women who do not use HRT [1, 2]. Consistent with these long-term observational studies have been randomized trials in which women who are recently menopausal, e.g., similar to the women in observational studies, when randomized to HRT versus placebo showed a reduction in total mortality. In a meta-analysis of 30 randomized controlled trials, a significant 39% reduction in total mortality was detected in women who were on average aged 54 years when randomized to HRT compared to placebo [3].

New epidemiological studies and clinical trials indicate that HRT reduce CVD incidence and mortality risk among recently menopausal women [2]. A large observational study with follow-up of almost half a million HRT users demonstrates that in estradiol-based HRT users, the risk for cardiac death was reduced up to 54% compared to the age-matched background population [4]. In absolute terms, of 1000 women using any HRT for at least 10 years, the risk reductions would mean 19 fewer cardiac deaths. Furthermore, the younger the women were at the initiation of HRT, the smaller was their CVD mortality risk [5]. These findings demonstrate that 60 years of age at the initiation of HRT is not a threshold age, but the earlier the HRT had been started, the smaller was the cardiac mortality risk (Fig. 19.1). This is in line with the fact that atherosclerotic changes start to develop already in premenopausal age. Thus, these data support the "timing hypothesis" but not the "window hypothesis" since cardiac mortality risk increase was not detected when HRT was initiated after 60 years of age.

T. S. Mikkola (✉)
Department of Obstetrics and Gynecology, University of Helsinki and Helsinki University Hospital, Helsinki, Finland
e-mail: tomi.mikkola@hus.fi

© International Society of Gynecological Endocrinology 2019
R. D. Brinton et al. (eds.), *Sex Steroids' Effects on Brain, Heart and Vessels*,
ISGE Series, https://doi.org/10.1007/978-3-030-11355-1_19

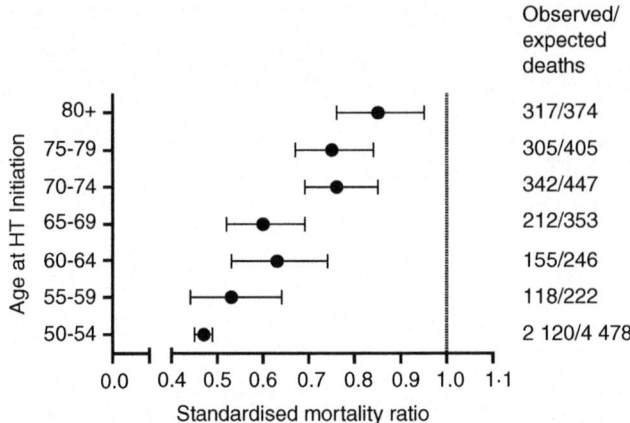

Fig. 19.1 Coronary heart disease mortality in women initiating HRT at different ages. The vertical dotted line denotes the risk in age-matched background population in Finnish women. Modified from Ref. [5]

In several sub-analyses of the WHI study, HRT appears to provide CVD protection if initiated close to menopause. Risk ratios of cardiac events were (HRT vs. placebo) 0.89, 1.22, and 1.71 for women randomized at <10 years, 10–19 years, and 20 or more years past menopause, respectively [6]. In the very recent WHI publication, total and cause-specific mortality during 18-year follow-up were reported [7]. When examined by 10-year age group comparing women aged 50–59 years to those aged 70–79 years, the ratios for all-cause mortality were 0.61 (95% CI, 0.43–0.87) during the intervention phase and 0.87 (95% CI, 0.76–1.00) during cumulative 18-year follow-up. Furthermore, younger women (aged 50–59 years) tended to have lower risk than older women for mortality due to CVD, particularly those with estrogen only treatment. These WHI results together with other recent data [2] uniformly witness for the cardioprotective effect of estradiol-based HRT regimens when initiated among recently menopausal healthy women.

19.2 Discontinuation of HRT and Cardiovascular Mortality Risk

Although many women need to treat vasomotor symptoms with HRT for several years, biannual or even annual HRT pause has become a routine practice to evaluate if a woman could manage without HRT. Long-term consequences of HRT discontinuation have been assessed, e.g., in the WHI study, revealing that 3 years after HRT cessation, the overall mortality was significantly increased in women originally assigned to estrogen + progestin treatment relative to those who were assigned to placebo and who were at least 80% compliant with intervention [8]. In the HERS post-trial 2.7-year follow-up, women originally assigned to estrogen had a 3.3-fold

Table 19.1 Risk of cardiac mortality in women during first post-HRT year in relation to HRT exposure duration and age at the HRT initiation or discontinuation, as compared with age-matched HRT users

HT exposure	≤5 years SMR (95% CI)	>5 years SMR (95% CI)
HT initiation		
<60 years	**1.42 (1.09–1.82)**	0.99 (0.89–1.11)
≥60 years	0.91 (0.75–1.09)	1.81 (0.51–1.21)
HT discontinuation		
<60 years	**1.55 (1.16–2.04)**	**2.13 (1.48–2.96)**
≥60 years	0.91 (0.76–1.09)	0.92 (0.82–1.03)

The numbers are standardized mortality ratios and confidence intervals (CI). When the CI does not overlap 1 the finding is significant (bold)

SMR standardised mortality ratio

Modified from Ref. [11]

higher rate of ventricular arrhythmia requiring resuscitation compared with those women assigned to placebo [9]. A recent large-scale population study showed that women who discontinued estradiol-based HRT compared to women who continued it had a greater risk of cardiac death within the first post-HRT year [10, 11]. Furthermore, these risk elevations were markedly higher in women who had been younger than 60 years at the initiation or discontinuation of HRT use (Table 19.1). Thus, discontinuation of postmenopausal HRT may be associated with increased risk of cardiac death during the first posttreatment year, particularly in women who discontinue HRT close to menopause. The deaths reflect only a minor part of total burden of these diseases, since for each woman who dies from cardiac cause, approximately 5–10 women will survive and continue living with different physical and mental incapacities. These findings question the safety of annual discontinuation practice to evaluate whether recently menopausal symptomatic women could manage without HRT.

19.3 Conclusions

New research data have accumulated after the original WHI publications, which uniformly indicate that estradiol-based HRT provide primary prevention of CVD and cardiac mortality. Although the treatment of vasomotor symptoms should remain the primary indication for HRT use, in order to get a concomitant cardiac benefit, HRT should be started soon after the onset of menopause. The safety of annual or biannual pausing to test the persistence of vasomotor symptoms is potentially dangerous, because acute withdrawal of HRT may predispose to cardiac events.

References

1. Grodstein F, Manson JE, Colditz GA, Willett WC, Speizer FE, Stampfer MJ. A prospective, observational study of postmenopausal hormone therapy and primary prevention of cardiovascular disease. Ann Intern Med. 2000;133(12):933–41.
2. Mikkola TS, Savolainen-Peltonen H, Venetkoski M, Ylikorkala O. New evidence for cardiac benefit of postmenopausal hormone therapy. Climacteric. 2017;20:5–10.
3. Salpeter SR, Walsh JME, Greyber E, Salpeter EE. Brief report: cronary heart disease events associated with hormone therapy in younger and older women - a meta-analysis. J Gen Intern Med. 2006;21(4):363–6.
4. Mikkola TS, Tuomikoski P, Lyytinen H, Korhonen P, Hoti F, Vattulainen P, Gissler M, Ylikorkala O. Estradiol-based postmenopausal hormone therapy and risk of cardiovascular and all-cause mortality. Menopause. 2015;22(9):976–83.
5. Savolainen-Peltonen H, Tuomikoski P, Korhonen P, Hoti F, Vattulainen P, Gissler M, Ylikorkala O, Mikkola TS. Cardiac death risk in relation to the age at initiation or the progestin component of hormone therapies. J Clin Endocrinol Metab. 2016;101:2794–801.
6. Rossouw JE, Prentice RL, Manson JE, Wu L, Barad D, Barnabei VM, et al. Postmenopausal hormone therapy and risk of cardiovascular disease by age and years since menopause. JAMA. 2007;297:1465–77.
7. Manson JE, Aragaki AK, Rossouw JE, et al. Menopausal hormone therapy and long-term all-cause and cause-specific mortality – the Women's Health Initiative randomized trials. JAMA. 2017;318:927–38.
8. Heiss G, Wallace R, Anderson GL, et al. Health risks and benefits 3 years after stopping randomized treatment with estrogen and progestin. JAMA. 2008;299:1036–45.
9. Grady D, Herrington D, Bittner V, et al. Cardiovascular disease outcomes during 6.8 years of hormone therapy: heart and estrogen/progestin replacement study follow-up (HERS II). JAMA. 2002;288:49–57.
10. Mikkola TS, Tuomikoski P, Lyytinen H, et al. Increased cardiovascular mortality risk in women discontinuing postmenopausal hormone therapy. J Clin Endocrinol Metab. 2015;100:4588–94.
11. Venetkoski M, Savolainen-Peltonen H, Rahkola-Soisalo P, Hoti F, Vattulainen P, Gissler M, Ylikorkala O, Mikkola TS. Increased cardiac death risk in the first year after discontinuation of postmenopausal hormone therapy. Menopause. 2018;25:375–9.

HT: Pharmacology Tailored to Women's Health

20

Sven O. Skouby

20.1 Introduction

As many as 80% of women experience subjective menopausal vasomotor symptoms (VMS), and in a number of cases, these are sufficiently unpleasant to significantly impair the quality of life [1, 2]. The frequency and severity of VMS peak in the late perimenopause and early postmenopausal years, with large ethnic and racial variation in prevalence, frequency, and severity of symptoms [3]. Obesity has been found to be a key risk factor for perimenopausal, but not postmenopausal VMS. Women with higher abdominal adiposity, particularly subcutaneous adiposity, are more likely to report VMS in the early and late perimenopause [4]. Recent genome-wide association studies (GWAS) have identified over 44 genetic variants that are associated with age of onset of natural menopause. Genes linked with menopause can be classified into three major groups: genes implicated in genome stability (DNA repair), immune function, and mitochondrial biogenesis. Biological and epidemiological data indicate that reproductive performance, age at menopause, and longevity are interlinked through common genetic factors, which play a pivotal role in DNA repair and genome maintenance, which has been linked before with the process of aging [5]. Studies also suggest a possible link between genetic polymorphisms and prevalence and severity of VMS. These involve variants in genes encoding estrogen receptor alpha [6, 7] and single-nucleotide polymorphisms involved in the synthesis and metabolism of estrogens, such as those affecting enzymes (like sulfotransferase and aromatase) related to synthesis of and conversion to more or less potent estrogens [8]. These polymorphisms may alter sex steroid hormone activity, but it is unknown whether these genetic determinants exert their effects centrally or peripherally [9]. Of note the decline in estrogen production has more

S. O. Skouby (✉)
Endocrinological and Reproductive Unit, Department of Obstetrics/Gynecology, Faculty of Health and Medical Sciences, Herlev Hospital, University of Copenhagen, Herlev, Denmark
e-mail: sven.olaf.skouby@regionh.dk; sos@dadlnet.dk

© International Society of Gynecological Endocrinology 2019
R. D. Brinton et al. (eds.), *Sex Steroids' Effects on Brain, Heart and Vessels*,
ISGE Series, https://doi.org/10.1007/978-3-030-11355-1_20

threatening long-term health implications in that it is closely associated with the development of osteoporosis and the increased risk of cardiovascular disease (CVD), the main cause of death in the Western world, and, as a consequence, a major public health issue. Abundant RCTs have demonstrated that estrogen represents the most effective treatment for menopausal symptoms including vasomotor, psychologic, and related issues including impaired cognition, sleep, and irritability, resulting in decreased quality of life [10, 11]. Higher doses are associated with enhanced efficacy. In women with an intact uterus, treatment with estrogen only is associated with an elevated risk of endometrial neoplasia with dose and duration of treatment directly related to the magnitude of this risk. When adequate progestogen is combined with estrogen, risk of endometrial neoplasia is not higher than in untreated women [11]. Oral and transdermal estrogen formulations have comparable efficacy in treating menopausal symptoms [12], and with the exception of estriol products, all systemic estrogen (17 beta estradiol and conjugated estrogen) formulations are approved for treatment of vasomotor symptoms.

However, the Women's Health Initiative (WHI) hormone therapy trials [13, 14], especially the trial involving estrogen plus progestin, completely changed the understanding of the risks and benefits of hormone therapy and reinforced the importance of assessing numerous outcomes. Cardiovascular disease risk was increased rather than decreased as was the risk of thromboembolic disease.

The relationship of hormone therapy to breast cancer was complex and confusing, and for the first time, differences in outcomes other than endometrial cancer risk were identified based on the administration of combination hormone therapy vs. estrogen only, with combination therapy increasing the likelihood of breast cancer and estrogen only seemingly having no effect. In addition, instead of a reduction in mortality, there was no significant effect on life expectancy among hormone users vs. nonusers. More questions than answers were raised including (a) why were the mortality results of previous cohort studies, e.g., the Nurses' Health Study [15], so different from the results of the WHI randomized trials; (b) why were the outcomes from combination therapy with estrogen plus progestin compared with estrogen only different; and (c) are there differences in the health benefits of hormone therapy for women based on the age or time since menopause when the hormone therapy was started. The only certainty is that controversy remained as to the risks and benefits of different hormone therapy preparations for women of different risk profiles.

20.2   The Present Tense: The Lesson Learned from the WHI

20.2.1   The Role of Personalized Medicine

Several clinical factors, including a women's age, time since menopause, baseline vascular health, risk for breast cancer, biomarker levels, and genetic predisposition, appear to modulate health outcomes on hormone therapy. As a consequence personalized medicine should be applied with special reference to tailoring HT including pharmacodynamics and pharmacokinetics of the different available hormonal agents because pharmacogenomics is one aspect of personalized medicine that has the potential to impact all areas of medicine, including HT. The goal of pharmacogenomics is to use genetic information to predict how an individual will respond to a drug, with the ultimate objective of aiding clinicians in selecting the right drug, in the right dose, at the right time, for every patient in order to ensure drug efficacy and to avoid adverse drug reactions. Estrogen is the most effective treatment for vasomotor and other symptoms related to menopause, and the current approach to individualizing HT includes consideration of the severity of the menopausal symptoms, a personalized risk assessment, and the patient's personal preferences [16]. Typically, dosing is targeted toward symptom relief, but there is significant variability in the doses required for symptom relief among women. For women experiencing primary ovarian insufficiency (<40 years) or early menopause (<45 years), estrogen therapy is needed not only for symptom management but also protection against the potential long-term adverse health consequences of early estrogen deprivation, including increased risk for cardiovascular disease, osteoporosis, dementia, parkinsonism, mood disorders, sexual dysfunction, and early death [17]. Environmental and biological factors may also impact menopausal symptoms, including body mass index, tobacco, alcohol or caffeine use, stress, anxiety, a history of recent abuse, or adverse childhood experiences [18]. Further work is required to understand the mechanisms by which these environmental and biologic factors affect menopausal symptoms. They may be independent variables or may be intertwined with genetic variation in gene-environment interactions. The strongest factors that have been found to modify CVD risk while taking HT and that appear to help identify better vs. worse candidates for HT use are age, time since menopause onset, LDL cholesterol and other lipid levels, metabolic syndrome, and Factor V Leiden genotype (Table 20.1) [19].

20.2.2 Influence of Age and Time Since Menopause

The WHI analyses reveal that age or time since menopause influences the relation between HT and CHD. In analyses pooling data across both trials, HT-associated RRs for CHD were 0.76 (95% CI 0.50–1.16), 1.10 (95% CI 0.84–1.45), and 1.28 (95% CI 1.03–1.58) among women who were <10, 10–19, and ≥20 years past the menopausal transition at study enrollment, respectively (p, trend = 0.02). Among women aged 50–59, estrogen only was associated with significant reductions in the secondary endpoint of coronary revascularization (RR = 0.55; 95% CI 0.35–0.86) and a composite endpoint of MI, coronary death, or coronary revascularization (RR = 0.66; 95% CI 0.44–0.97), but CHD risk reductions were not seen for ages 60–69 or 70–79. Overall, HT appeared to have a beneficial or neutral effect on CHD in women closer to menopause (who are likely to have healthier arteries) but a harmful effect in later years [20]. In the Early Versus Late Intervention Trial with Estradiol (ELITE), 643 postmenopausal women free from cardiovascular disease were stratified according to time since menopause (<6 years [early] vs. ≥10 years [late]) and were randomly assigned to receive either estrogen such as 17β-estradiol (E2) (plus micronized progesterone vaginal gel for women with a uterus) or placebo

Table 20.1 Selected biomarkers to aid risk stratification for HT decision-making (Adapted from [19])

Biochemical markers:
• Lipids (serum LDL cholesterol, LDL/HDL ratios, triglyceride levels, Lp(a), 27-OH-cholesterol, apolipoprotein levels)
• Inflammatory markers (high-sensitivity C-reactive protein [hsCRP], interleukin-6, tumor necrosis factor alpha, leukocyte count)
• Adipokines (adiponectin, leptin, retinol binding protein-4 [RBP4])
• Endothelial markers (E-selectin, P-selectin, ICAM, VCAM)
• Glucose tolerance markers: fasting glucose, insulin, HOMA-IR, IGF-1, and biomarkers of metabolic syndrome
• Matrix metalloproteinases
• Hemostatic markers (D-dimer, factor VIII, von Willebrand factor, homocysteine, fibrinogen, tissue factor pathway inhibitor or acquired activated protein C resistance)
• Sex steroid hormone levels, sex hormone binding globulin level
Genetic markers:
• Factor V Leiden
• Glycoprotein IIIa leu33pro
• Gene variants in ABO blood group
• Estrogen and progesterone receptor polymorphisms
• Gene variants related to sex hormone biosynthesis
• Gene variants related to sex hormone metabolism
• Gene variants related to sex hormone signaling
• Genome-wide association studies (GWAS) and exome sequencing for gene discovery

over a median of 5 years. The primary outcome was atherosclerosis progression measured by means of ultrasonography such as carotid-artery intima-medial thickness (CIMT). As compared with placebo, estrogen treatment resulted in a significantly lower rate of atherosclerosis progression among early postmenopausal women but not among late postmenopausal women. The results were similar regardless of whether the women also received progesterone [21]. There was no significant difference between estradiol and placebo in either the early or the late postmenopause stratum with regard to a secondary outcome, measurement of atherosclerosis by cardiac computerized tomography (CT) at the end of the study; however, this assessment was performed in only a subset of women, and no baseline measures were available. These data are of keen biologic interest, because they suggest that favorable pharmacodynamic responses of receptors in the vasculature to estrogen may be lost with lack of exposure to estrogen and of note prior to the initiation of the HT, genetic variations in the innate immunity pathway were found to be associated with CIMT and coronary arterial calcification (CAC) [22].

20.2.3 Low Dose Versus High Dose

The primary indication for HT is relief of vasomotor symptoms. Individual risks and benefits should be weighed, and the lowest effective hormone dosage be chosen. For many women, low-dose (<2 mg oral E2/<100 g transdermal E2) or ultralow-dose HT (<1 mg oral E2/<50 mcg E2) may be sufficient to decrease vaso-motor symptoms, but not necessarily to guarantee fracture prevention. Low- and ultralow-dose combined HT has been successfully used in clinical trials but has not been introduced for general use until 2011 [23]. Since then, fixed oral combined ultralow-dose HT containing 17β-E2 has been available as well as patches with varying low-dose 17β-E2. Efficacy and safety were assessed in a 52-week, random-ized placebo-controlled trial in 313 postmenopausal healthy women aged 54 years on average. Participants were randomized to (1) 0.5 mg 17β-E2 combined with 2.5 mg dydrogesterone, (2) 1 mg 17β-E2 combined with 5 mg dydrogesterone, or (3) placebo. Both ultralow-dose and low-dose HT significantly reduced moderate to severe vasomotor symptoms [24]. Similarly, the 24-week, randomized, placebo-controlled trial CHOICE demonstrated a significant reduction of vasomotor symp-toms by 0.5 mg 17β-E2 combined with either 0.1 mg or 0.25 mg norethindrone acetate (NETA), in 577 postmenopausal healthy women aged 55.5 years on average [25]. Possibly, ultralow-dose HT might be a compromise for those women who are more critical toward HT but in whom alternative and complementary medicine strategies have not been successful. Comparable to standard-dose and low-dose HT, bleeding events may occur when initiating ultralow-dose HT and may require indi-vidual dosage adjustments. For women treated with high- or standard-dose HT, switching progressively to low-dose and then to ultralow-dose HT may be a good way to lower hormone dosage without compromising vasomotor symptom relief before stopping HT as soon as it is needed no more. To date, there are no direct head-to-head trials comparing long-term safety of standard-dose, low-dose, and ultralow-dose HT. It appears reasonable to assume that a lower hormone dosage would be associated with fewer estrogenic and especially progestogenic side effects as well as fewer safety concerns, but this has not been conclusively demonstrated. So far, for example, the Nurses' Health Study has demonstrated a lack of increased risk of stroke for ultralow-dose treatment with conjugated estrogens (CEE) [26]. In a nested case-control study based on the United Kingdom's General Practice Research Database, no increased risk of stroke has been observed in users of trans-dermal HT containing low doses of estrogen, whereas, in users of oral HT, risk was dose-dependent. A more recent review has shown that transdermal estrogens are not associated with a higher risk of recurrent venous thromboembolism among post-menopausal women and that, for oral HT, the dose of estrogens is an important determinant of the thrombotic risk among postmenopausal women using HT [27]. However, until there are clinical studies demonstrating a better long-term safety profile for low-dose or ultralow-dose HT, risks associated with long-term standard-dose HT are most wisely also applicable to ultralow-dose HT despite the biological discrepancies.

20.2.4 Estrogen only Therapy

Looking at the main results from the Heart and Estrogen/progestin Replacement Study (HERS) [28] and the WHI [20], most participants were postmenopausal

American women with at least some degree of comorbidity, and mean participant age in most studies was over 60 years. In relatively healthy postmenopausal women combined continuous HT increased the risk of a coronary event (after 1 year's use: from 2 per 1000 to between 3 and 7 per 1000), venous thromboembolism (after 1 year's use: from 2 per 1000 to between 4 and 11 per 1000), and stroke (after 3 years' use: from 6 per 1000 to between 6 and 12 per 1000). Estrogen only HT increased the risk of venous thromboembolism (after 1–2 years' use: from 2 per 1000 to 2–10 per 1000; after 7 years' use: from 16 per 1000 to 16–28 per 1000), stroke (after 7 years' use: from 24 per 1000 to between 25 and 40 per 1000), but reduced the risk of breast cancer (after 7 years' use: from 25 per 1000 to between 15 and 25 per 1000) and did not increase the risk of coronary events at any follow-up time.

Analysis of the entire follow-up period (i.e., intervention plus post-intervention phases) of the WHI estrogen only trial also found more favorable effects for myocardial infarction (MI) and CHD in younger, compared with older, women. For MI, the RRs associated with randomization to estrogen only were 0.54 (0.34–0.86), 1.05 (0.82–1.35), and 1.23 (0.92–1.65) for ages 50–59, 60–69, and 70–79, respectively (p, interaction = 0.007). Results were similar for CHD [20].

20.2.5 Progestins Not Only One Class

Progesterone and progestogens are nonselective ligands for the progesterone receptor and bind also with other steroid receptors, with agonistic or antagonistic effects according to the structure of the molecule. Their half-life and metabolism are also different, progesterone being rapidly degraded with a short half-life. Progestogen compounds of combined estrogen-progestogen therapy include both progesterone (the bioidentical compound synthesized and secreted by the ovary) and synthetic compounds named progestins, which are derived from either progesterone (pregnanes and 19-norpregnanes) or testosterone (19-nortestosterone). Pregnane derivatives consist of different molecules, including dydrogesterone, medrogestone, chlormadinone acetate, cyproterone acetate, and medroxyprogesterone acetate (MPA). Norpregnane derivatives include nomegestrol acetate, promegestone, trimegestone, and nestorone. Finally, nortestosterone derivatives consist of ethinylated derivatives, nonethinylated derivatives, spironolactone derivatives, and tibolone. Nortestosterone ethinylated derivatives are composed of estranes (including especially norethisterone acetate) and gonanes, which are preferentially used in contraceptive pills. Nortestosterone nonethinylated derivative (dienogest) and spironolactone derivative (drospirenone) are also used in contraception.

As an HT compound, progestogens are always combined with estrogens and are almost exclusively administered by the oral route. However, across countries, medical practices regarding HT use may present important differences in terms of chemical structure and route of administration. In France, women are preferentially prescribed transdermally administered 17β-E2 combined with micronized progesterone. By contrast, oral CEE combined with MPA are often used in the United States.

20.2.6 Differential Effects of Progestogens on Thrombosis Risk

As progestogens consist of several compounds with different pharmacologic properties and all, when added to estrogens for women with an intact uterus, reduce the increased risks of endometrial hyperplasia and cancer, randomized controlled trials that are able to assess the main effects of a progestogen or to compare different progestogens are scarce. In the PEPI (Postmenopausal Estrogen/Progestin Interventions) trial, MPA was administered either sequentially or continuously, and these two hormone regimens were compared with micronized progesterone or no progestogen. Results showed similar changes in fibrinogen across different active groups, with neither an effect of addition of a progestogen nor a specific effect of different chemical structures [29]. A few years later, Lobo et al. [30] conducted a large trial with different doses of CEE alone or combined with MPA and did not highlight any evidence for a specific effect of MPA on hemostatic parameters. At the same time, van Baal et al. [31] and Post et al. [32, 33] investigated the impact of dydrogesterone and trimegestone, a pregnane and a norpregnane derivative, respectively. Here, they also found no difference in their effects on hemostasis and pooled the two groups receiving opposed oral estrogens for some specific analyses. In another study, the main effect of gestodene, a testosterone derivative, was assessed by comparing changes in hemostatic parameters between two arms consisting of oral estrogens either alone or combined with this progestin [34]. This was the only study that found a decrease in protein C in the opposed oral estrogen group but not in the estrogen only group.

Overall, randomized controlled trials did not consistently detect any specific effect of progestogen on hemostasis among postmenopausal women using oral estrogens. Nevertheless, this absence of association does not necessarily imply that progestogens have no effect. It could be partly explained by a lack of statistical power and/or a dilution effect caused by the concomitant use of oral estrogens that activate blood coagulation by themselves and might then hide the specific effect of progestogens. A cross-sectional study on postmenopausal HT and hemostasis suggested that norpregnane derivatives and micronized progesterone could have a differential effect on APC resistance and blood coagulation activation when combined with transdermal estrogens [35]. In addition, clinical data support a differential effect of pharmacologic classes of progestogens on thrombotic risk [36, 37]. Further data on the biological and clinical effects of progestogens are therefore needed, especially in the context of transdermal estrogen use.

20.2.7 Oral Versus Non-oral Administration Forms

As already pointed out, estrogen dose and routes of administration vary in regard to their risks. Lower doses are associated with less adverse effects like breast tenderness or uterine bleeding and may have a more favorable risk-benefit ratio than standard doses. Transdermal estrogen is preferred to the oral route, as the latter is subject to first-pass hepatic metabolism which promotes prothrombotic hemostatic changes in factor IX, activated protein C resistance, and tissue-plasminogen activator [38]. Furthermore, observational data from the Estrogen and Thromboembolism Risk (ESTHER) multicenter case-control study of thromboembolism among postmenopausal women demonstrated an odds ratio for venous thromboembolism in users of oral estrogen to be 4.2 (95% CI, 1.5–11.6) and 0.9 (95% CI, 0.4–2.1) for transdermal estrogen, compared to nonusers [36]. In accordance, 22 studies were included in meta-analyses (nine case-control studies, nine cohort studies, and four randomized controlled trials). As compared to control groups, VTE risk was not increased with non-oral HT, including users of estrogens and estrogens plus progestins (OR 0.97 [0.9–1.06]), non-oral estrogen therapy (ET)-only (OR 0.95 [0.81–1.10]), and non-oral combined estrogen-progestin therapy (OR 0.92 [0.77–1.09]). Conversely, increased risk of VTE was observed as compared with control groups in users of oral HT, including users of estrogens and estrogens plus progestins HT (OR 1.72 [1.47–2.01]), oral ET-only (OR 1.43 [1.34–1.53]), and combined oral estrogen-progestin HT (OR 2.35 [1.9–2.9]). The comparison of non-oral vs. oral HT showed increased VTE risk with oral HT (OR 1.66 [1.39–1.98]) [39]. The authors consider the quality of the evidence produced in their meta-analyses which is low to moderate, and further clinical trials are needed to sort out the impact of different types of progestin and different estrogen doses and administration routes on VTE risk. However, this approach has been endorsed by the American College of Obstetricians and Gynecologists, as gynecologists were recommended to take into consideration the possible thrombosis-sparing properties of transdermal forms of estrogen therapy [40].

20.3 Conclusion

Ideally, HT should be initiated in the perimenopause or early postmenopause, but not 10 or more years after menopause as atherosclerotic changes are likely to have occurred by then, increasing, for example, the risk of myocardial infarction. However, the choice of a particular modality should be guided by the patient's risk profile, other symptoms, and preferences considered for each patient during the decision-making. We have to date wider repertoire of agents for successful treatment than ever. This report has focused on vascular health and reviewed the evidence on the role of pharmacology and pharmacogenomics in tailoring the use of hormone therapy to appropriate candidates in order to develop a personalized risk-benefit prediction model that takes into account clinical and genetic factors. The proposed personalized approach to HT decision-making has also the potential to improve the quality of health care including also "patient-centered" outcomes such as sense of well-being and quality of life. However, due to the complexity of both the estrogen pharmacodynamic and pharmacokinetic pathways, and the many additional variables reviewed here that may be of importance, large studies will be required to develop genetically based algorithms for estrogen administration/dosing.

US Preventive services Task Force (USPSTF) process. The introduction of continuous combined ultra-low-dose MHT enlarge our possibilities to individualize the treatment of symptomatic postmenopausal women. Thus, the risk can be avoided of serum hormone fluctuations arising from the previous practice of splitting tablets or cutting patches to reduce the hormone dosage of low-dose MHT.

Author Statement *Funding*: Author states no funding involved.
Conflict of Interest: Author states no conflict of interest.
Material and Methods: Informed consent is not applicable.
Ethical Approval: The conducted research is not related to either human or animal use.

References

1. Oldenhave A, Jaszmann LJB, Haspels AA, Everaerd WTAM. Impact of climacteric on well-being: a survey based on 5213 women 39 to 60 years old. Am J Obstet Gynecol. 1993; 168:772.
2. Santen RJ, Allred DC, Ardoin SP, Archer DF, Boyd N, Braunstein GD, et al. Postmenopausal hormone therapy: an Endocrine Society scientific statement. J Clin Endocrinol Metab. 2010;95:s1.
3. EB G, Colvin A, Avis N, Bromberger J, GA G, Powell L, et al. Longitudinal analysis of the association between vasomotor symptoms and race/ethnicity across the menopausal transition: study of women's health across the nation. Am J Public Health. 2006;96(7):1226–35. Available from: http://search.ebscohost.com/login.aspx?direct=true&AuthType=ip,uid&db=r zh&AN=106335023&site=ehost-live&scope=site.
4. Thurston RC, Sowers MR, Sutton-Tyrrell K, Everson-Rose SA, Lewis TT, Edmundowicz D, et al. Abdominal adiposity and hot flashes among midlife women. Menopause. 2008;15(3):429–34.
5. Laven JS, Visser JA, Uiterlinden AG, Vermeij WP, Hoeijmakers JH. Menopause: genome stability as new paradigm. Maturitas. 2016;92:15–23. Available from: https://www.ncbi.nlm.nih. gov/pubmed/27621233.
6. Crandall CJ, Crawford SL, Gold EB. Vasomotor symptom prevalence is associated with polymorphisms in sex steroid-metabolizing enzymes and receptors. Am J Med. 2006;119(9 SUPPL. 1):S52.
7. Malacara JM, Pérez-Luque EL, Martínez-Garza S, Sánchez-Marín FJ. The relationship of estrogen receptor-α polymorphism with symptoms and other characteristics in post-menopausal women. Maturitas. 2004;49(2):163–9.
8. Rebbeck TR, Su HI, Sammel MD, Lin H, Tran TV, Gracia CR, et al. Effect of hormone metabolism genotypes on steroid hormone levels and menopausal symptoms in a prospective population-based cohort of women experiencing the menopausal transition. Menopause. 2010;17(5):1026–34. Available from: http://www.embase.com/search/result s?subaction=viewrecord&from=export&id=L359724663%5Cn, https://doi.org/10.1097/ gme.0b013e3181db61a1%5Cn, http://sfx.library.uu.nl/utrecht?sid=EMBASE&issn=1072371 4&id=doi:10.1097%2Fgme.0b013e3181db61a1&atitle=Effect+of+hormo.
9. Thurston RC, Joffe H. Vasomotor symptoms and menopause: findings from the study of women's health across the nation. Obstet Gynecol Clin North Am. 2011;38:489–501.
10. Consensus NIH. Statements S. NIH State-of-the-Science Conference Statement on management of menopause-related symptoms. NIH Consens State Sci Statements. 2005;22(1):1–38. Available from: https://www.ncbi.nlm.nih.gov/pubmed/17308548.
11. Pinkerton JAV, Aguirre FS, Blake J, Cosman F, Hodis H, Hoffstetter S, et al. The 2017 hormone therapy position statement of the North American Menopause Society. Menopause. 2017;24:728–53.
12. Schnatz PF, Pinkerton JV, Utian WH, Appt SE, de Villiers TJ, Henderson VW, et al. NAMS 3rd Utian Translational Science Symposium, October 2016, Orlando, Florida A conversation

about hormone therapy: is there an appropriate dose, route, and duration of use? Menopause. 2017;24(11):1221–35.

13. Rossouw J, Anderson G, Prentice R. Women's Health Initiative Investigators. Risks and benefits of estrogen plus progestin in healthy postmenopausal women. JAMA. 2002;288(3):321–33.

14. Anderson G, Limacher M, Assaf A, Bassford T, Beresford S, Black H, et al. Effects of conjugated equine estrogen in postmenopausal women with hysterectomy: the Women's Health Initiative randomized controlled trial. N Engl J Med. 2004;350(12):1189–99. Available from: https://www.pubmedcentral.nih.gov/articlerender.fcgi?artid=2861441&tool=pmcentrez&rend ertype=abstract.

15. Stampfer MJ, Colditz GA, Willett WC, Manson JE, Rosner B, Speizer FE, et al. Postmenopausal estrogen therapy and cardiovascular disease. Ten-year follow-up from the nurses' health study. N Engl J Med. 1991;325(11):756–62. Available from: https://www.ncbi.nlm.nih.gov/pubmed/1870648.

16. Kaunitz AM, Manson JE. Management of menopausal symptoms andrew. Obstet Gynecol. 2015;126:859.

17. Faubion SS, Kuhle CL, Shuster LT, Rocca WA. Long-term health consequences of premature or early menopause and considerations for management. Climacteric. 2015;18:483.

18. Moyer AM, Miller VM, Faubion SS. Could personalized management of menopause based on genomics become a reality? Pharmacogenomics. 2016;17:659.

19. Manson JE. The role of personalized medicine in identifying appropriate candidates for menopausal estrogen therapy. Metabol Clin Exp. 2013;32:s15.

20. Manson JE, Aragaki AK, Rossouw JE, Anderson GL, Prentice RL, LaCroix AZ, et al. Menopausal hormone therapy and long-term all-cause and cause-specific mortality. JAMA. 2017;318:927.

21. Hodis HN, et al. Vascular effects of early versus late postmenopausal treatment with estradiol. N Engl J Med. 2016;374:1221.

22. Miller VM, Jenkins GD, Biernacka JM, Heit JA, Huggins GS, Hodis HN, et al. Pharmacogenomics of estrogens on changes in carotid artery intima-medial thickness and coronary arterial calcification: Kronos early estrogen prevention study. Physiol Genomics. 2016;48:33.

23. Stute P, Becker H-G, Bitzer J, Chatsiproios D, Luzuy F, von Wolff M, et al. Ultra-low dose – new approaches in menopausal hormone therapy. Climacteric. 2015;18:182.

24. Stevenson JC, Durand G, Kahler E, Pertyński T. Oral ultra-low dose continuous combined hormone replacement therapy with 0.5 mg 17β-oestradiol and 2.5 mg dydrogesterone for the treatment of vasomotor symptoms: results from a double-blind, controlled study. Maturitas. 2010;67:227.

25. Panay N, Ylikorkala O, Archer DF, Gut R, Lang E. Ultra-low-dose estradiol and norethisterone acetate: effective menopausal symptom relief. Climacteric. 2007;10:120.

26. Grodstein F, Manson JE, Colditz GA, Willett WC, Speizer FE, Stampfer MJ. A prospective, observational study of postmenopausal hormone therapy and primary prevention of cardiovascular disease. Ann Intern Med. 2000;133:933.

27. Olié V, Plu-Bureau G, Conard J, Horellou MH, Canonico M, Scarabin PY. Hormone therapy and recurrence of venous thromboembolism among postmenopausal women. Menopause. 2011;18:488.

28. Hulley S, Grady D, Bush T, Furberg C, Herrington D, Riggs B, et al. Randomized trial of estrogen plus progestin for secondary prevention of coronary heart disease in postmenopausal women. Heart and Estrogen/progestin Replacement Study (HERS) Research Group. JAMA. 1998;280:605.

29. Stefanick ML. Estrogen, progestogens and cardiovascular risk. J Reprod Med. 1999;44:221.

30. Lobo RA, Bush T, Carr BR, Pickar JH. Effects of lower doses of conjugated equine estrogens and medroxyprogesterone acetate on plasma lipids and lipoproteins, coagulation factors, and carbohydrate metabolism. Fertil Steril. 2001;76:13.

31. Van Baal WM, Emeis JJ, Van Der Mooren MJ, Kessel H, Kenemans P, Stehouwer CDA. Impaired procoagulant-anticoagulant balance during hormone replacement therapy? A randomised, placebo-controlled 12-week study. Thromb Haemost. 2000;83:29.

32. Post MS, Rosing J, Van Der Mooren MJ, Zweegman S, Van Baal WM, Kenemans P, et al. Increased resistance to activated protein C after short-term oral hormone replacement therapy in healthy post-menopausal women. Br J Haematol. 2002;119:1017.

33. Post MS, Van Der Mooren MJ, Van Baal WM, Blankenstein MA, Merkus HMWM, Kroeks MVAM, et al. Effects of low-dose oral and transdermal estrogen replacement therapy on hemostatic factors in healthy postmenopausal women: a randomized placebo-controlled study. Am J Obstet Gynecol. 2003;189:1221.

34. Post MS, Christella M, Thomassen LGD, Mooren van der MJ, Baal van WM, Rosing J, et al. Effect of oral and transdermal estrogen replacement therapy on hemostatic variables associated with venous thrombosis: a randomized, placebo-controlled study in postmenopausal women. Arterioscler Thromb Vasc Biol. 2003;23:1116.

35. Canonico M, Alhenc-Gelas M, Plu-Bureau G, Olié V, Scarabin PY. Activated protein C resistance among postmenopausal women using transdermal estrogens: importance of progestogen. Menopause. 2010;17:1122.

36. Canonico M, Oger E, Plu-Bureau G, Conard J, Meyer G, Lévesque H, et al. Hormone therapy and venous thromboembolism among postmenopausal women: impact of the route of estrogen administration and progestogens: the ESTHER study. Circulation. 2007;115:840.

37. Canonico M, Fournier A, Carcaillon L, Olié V, Plu-Bureau G, Oger E, et al. Postmenopausal hormone therapy and risk of idiopathic venous thromboembolism: results from the E3N cohort study. Arterioscler Thromb Vasc Biol. 2010;30:340.

38. Lowe GDO, Upton MN, Rumley A, McConnachie A, O'Reilly DSJ, Watt GCM. Different effects of oral and transdermal hormone replacement therapies on factor IX, APC resistance, t-PA, PAI and C-reactive protein: a cross-sectional population survey. Thromb Haemost. 2001;86:550.

39. Rovinski D, Ramos RB, Fighera TM, Casanova GK, Spritzer PM. Risk of venous thromboembolism events in postmenopausal women using oral versus non-oral hormone therapy: a systematic review and meta-analysis. Thromb Res. 2018;168:83–95. https://doi.org/10.1016/j.thromres.2018.06.014.

40. American College of O, Gynecologists. ACOG committee opinion no. 556: Postmenopausal estrogen therapy: route of administration and risk of venous thromboembolism. Obstet Gynecol. 2013;121:887.

Index

The manufacturer's authorised representative in the EU is Springer
Nature Customer Service Centre GmbH, Europaplatz 3, 69115 Heidelberg,
Germany. If you have any concerns regarding our products, please
contact ProductSafety@springernature.com

Printed and bound by CPI Group (UK) Ltd, Croydon, CR0 4YY
23/04/2026
02095586-0002